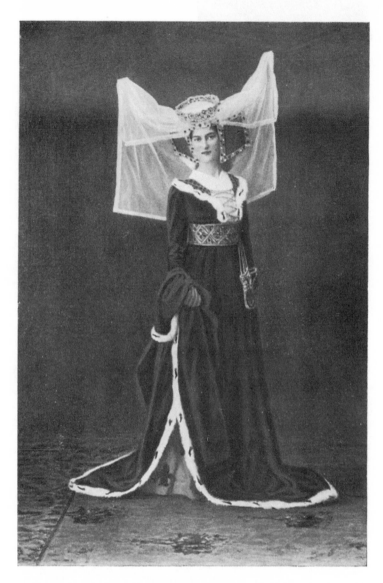

LADY, *temp.* HENRY VI.

Head-dress.—The horned; note the coronet and the size of the cauls.

Robe.—The short-waisted, train in front and behind, V-shaped opening in bodice.

Cincture.—Very broad, from which depends the gypcière.

Underdress.—Decorated with heraldic designs.

(Photographed direct from examples used in the Author's lecture upon "Mediæval Costume and Head-dresses.")

BRITISH COSTUME
from Earliest Times to 1820
with 468 illustrations

Mrs. Charles H. Ashdown

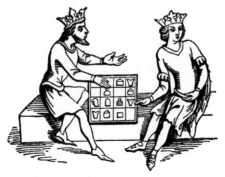

DOVER PUBLICATIONS, INC.
Mineola, New York

Published in Canada by General Publishing Company, Ltd., 30 Lesmill
Road, Don Mills, Toronto, Ontario.

Bibliographical Note

This Dover edition, first published in 2001, is an unabridged republication
of the book originally published in 1910 under the title *British Costume during XIX Centuries (Civil and Ecclesiastical)* by T. C. & E. C. Jack, Ltd., London.
The only significant alteration consists in retaining the nine color plates in
black and white in their original positions in the book, as well as reproducing
them all in full color on the covers.

DOVER *Pictorial Archive* SERIES

Library of Congress Cataloging-in-Publication Data

Ashdown, Charles H., Mrs.
    [British costume during XIX centuries (civil and ecclesiastical)]
    British costume from earliest times to 1820 / Mrs. Charles H. Ashdown.
        p. cm.
    Originally published: British costume during XIX centuries (civil and
ecclesiastical). London : T.C. & E.C. Jack, 1910.
    "The only significant alteration consists in retaining the nine color plates
in black and white in their original positions in the book, as well as repeat-
ing them all in full color on the covers"—T.p. verso.
    Includes index.
    ISBN 0-486-41813-8 (pbk.)
    1. Costume—Great Britain—History. I. Title.

GT730 .A7 2001
391'.00942—dc21

                                                                    2001032304

Manufactured in the United States of America
Dover Publications, Inc., 31 East 2nd Street, Mineola, N.Y. 11501

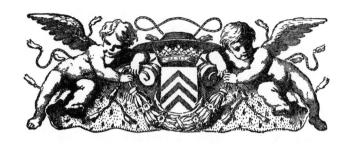

THIS BOOK

IS AFFECTIONATELY DEDICATED TO

MY HUSBAND

TO WHOSE INVALUABLE HELP AND ENCOURAGEMENT

DURING THE PRODUCTION OF THIS WORK I AM

MUCH INDEBTED

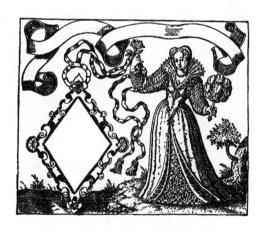

PREFACE

Books upon costume are to a certain extent plentiful, but those long-suffering individuals who have occasion to search them frequently, or possess the wish to grasp and thoroughly comprehend the exact style prevailing during a particular period in, say, the Middle Ages, can fully testify to the complete confusion prevailing in the majority of works upon the subject. Thus, styles which were in vogue for only a short period are vaguely defined as fourteenth century, Plantagenet, or Edwardian, as the case may be, while the approximate time when any costume died out — which is just as important as its introduction — is practically never alluded to.

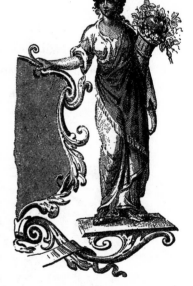

It was with a humble but earnest endeavour to rectify this condition of things, and to introduce some degree of order and method, whereby definite styles could be appropriated to definite periods, that I began a course of methodical research in the manuscript department of the British Museum to verify years of previous work, and the result

will, I hope, be appreciated by those who are interested
in the subject. The method and general arrangement
followed is similar to that carried out in the companion
volume upon "Arms and Armour" by my husband, which
has received many encomiums for its definiteness and lucidity.
For the first time a system of classifying the costume of the
ladies according to the head-dress which prevailed has been
attempted, and it is hoped with success. There is undoubtedly a great revival of interest in the wearing apparel
of our ancestors at the time of writing, possibly owing to
the numerous Pageants which have been held during the
past few years, and it should be hailed with satisfaction;
for if they have led to costumes being produced which are
historically correct, much educational work will have been
accomplished. To the earnest student, however, there have
been many occasions for regret when painful anachronisms
have appeared upon the arena, but these have been growing
less year by year.

With some notable exceptions the representation of
historical costume upon the stage is still almost in its infancy, so far as the periods anterior to the Tudor are concerned, and this is most sincerely to be deplored, inasmuch
as mediæval costume has a charm and grace of its own which
is quite unknown to post-Reformation dress. By actual experience I have found upon more than one occasion that an
audience pays much more critical and appreciative attention
to a play which is costumed strictly in accordance with
historical detail, and as such is duly advertised, than to one
dressed in a pot-pourri of stage dresses, which are invariably
a réchauffé of costumes authentic, conjectural, and mythical.
The idea prevailing among stage costumiers that a dress

cannot be striking without multitudinous furbelows is doubtless responsible for many of the lamentable mistakes so frequently seen, and the manager of a theatre who insists upon rigid adherence to historical accuracy in preference to the "effectiveness" at one time chiefly aimed at, richly deserves the warmest thanks of the community. In the illustrations of books, too, there is much to be done before satisfactory work is achieved, and this remark also applies specially to costumes ante-dating the Tudor period. Perhaps the most earnest workers in the realm of truth are the many artists who ransack every available authority in the sincere endeavour to produce pictures combining beauty with absolute truthfulness, though some are beguiled into representing both civil and military dress by the fantastic illustrations of certain fifteen century illuminators of manuscripts, who revelled in imagery and depicted impossibly fantastic costumes, which are eagerly followed by stained-glass window artists, wood-carvers, sculptors, and modern-day illuminators.

I take this opportunity of expressing my indebtedness to the custodians of the Manuscript Department of the British Museum and Printed Books Department; also to those at South Kensington Museum and the National Gallery; to the curators of the Public Libraries at Eastbourne, Whitby, Nottingham, St. Albans, Brighton, St. Heliers, &c.

My thanks are also due to H. J. Toulmin, Esq., E. P. Debenham, Esq., W. M. Myddelton, Esq., to those ladies and gentlemen who have kindly acted as models for the coloured illustrations, and to my husband for kind revision of proofs.

(MRS.) CHARLES H. ASHDOWN.

Monastery Close,
    St. Albans, Herts.

CONTENTS

FIRST PART: CIVIL

CONTENTS

LIST OF COLOURED ILLUSTRATIONS*

---

*For this edition, the color plates listed above appear in black and white in their original positions, as well as in color on the covers.

FIRST PART: CIVIL

CHAPTER I

THE BRITONS

THE subject of British costume naturally commences with the garments worn by the primitive inhabitants of these Islands, but, as might be anticipated, the necessary particulars for describing the dress of the Ancient Britons are extremely meagre, and even when given are in many parts almost hopelessly obscure. Of definite descriptions anterior to the date of the first Roman invasion there are practically none extant, and even after Cæsar's two visits the references to such matters as dress and adornments for the person are scanty and unsatisfactory. We know that the constant intercourse between the Southern coast of Britain and the mainland naturally led to a higher degree of civilisation being existent along the southern littoral than in the Midland and Northern districts; and thus, while the inhabitants of Trent enjoyed the full benefit of that intercourse, the dwellers of Strath-Clyde were still plunged in the depth of barbarism. Arguing from analogy, we should expect the latter to have been clothed in what may be termed man's primitive attire, namely, the skins of the beasts struck down in the chase, or those of domestic animals slaughtered for food. This assumption is confirmed by Cæsar, who states in his Commentaries, "that those within the country went clad in skins," while the Southern Britons were clothed like the Gauls. This condition of things must have lasted for centuries, for even after the Roman occupation we read of the Northern tribes as being but little removed from savages. As we have the authority of Cæsar and other ancient writers for asserting that the Southern Britons were similar in manners, customs, and dress to the Gauls, any contemporary knowledge of the latter would naturally apply to the former. Thus the Gaulish methods for spinning, weaving wool, dressing, and dyeing had been copied by the men of Trent, and, according to the evidence of Diodorus Siculus, Strabo, and Pliny, certain trade secrets in the art of dyeing had also been communicated. The parti-coloured cloth worn by the Gauls was also manufactured in Britain, and appears to have been very characteristic of that period. It was composed of strands of wool dyed in different colours, and afterwards woven in such a manner that the resulting fabric presented a chequered or parti-coloured appearance, and may have been the prototype of the Scottish plaid. Respecting the dress of Boadicea, who flourished more than a hundred years after the Cæsarean invasions, we are informed by Dion Cassius that she wore " a tunic of several colours all in folds, and over it, fastened by a fibula or brooch, a robe of coarse stuff." This tunic was evidently made of what may be termed the national cloth, and the cloak of common fustian, which all nations emerging from barbarism appear to have the faculty of manufacturing.

THE DRUIDS

The Druidical priests were clad in white voluminous robes reaching to the feet, and consisting of two essential parts, the robe proper and the cloak.

Robe.—This garment was similar to a sleeveless dressing-gown reaching to the feet, but with no collar. We have no knowledge of the material of which it was made, but it was probably of wool, and of special manufacture. A bas-relief found at Autun in France represents two Druids (Fig. 1), and from the many folds delineated in each of these robes they were evidently of a soft material.

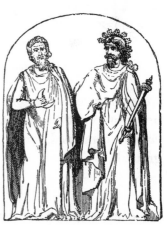

FIG. 1.—Druids from bas-relief found at Autun.

Cloak.—From the illustration it will be gathered that this was peculiarly ample, inasmuch as some parts reach to the ground. Of the form and dimensions of this garment no data are extant, but practical experience has discovered that if it be cut somewhat like a Roman toga it will give when draped an appearance very similar to that shown in the figure. The Druid upon the right is crowned with an oak garland and bears a sceptre; while the one upon the left carries a sacred symbol, the crescent, in his hand. At important ceremonials the Arch-Druid wore a torque or breastplate of a peculiar shape (shown in Fig. 2). The broad lower portion rested upon the chest, and the two bosses reached on either side to the ears, while upon his head a tiara was worn with diverging rays. These ornaments were all of gold, and engraved. Respecting the

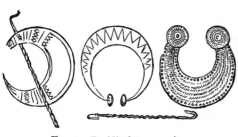

minor priestly orders, the Bards or Singers were habited similarly to the Druids, but in cloth of a sky-blue colour, symbolical of peace. The Ovates, a class professing erudition,

FIG. 2.—Druidical torques, &c.

were in green, a colour signifying learning. The lowest order of priests or novitiates wore garments of the three colours combined, presumably spots of colour on a white ground.

CIVIL DRESS: THE MEN

The Tunic.—The men were habited in a loose-fitting sleeveless tunic, confined at the waist by a belt. Diodorus tells us the Belgic Gauls wore dyed tunics beflowered with all manner of colours, and possibly the Britons may have imitated them. The tunic partly covered the *braccæ,* or trousers, an article of apparel by which all barbaric nations seem to have been distinguished from the Romans. They reached from the waist to the feet, and were either close-fitting or loose; if the latter, they were partly confined by bandages passed round the limb at wide intervals. By the use of the term " braccæ," signifying spotted, we may infer that these garments were fashioned from the native cloth, the predominating colour in which was red.

The Sagum was a cloak dyed blue or black, which had superseded the skins still worn by the inhabitants of the interior. The hair was long, and fell in curls down the back; the face was clean shaven, except for the moustache, which was apparently cultivated to its utmost extent, and occasionally reached to the chest. Probably no covering for the head was in use.

THE WOMEN

The dress of the women consisted of a long loose-fitting sleeveless garment, confined at the waist, over which was worn a cloak or skin, the head as a rule being left uncovered.

With respect to the inhabitants of the interior, we can only surmise that they were dressed in skins, and consequently no definite fashions prevailed.

A national characteristic appears to have been the staining of the skin with woad, which is referred to by many ancient writers. From some we should gather that this was a system of tattooing similar to that practised by the Maori, while others infer that the whole skin was stained with the colour so as to give a bluish-green appearance. Both Herodotus and Isidorus concur in stating that the skin was punctured by needles and the colour afterwards rubbed in. Pliny asserts that this was done during infancy by the British wives and nurses. We may therefore safely assume that the Britons carried indelible designs upon their bodies, which were calculated to add to their ferocious aspect in war. The articles of personal adornment consisted of armlets, bracelets, rings, collars, and necklaces of twisted wire, made of gold, silver, and the commoner metals and alloys.

CHAPTER II

THE SAXON PERIOD, *c.* 460 TO 1066

WITH the advent of this period we leave to a certain
extent the region of conjecture, and enter within the
bounds of certainty, inasmuch as the material for recon-
structing the Saxon Period is of a much more tangible
character than that afforded by the British. There are
practically three authorities from which we derive information, namely, the Sagas, the contents of Saxon barrows,
and the MSS. Unfortunately the Sagas deal as a rule
with the heroic deeds of Scandinavian heroes, and although
they furnish us with what may be termed minute details
of military equipment, there are practically no references
of any value to the civil or ecclesiastical garments of the
men, or to the costume of the women. The second source,
the Saxon barrows, only affords us information concerning
the gold, silver, and other ornaments, together with the
military arms of our Saxon ancestors; and although this
is valuable to a great extent, we have to rely finally for
precise knowledge of dresses and decorations to the many
priceless manuscripts which are preserved in the British
Museum and elsewhere. The Saxons commenced their
conquests during the fifth century, but it was not until
the year 720 that the earliest MS. preserved to us saw
the light; there are consequently more than two centuries
during which we have no reliable details. Spelman, in his

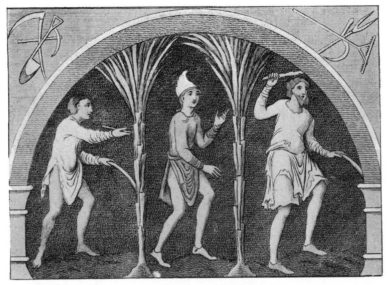

FIG. 3.—Saxon rustics.

No. 1. (Harl. MS. 603.)   No. 2. (Cott. MS. Claudius B iv.)   No. 3. (Bod. MS. Junius xi.)

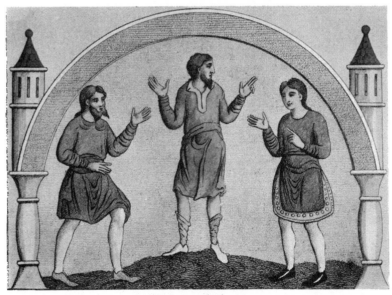

FIG. 4.—The Saxon tunica.

No. 1. (Cott. MS. Claud. B iv.)   No. 2. (Bod. MS. Junius xi.)   No. 3. (Cott. MS. Claud. B iv.)

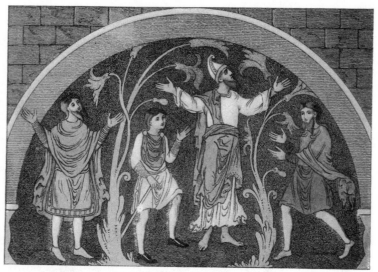

FIG. 5.—Saxon mantles.

No. 1. (Cott. MS. Claudius B iv.)　　No. 2. (Cott. MS. Claudius B iv.)
No. 3. (Bod. MS. Junius xi.)　　　　No. 4. (Cott. MS. Claudius B iv.)

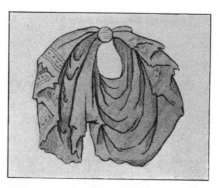

FIG. 6.—The Saxon mantle.　(Cott. MS. Tiberius C vi.)

"Councils," refers to a meeting at the end of the eighth century, in which a speaker chides the Saxons for the manner in which they wore their dress, intimating that the nation had changed its style of clothing upon its conversion to Christianity. As a consequence, the description of the Saxon dress must be accepted as that which prevailed after the time of St. Augustine, and not to that worn before 597.

SAXON CIVIL COSTUME: THE MEN

The garment worn next to the skin, or the *just-au-corps*, appears to have been universal among all ranks, even to the humblest, who at times possessed no other clothing. For example, the Saxon rustic shown in Fig. 3, Pl., No. 1, taken from Harl. MS. 603, dating from the reign of Harold II., is thus habited, and a still earlier example, No. 2, possesses but one garment. Of course it may be claimed that these figures are dressed in tunics. It was always made of linen, the wearing of a woollen garment next the skin being enjoined at that period as a severe penance.

The Tunica.—This was of two kinds—the short, which was practically worn by all classes of people, and the long, which was generally considered as a mark of superior rank. The short tunica in the earlier period was simply provided with an opening for the passage of the head (Fig. 4, Pl., No. 1), but in later examples it was open for a short distance from the neck, and laced up in front when adjusted, No. 2. The sleeve was cut with the garment, having one seam only, and a very marked peculiarity of Saxon sleeves, which may even be traced for nearly two centuries after the period, is the extraordinary rucking upon the forearm. This is explained by the fact that, during cold weather, the sleeves could be drawn over the hands to provide warmth. The hem reached to just below the knees, and subsequently became decorated with a worked border, which was carried up the two sides where the openings occurred, as in No. 3. Around the waist a girdle was worn, seldom shown in the engravings, inasmuch as the tunica was pulled up through it, and fell in folds over it, giving the strange appearance which is such a marked feature of the waist. When indulging in very violent exercise, such as sword-play, throwing the lance, &c., more of the tunica worked up through the girdle on the right side than on the left, thus giving a slanting appearance to the hem. This striking point was promptly copied by the ladies (Fig. 21, Pl.). The lavish ornamentation bestowed upon the garment in the later part of the period is indicated in No. 3. The tunica was not always cut up at the side. It is perfectly permissible to suppose that the smock-frock, or carter's gown, of the present day, with its peculiar needlework, may be a direct descendant of the Saxon tunica.

The Mantle.—Probably the most distinctive feature of the Saxons of both sexes was the mantle, flowing in graceful folds, and in sweeping curves of beauty. It was not always adjusted after a stereotyped fashion, but much was left to individual taste; the mode of fastening, however, was either in the centre of the chest, or upon one or both shoulders. The shape of this mantle was that shown in Fig. 5, Pl., No. 1; although plain in the earlier years,

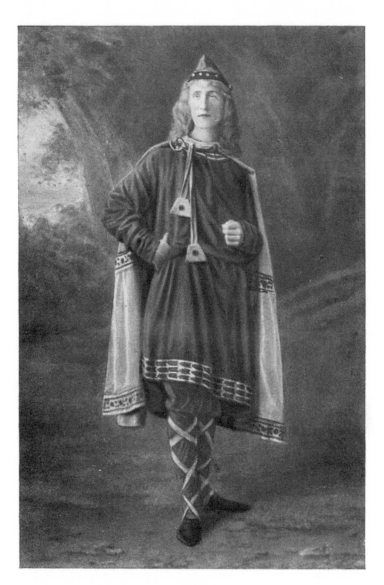

SAXON

Head-gear.—Banded Phrygian cap.
Cloak.—Of blue cloth embroidered.
Tunica.— Green cloth embroidered.
Stockings.—Red cloth cross-gartered yellow.

(Photographed direct from examples used in the Author's lecture upon
    "Mediæval Costume and Head-dresses.")

it finally became decorated (Fig. 6, Pl.). An example in which it is shown fastened upon the chest is given in Fig. 7, Pl., where it is very voluminous ; upon both shoulders in Fig. 5, Pl., No. 2, and upon one shoulder in Fig. 9, Pl. Occasionally the mantle was made in a circular form, with a hole for the head not placed in the centre, as shown in Fig. 5, Pl., No. 1. Upon comparing Fig. 5, Pl., No. 4, which is of the eighth century, with No. 2, which dates from the

tenth, it will be gleaned that the mantle eventually became much smaller; but this must not be taken as universal, inasmuch as persons of distinction and elderly people frequently wore mantles of great length, sometimes reaching the ground, over the long tunicas which they also affected. The method of fastening the mantle was generally by means of fibulæ or brooches, often of very elaborate workmanship.

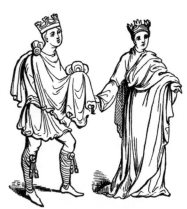

FIG. 8.—Method of fastening cloak by a ring. (Harl. MS. 603.)

As a proof that the old method used by the Druids for fastening the mantle had not fallen into disuse, we give an illustration from the Harl. MS. 603 (Fig. 8), where the mantle is distinctly seen to be pulled up through a ring on the right shoulder (see also Fig. 9, Pl.). That the fastening was not always undone when it was removed is proved by an illustration in the above MS. representing the encounter between David and Goliath, in which David has thrown his mantle upon the ground still fastened with the brooch (Fig. 6, Pl.).

The Stockings.—All Scandinavian nations wore short trousers reaching to mid-thigh, and the stockings of thin cloth were frequently made sufficiently long to join them; but the prevailing mode, and one which lasted for many years, was to wear short stockings reaching nearly to the knees, where they finished generally in the shape of the top part of a Hessian boot (Fig. 10, Pl.), but occasionally passed horizontally round the leg, and even at times downwards from the back. Where no stockings are seen it invariably signifies that the long variety were used, the upper part not being visible. The exception to this was the rustic, who is very rarely shown with any stockings at all.

The Cross-Gartering.—Like the Franks, Normans, and other Northern nations of Europe, the Saxons affected a style of cross-gartering which was often very elaborate. It consisted of strips of cloth of various colours, or, in the case of soldiers, strips of leather bound round the leg so as to form a pattern, and always terminating below the knee (Fig. 10, Pl.). In the case of persons of rank an ornament is some-times shown at the knee (Fig. 11, Pl.).

The Shoes.—The general form of foot-gear was a low shoe, fastening up the front or the sides; occasionally

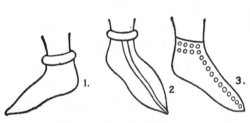

FIG. 12.—Late Saxon boots.

a boot is shown, as in Fig. 12. The shoes appear to be universal, even the Saxon rustic being provided with them, although, as we have seen, he wore them without stockings.

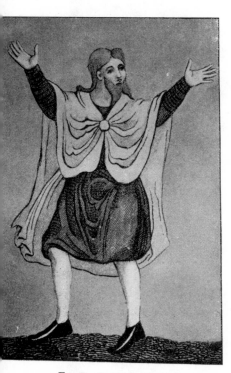

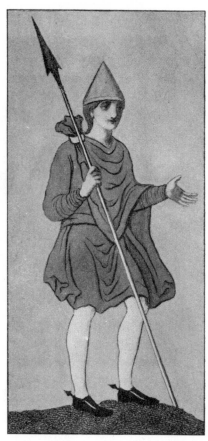

Fig. 7.—Saxon mantle.
(Cott. MS. Claudius B iv.)

Fig. 9.—The Saxon mantle, showing method of
fastening. (Cott. MS. Claudius B iv.)

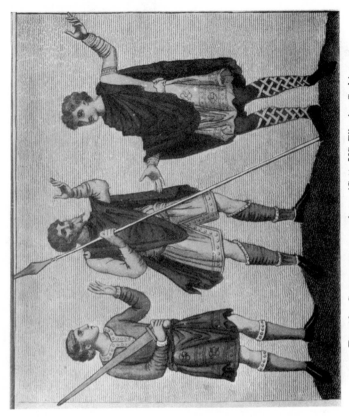

Fig. 10.—Saxon cross-gartering. (Cott. MS. Tiberius C vi.)

The Cap.—As a general rule the Saxons went bare-headed, but what may be termed the national covering was a cap of the Phrygian shape, made of leather or skin, with the hair outside in the case of the lower classes; and of cloth, more or less decorated with embroidery, among the upper. The same cap, strengthened with bands of steel, covered the head of the warrior. The pattern of this cap varied considerably, sometimes being high (Fig. 4, Pl., No. 3), or low with a comb (Fig. 9, Pl.). A circular variety is shown upon a representation of King David. The members of the Witan and other personages of distinction affected a sugar-loaf cap, and we also find Saxon soldiers with a helmet of this shape (Fig. 9, Pl.).

The Saxon men delighted in having long and flowing hair, in which they took a particular pride; only the very lowest classes had it cropped short. The beard was worn long and flowing, and a remarkable feature was the bifid form, which is so strongly emphasised in illuminations (Figs. 13 and 14, Pls.). Although in many of these the beard and also the hair is rendered of a distinctly blue colour, it must not be imagined that a style prevailed for dyeing the hair, such a feature, if habitual, would certainly have been mentioned by contemporary writers.

THE WOMEN

THE HEAD-RAIL HEAD-DRESS TO 1066

A remarkable feature of the costume of Anglo-Saxon ladies was the astonishing persistence of one particular style of dress over so many centuries. The earliest pictorial representation does not vary to any marked extent from the latest; practically the only alteration of any importance appears in the head-gear.

The Head-rail.—This distinctive covering in the earlier form consisted of a piece of material—silk, cloth, or linen according to the social status of the wearer—which was approximately 2½ yards in length and ¾ yard wide. Its method of adjustment was to place one end of the rail loosely on the left shoulder, pass it over the head down to the right shoulder, under the chin, and round the back of the neck, and over the right shoulder again; the free end could either be left hanging loosely down in front, or the chest might be completely covered by taking one corner of the loose end and passing it over the left shoulder again (Fig. 15, Pl.). A variation of this mode is perceived in the latter part of the period whereby the neck is exposed. In this case the rail was made only half its original length; the centre is placed upon the forehead and the two ends allowed to hang freely on either side (Fig. 15, Pl.). In order to keep the rail in position during gusty weather, and also perhaps for ornamentation, a narrow circlet seems to have been worn at times over it. An example of this occurs in Cott. MS. Vespasian A viii. (Fig. 16). The rail was of various colours, but apparently never white.

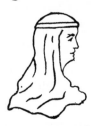

FIG. 16.—The head-rail. (Cott. MS. Vesp. A viii.)

The Hair.—Of the coiffure worn under the head-rail we have no illustration. The Bishop of Sherborne, who wrote in the eighth century, particularly mentions a woman having her twisted locks delicately curled by an iron; another is mentioned in the Anglo-Saxon poem of " Judith "

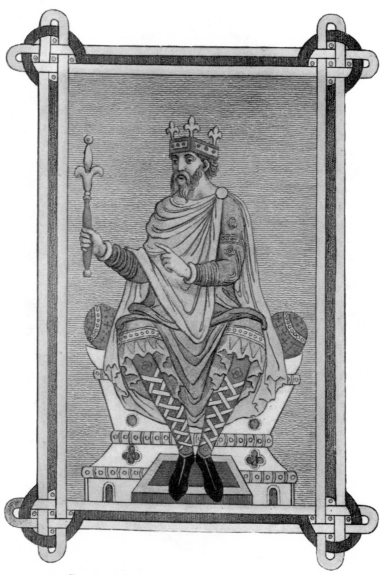

Fig. 11.—A Saxon monarch. (Cott. MS. Tiberius C vi.)

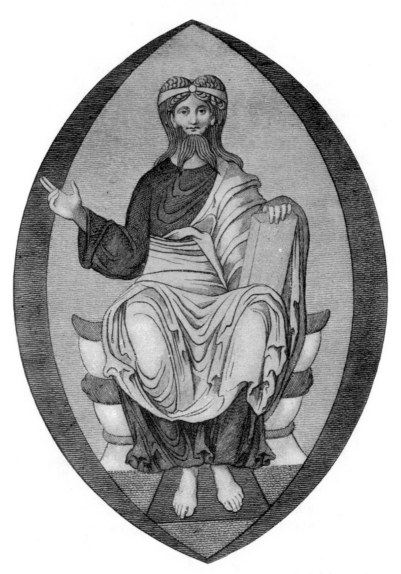

FIG. 13.—The Saxon bifid beard. (Cott. MS. Claudius B iv.)

as having twisted locks; while from analogy with the continental nations, we may infer that they wore the hair in long plaits. Among the jewellery mentioned in wills of that period, golden head-bands and half circlets occur, and from this one may gather that, although the head was always covered at home and abroad, the hair was by no means neglected. The term "fair-haired Saxons" has led many astray when repro-ducing costume for female Saxon characters, and numerous examples have been seen upon the arenas of pageants of hair freely exposed. In the case of children this might be allowed, but certainly not with regard to adults. So rigorously is this rule en-forced in all illuminations, that we have every right

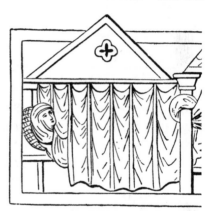

Fig. 17.—Saxon lady in head-rail after re-tiring to rest. (Cott. MS. Claud. B iv.)

to suppose that it was a disgrace for a woman to appear in public with her head uncovered. So deeply sensitive was the Saxon woman with regard to this rule, that, as may be seen in Fig. 17, from Cott. MS. Claudius B iv., they wore the rail even after they had retired to rest, and a similar example may be noticed in the interesting wood-cut from the Saxon MS. of Cædmon (Fig. 18). There are examples, we may add, of women with their hair exposed, but they always represent questionable characters, such as public dancers, minstrels, &c. (Fig. 19).

The Kirtle.—Respecting this garment we have no illustrations given; it was an article of dress corresponding to a combined petticoat and bodice of the present day. It is quite possible, however, that this garment is intended to

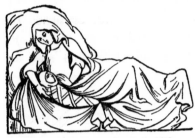

be shown in the representation of the Virgin Mary in Cott. MS. Vesp. A viii., dating from 966, being a grant of privileges made by King Edgar to Winchester. The gunna is seen looped up, and the kirtle, of a darker colour,

FIG. 18.—Saxon mother and child.

appears underneath. It is quite open to argument, however, that these may be the gunna and tunica respectively.

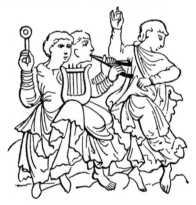

FIG. 19.—Saxon dancing-girl and minstrels.
(Cott. MS. Cleopatra C viii.)

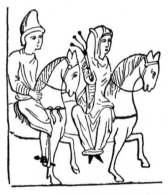

FIG. 20.—Anglo-Saxons on a journey, illustrating the side-saddle for ladies.
(Cott. MS. Claudius B iv.)

Incidentally it may be mentioned that the ladies always rode side-saddle, as in the fashion shown in the accompanying sketch (Fig. 20) from Cott. MS. Claudius B iv.

The Gunna.—The English term "gown" is a direct derivative from this Saxon word. The garment was fairly tight-fitting, but long and flowing round the feet. It was furnished with tight sleeves, which were very long and puckered upon the forearm. In the earlier centuries the gunna was plain, and only ornamented by a band of embroidery round the hem, but in the tenth and eleventh centuries the material itself was at times covered with a design, often very elaborate.

The Tunica.—This article of dress, which roughly corresponded with that worn by the men, was a very characteristic Saxon garment. The sleeves invariably reached to the elbows, and had large openings. The shape at the neck was probably like that of the man, being encircled with a piece of embroidery, the latter being carried down the front, where it joined another piece which passed round the hem. A girdle as a rule confined the waist. It will be noticed by reference to Fig. 21, Pl., adapted from Harl. MS. 2908, that the marked peculiarity of the lower hem of the man's tunic, in working up on the right side, has been faithfully imitated in the dress. As this is the first example noted in this work of the imitation of features in the masculine dress by the ládies, we may say that it is of constant occurrence in all ages, and that we shall meet with many examples during the mediæval and later periods. It is the fashion, which has almost become stereotyped at the present day, to complain of the ladies copying the dress of the men; but surely we may argue, that what has always been we should expect to prevail now, and there is no guarantee for its discontinuance in the future. After all, it is a compliment, for imitation is the sincerest form of flattery.

The Mantle.—This covering for the shoulders was made after the fashion of the ecclesiastical chasuble, but with more material in it, which gave it the graceful folds not seen in the priestly vestment (Fig. 21, Pl.). They were frequently very handsomely embroidered.

The Travelling Cloak was of varying designs, of which two may be seen in Fig. 22, taken from Cott. MS. Claudius B iv.

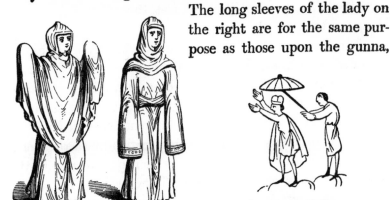

The long sleeves of the lady on the right are for the same purpose as those upon the gunna,

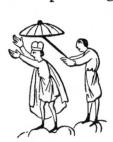

FIG. 23.—Anglo-Saxon
umbrella.   (Harl.
MS. 603.)

FIG. 22.—Travelling cloaks.
(Cott. MS. Claudius B iv.)

namely, to protect the hands during cold weather. The umbrella was not unknown to the Anglo-Saxons; it was of peculiar shape, as shown in Fig. 23.

The Shoes.—These are but seldom seen in any illustrations, but when they do appear they are invariably black, and close-fitting.

THE DANES

The advent of the Danes did not affect the Saxon dress to any appreciable extent. They wore garments of the same pattern, and it was only by the colours that they could

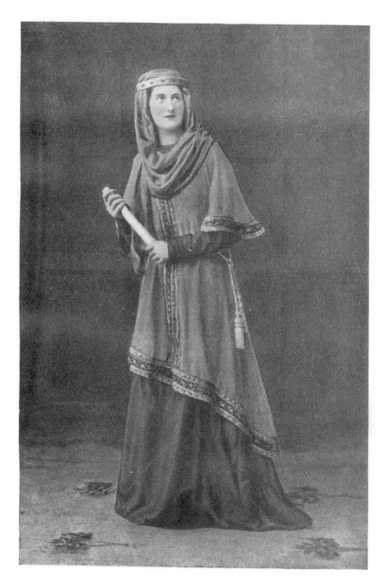

SAXON LADY

Head-rail.—Soft green silk with jewelled band.
Tunica.—Of blue woollen material, edged with embroidery.
Gunna.—Red cloth.

(Photographed direct from examples used in the Author's lecture upon
    "Mediæval Costume and Head-dresses.")

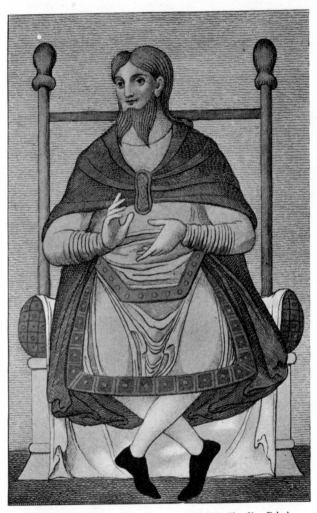

FIG. 14.—The Saxon bifid beard.   (Cott. MS. Claudius B iv.)

be distinguished.   We glean from Saxon writers that black
was the prevailing hue.   The short period which marked

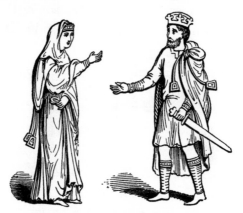

FIG. 24.—Queen Alfgyfe and King Canute.

their stay in England is very deficient in authorities upon

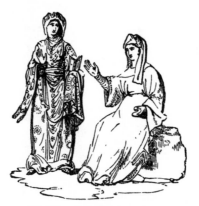

FIG. 25.—Anglo-Saxon costume.

Figure on left from Benedictional of St. Ethelwold.
Figure on right from Abbot Elfnoth's Prayer Book.   (Harl. MS. 2908.)

costume, but the references in Saxon writers to "the black
Danes" leads us to suppose that it was their favourite

colour. Certain it is that they sailed under the black banner, the raven being their emblem, as befitted Northern pirates; but no superstition was attached to the colour, as we find that soon after their conquests in England they

(Cott. MS. Nero D iv., A.D. 720.)

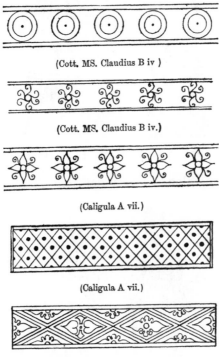

(Cott. MS. Claudius B iv)

(Cott. MS. Claudius B iv.)

(Caligula A vii.)

(Caligula A vii.)

FIG. 26.—Saxon embroidery.

became as gay in their clothing as their neighbours. They were extremely proud of their long hair, which they regularly combed once a day; as this is related by a Saxon writer, we may infer that the latter was not quite so careful in his toilet. The hair of King Canute descended upon his shoulders, and that of many of his courtiers to their waists.

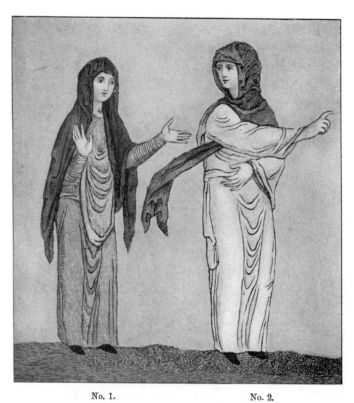

No. 1.   No. 2.

Fɪɢ. 15.—The Saxon head-rail.   (Cott. MS. Claudius B iv.)

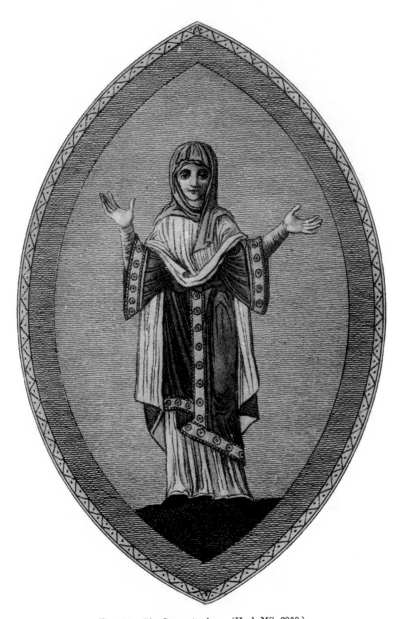

Fig. 21.—The Saxon tunica. (Harl. MS. 2908.)

The full-length figures of Canute and his Queen Alfgyfe are reproduced from the manuscript Register of Hyde Abbey (Fig. 24); the only noteworthy feature with regard to the King is the way in which the mantle is fastened by a cord having two large pendants or tassels at the extremities. This feature is also seen depending from the cloak of the lady, who wears a golden circlet, indicative of her rank, under the head-rail. The reign of Edward the Confessor

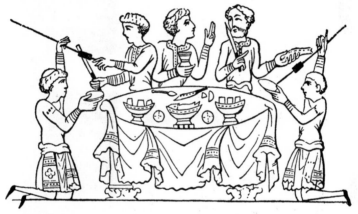

FIG. 27.—Anglo-Saxons at dinner.   (Cott. MS. Tiberius C vi.)

witnessed the introduction into England of the Norman style of dress by many of those attending his court, and we know it to be one of the principal causes of the disaffection which prevailed throughout the country among the Saxon nobility. This period also saw the introduction of new textiles and fresh designs, but the materials, which were essentially Saxon, consisted of linen, cloths of various textures, and silk, which was known to them as early as the eighth century. Their knowledge of embroidery was remarkable, and the figure given here, taken from the Bene-

dictional of St. Ethelwold, must have been extremely beautiful (Fig. 25), for she wears an embroidered scarlet mantle
over a gunna of gold tissue or cloth of gold. The veil and
shoes are also of the latter costly material. Appended are

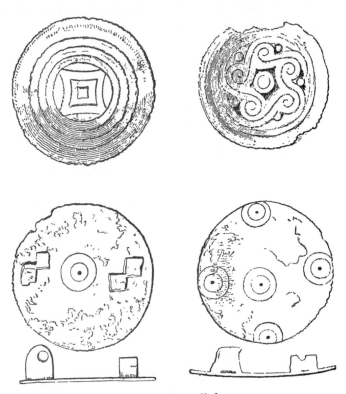

FIG. 28.—Saxon fibulæ.

a few examples of the designs upon characteristic **Saxon**
embroidery, with the sources from which they are obtained
(Fig. 26). In order to demonstrate the passion for embroidery, Fig. 27 has been reproduced from MS. Tiberius
C vi., which shows that not only did the upper classes

make extensive use of this method of ornamentation, but they also permitted its use among their servitors.

Ornaments, &c.—In the excavation of Saxon barrows many articles relating to the toilet and dress of both sexes have come to light, and there is hardly a museum in the

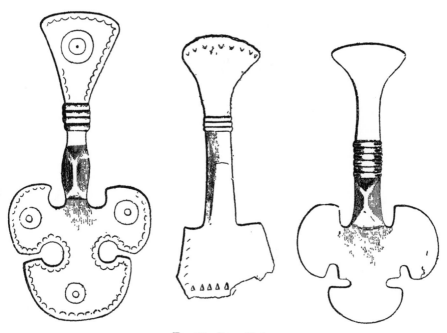

FIG. 29.—Saxon fibulæ.

country which does not contain examples. With such a wealth of material to hand, it is somewhat difficult to select specimens for illustration, but those found at a Saxon bury-ing-place near Banbury are typical (Figs. 28, 29, 30) of the fibulæ unearthed; they were generally disclosed in couples, each two corresponding to the right and left shoulders. They were mostly concave, and made of copper gilt, pure copper, and brass. The pin shown is of brass, and the ring made of silver wire (Figs. 31, 32). Two bracelets were discovered upon the arms of the skeleton of a woman, consisting of plates of metal which had been sewn on leather straps. Here also a comb was disinterred; it is of bone with iron rivets, and the teeth were apparently in the same condition when buried as they now appear (Fig. 33). Most of the skeletons had from four to twenty-six beads round the neck, of amber, glass, jet, various stones, and coloured clay, some with designs upon them. The most costly of the ornaments found are the fibulæ, and some have been discovered of the most beautiful character, made of gold set with garnets and other stones, with pins for affixing them. When it is remembered that the Saxon costume was essentially loose-fitting, the use of fibulæ for fastening the various parts will be at once perceived, and as many as four or five of these brooches have been found in one grave (Fig. 34). It is interesting to note that a Saxon lady was interred in full costume, with all her jewellery, no matter how costly, similarly to the warrior who was buried with his weapons, shield, &c. There are distinct characteristics

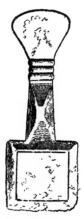

Fig. 30.—Saxon fibula.

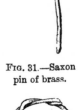

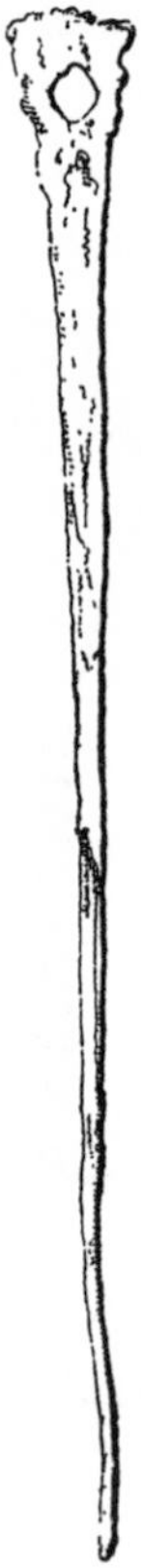

Fig. 31.—Saxon pin of brass.

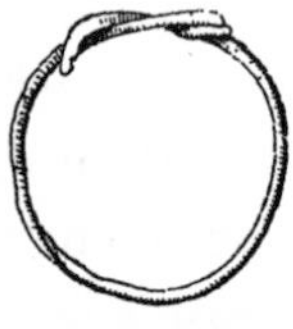

Fig. 32.—Saxon ring of silver wire.

pertaining to the fibulæ found in various parts of the

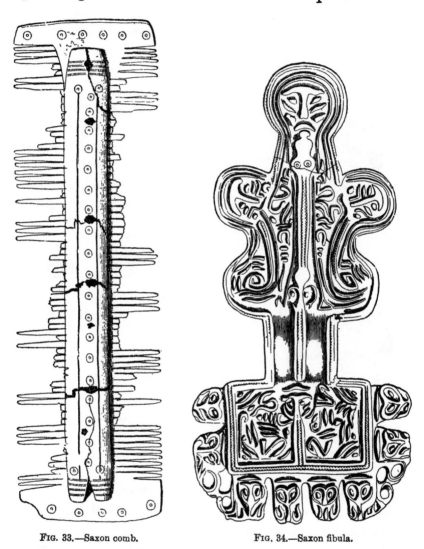

FIG. 33.—Saxon comb.   FIG. 34.—Saxon fibula.

country.   For instance, a circular fibula shaped like a small saucer is found in Oxfordshire and the adjacent counties (Fig. 35); it is always of brass and strongly gilt; in the Midland counties and East Anglia, bronze fibulæ of the pattern shown in No. 3, a smaller kind, as in No. 6, comes from Kent, where No 1, of gold, garnets, and turquoise embedded in mother-of-pearl, was also unearthed, probably the finest ever found. Pendent ornaments like earrings are

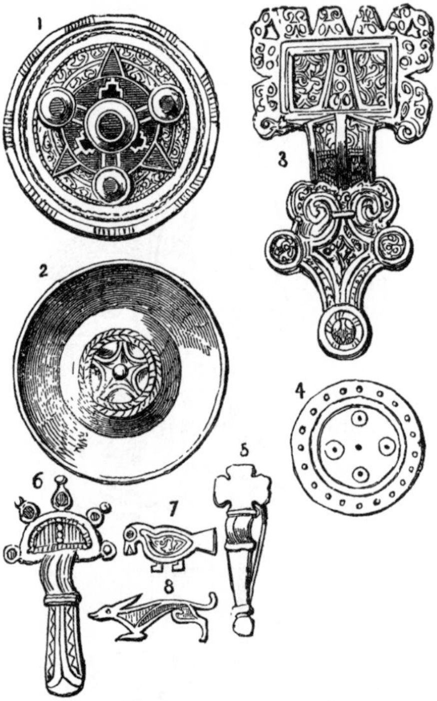

FIG. 35.—Anglo-Saxon fibulæ.

1 and 6. South Saxon. 2. South Midlands.
3 and 5. East Anglia and east part of Mercia.
4. Cambridgeshire. 7. Isle of Wight.
8. Roman.

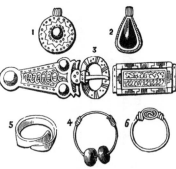

FIG. 36.—Anglo-Saxon buckle, rings, and earrings.

sometimes discovered, together with buckles, rings, &c. (Fig. 36). Many Saxon ladies appear to have been buried with chatelaines hanging from the waist-belt, from which depended scissors, combs, tweezers, knives in decorated sheaths, keys, &c.; and with purses also hanging from the same belt.

CHAPTER III

THE NORMAN PERIOD

WILLIAM THE CONQUEROR, 1066-1087

BEFORE proceeding with the main subject of this chapter, it may be advisable to say a few words of explanation respecting historical manuscripts, and the methods of delineation pursued by mediæval artists. We find that very few persons, apart from those in touch with the actual books, have the least idea what, say, "Cott. MS. Nero D vii." implies; and as references have already been made, and will frequently be met with in succeeding chapters, the explanation may probably be acceptable. It is the method adopted in the British Museum, the Bodleian Library, and other institutions for cataloguing the manuscripts in their possession. Thus "Cottonian MS." signifies that the manuscript is part of the collection presented to the nation by Sir John Cotton in 1700; "Nero," simply refers to a bust of that Emperor which stood over the bookcase in the original collection; "D" is the fourth shelf (in alphabetical order); and "vii." is the place occupied by the book along the shelf. Similarly "Roy. MS. C vii." refers to the bequest of manuscripts by King George II. in 1757, and "Add. MSS." refers to the large collection which has been acquired by Government grants.

With respect to the methods of delineation by mediæval

artists, it must be remembered that the latter were totally
ignorant of any style of costume other than that prevailing
in their own period. The dress of the Greek and the
Roman was as much a mystery to them as was that of the
Jew at the time of our Lord ; and as the manuscripts
they wrote and illuminated invariably related to sacred or
classical subjects, there was no alternative but to place
the various characters in the dress of the period. To our
eyes it would appear incongruous to represent Pontius
Pilate habited in the garb a gentleman assumes when pro-
menading Regent Street, or Joshua attired in the immaculate uniform of an officer in the Coldstream Guards ; but
to those who lived in the Middle Ages these anachronisms
presented no ludicrous features. Thus Moses appeared in
the Saxon period (Add. MSS. 10,546) in the dress of a
Thegn, while in Sloane MS. 846, written towards the
close of the thirteenth century, the lawgiver appears in
chain mail and plate, armed with sword and spear, and
prancing upon a gaily caparisoned charger. This custom
prevailed until the close of the fifteenth century, and it
affords us the finest and most reliable examples of all
kinds of costume, the most minute details being faithfully
reproduced. As a further example we will cite one of
common knowledge. King Arthur of the Round Table is
invariably represented in full plate armour of the fifteenth
century, at which period the manuscripts were written ;
as is well known, he was a British prince who died in the
sixth century.

With the advent of the Norman Period we find no
startling changes in costume, inasmuch as the Normans
of both sexes were habited somewhat similarly to those

of the conquered race. There were, however, minute peculiarities which distinguished the Normans, and these had been adversely commented upon by the elder Saxons in the reign of Edward the Confessor when they perceived the younger generation imitating the speech, manners, and garb of the Normans at the King's Court. " They shortened their tunics and trimmed their hair; they loaded their arms with golden bracelets, and entirely forgot their usual simplicity," is recorded by monkish chroniclers.

THE MEN

The essential garments affected by the Normans were the tunic, the super-tunic, and the mantle.

The Tunic was a garment worn next to the skin by the lower classes, and over the *just-au-corps* among the upper. It was made of linen or fine cloth, and at the time of the Conquest did not reach below the knees, and was furnished with short sleeves. Among the upper classes this garment is never visible, and it is simply from representations among the humbler people that we are aware of its existence.

The Super-Tunic.—This garment was similar to the tunica of the Saxons, but was worn much shorter; it is shown upon the Bayeux Tapestry, reaching to the knees. The sleeves were tight to the arms and long, terminating at the wrist with a small cuff. Embroidery was used at the neck and also round the hem.

The Mantle.—This differed but slightly from the Saxon; it was more voluminous, and in the early period was frequently longer than the tunic. It fastened up the front, or on either shoulder, precisely the same as in the previous period.

The Cap.—Upon the head of the civilians appears a small flat cap, with a band round the forehead (No. 1, Fig. 37); No. 2 is a very prevalent round skull-cap; No. 3 exemplifies the Norman pattern of the Phrygian shape,

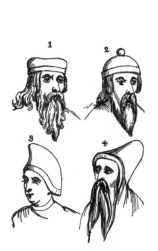

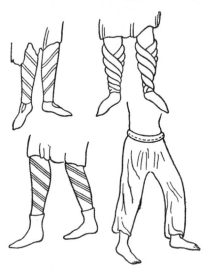

FIG. 37.—Norman head coverings.

FIG. 38.—Early Norman stockings, boots, &c.

which, as will be seen by comparison, differs from the Saxon by coming well down the back of the head; in No. 4 we note a variety of the cowl as usually worn; and in the four, almost every variety of head-gear is comprised.

The Chausses.—The tight coverings for the lower limbs worn by the Normans were continuous as far as the waist, and termed chausses; at times they were furnished with laces, in order to draw them closer to the body. Over these, various systems of cross-gartering were used (Fig. 38).

The Shoes.—The Bayeux Tapestry exhibits the plainest form of shoes worn by all persons represented upon it, no

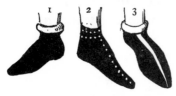

FIG. 39.—Shoes of the later Saxon and early Normans.

Centre example from Harl. MS. 2908.
The others from Cott. MS. Tiberius C vi.

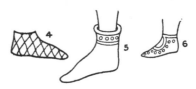

FIG. 40.—Norman boots and shoes.

ornamental work being discernible upon any character. They are similar to Nos. 1 and 2 in Fig. 39, but are generally represented without the projecting border round the top. The colours shown are yellow, blue, green, and red. As the period progressed they wore also short boots reaching above the ankle, with a plain band round the tops. The styles, however, became more elaborate, and some further examples are shown in Fig. 41.

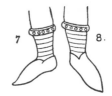

FIG. 41.—Norman shoes.

THE WOMEN

THE COUVRE-CHEF HEAD-DRESS, 1066–1100

During the reign of William the Conqueror the dress of the ladies to a great extent preserved the simplicity which characterised it upon their first landing in England. In the very few illuminations and descriptions which have come down to us from that period, we find no very marked deviation from the dress of the Saxon ladies; in fact the representation of one will, for all practical purposes, serve for the other. We may remark, however, that the covering for the head, although precisely the same as the Saxon head-rail, was dignified with a new name, and became the *couvre-chef*.

CHAPTER IV

THE NORMAN PERIOD (*continued*)

WILLIAM II., 1087–1100. HENRY I., 1100–1135. STEPHEN, 1135–1154

Civil Costume of the Men.—The reigns of these monarchs were distinguished by a love of display and ostentation in dress in remarkable contradistinction to that of the warlike Conqueror. King Rufus was fond of dressing in gorgeous apparel, and the rich Norman noblemen, battening upon the proceeds of their newly acquired English estates, were not one whit behind in following the example of their royal leader.

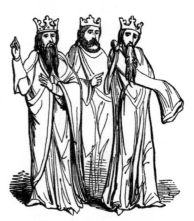

FIG. 42.—Regal costume.
(Cott. MS. Nero C iv.)

The Tunics, we are informed, were made so long and full that they lay upon the ground and cumbered the heels of the wearers (Fig. 42).

The Super-Tunic was considerably lengthened, and the sleeves so developed as to cover the hands. In addition to the rich embroidery used upon the dress at the time of William I., the material of the garments now showed signs of ornamentation, especially during the latter part of the reign of Rufus, when the Oriental feeling began to develop.

The Crusades exerted an influence upon the costume of the Western nations of Europe which cannot be too strongly accentuated. For many years before the First Crusade in 1096 a more or less constant intercourse with Eastern nations had prevailed, by reason of the numerous pilgrims who had visited the Holy Sepulchre; but when streams of men constantly poured backwards from the battle-fields of Palestine, wounded, or sick, or tired of the struggle, they brought with them such overwhelming stores of Oriental taste and Eastern culture, that the costume prevailing in their own land appeared to them simple and barbaric. Among the many beautiful materials brought home from the Orient, it is probable that *samite* found a place; it was sometimes entirely composed of silk, but frequently was interwoven with threads of gold and silver, and much embroidered or otherwise embellished with gold in a very costly manner. This material was chiefly dedicated to sacred uses; but it was not confined to the Church however, for we know it was used by the Norman monarchs, the nobility, and ladies of high rank on particular occasions, when more than an ordinary display of pomp was required. It is highly probable that many other rich materials mentioned in the thirteenth century were introduced at this time, although they are not distinctly identified by name.

The Mantle of the period was worn short or long, according to the length of the super-tunic; among the nobility it was made of the finest cloth, and lined with rich furs.

The Cap.—During this period a modified form of the Phrygian shape was worn (Fig. 43, No. 1); but during inclement weather, or when travelling, a cloak, to which was attached a hood of the Phrygian shape, was in use, and was called by the Normans the *Capa* (No. 2). An illumination of this date exhibits another kind of hat which prevailed (No. 3), similar to the cap worn by the modern carter.

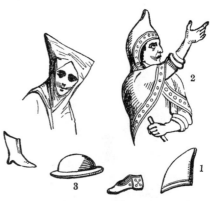

The Shoe.—The extravagance in dress in the time of King Rufus was also exemplified in the shoes, for the twist

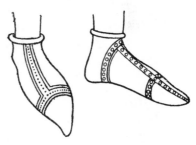

Fig. 43.—Head-dresses, &c., c. 1100. From Cott. MS. Nero C iv., &c.

given to the pointed toe of the boot during the reign of his father developed to an amazing extent during the reign of Rufus, while under Henry I. and Stephen the

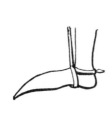

Fig. 44.—Shoe, *temp.* Rufus.

Fig. 45.—Norman shoes.

pike-toed boots and shoes excited the wrath of the monastic historians. The ecclesiastics were strictly forbidden to copy the monstrosities which they condemned. One variety, termed *Pigacia,* had points like a scorpion's tail, while we are told that a courtier stuffed his with tow, and caused them to curl round like a ram's horns,

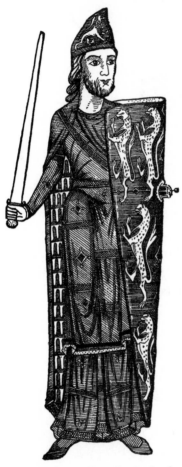

thereby eliciting much admiration from his companions. The general form may be gleaned from Fig. 44, taken from the seal of Richard, Constable of Chester in the reign of Stephen, which, though military, sufficiently exhibits it. They are now no longer shown black as in the previous reign, but invariably in colour, and decorated with bands (Fig. 45). Cross-banded chausses continued to be in use, although they are seldom visible by reason of the long garments. The brother of Rufus bore the name of Curt-Hose, but historians differ as to the reason for this appellation. It may be, however, that Robert, with soldier-like simplicity, refused to wear the exaggerated monstrosities he saw around him, and so obtained the nickname. It is worth remembering that for

FIG. 46.—Taken from the tomb of Geoffrey Plantagenet, Count of Anjou.

various reasons the civil, military, and ecclesiastical costumes, both in England and upon the Continent, were

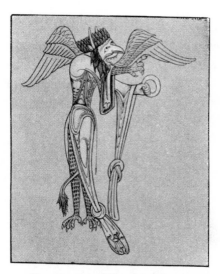

FIG. 48.—From Cott. MS. Nero C iv.

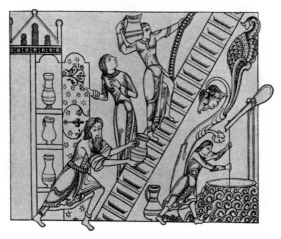

FIG. 57.—A Norman butler and his subordinates.
(Cott. MS. Nero C iv.)

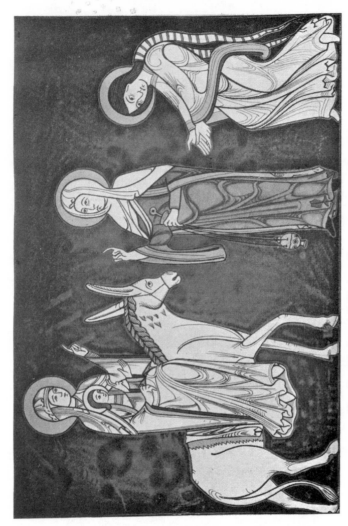

FIG. 51.—Virgin and Child, &c.   Norman costume.   (Nero C iv.)

precisely similar during the whole of the twelfth century, and that a distinct national costume, so far as civil dress is concerned, was not evolved by the English until the reign of Edward III. A typical example of this is shown in the preceding figure of Geoffrey Plantagenet, Count of Anjou, dating from the middle of the twelfth century, who is represented in a Phrygian cap, a mantle lined with fur, and a close-fitting super-tunic over a long tunic which reaches the ground. The long hair flowing upon the shoulders is very characteristic of the period (Fig. 46).

THE WOMEN

The Coif-de-mailles Head-dress, 1100–1150

The eccentricities in costume displayed by the nobles in the time of Rufus were speedily imitated by the ladies, who, however, proceeded to such extremes that they finally evolved a dress so fantastic and grotesque that it has seldom been exceeded. The long hanging sleeves of the nobles appear to have given the cue to the gentler sex (Fig. 47), who forthwith commenced to exhibit a perfect craze for lengthening every part of their garments which permitted.

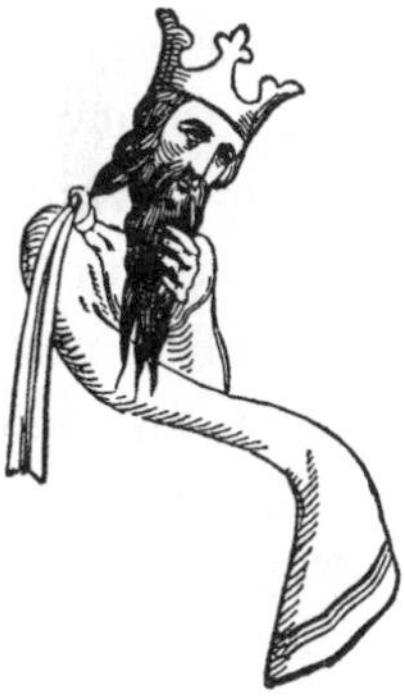

The *Robe* was more tight-fitting than in the preceding reign, and was lengthened to such a preposterous extent that it lay in great folds upon the ground. In the

Fig. 47. — The sleeve, c. 1100. (Cott. MS. Nero D iv.)

Cott. MS. Nero C iv. a representation of his Satanic majesty is given in the form of a woman—a compliment to the ladies which the monastic illuminators were very fond of paying. It is given here in Fig. 48, Pl., and affords a very fair

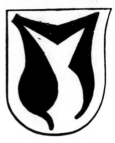

idea of the length of the prevailing skirts, inasmuch as it is seen to be knotted, and yet lying upon the ground. The sleeve also manifests the lengthening tendency, and is duly knotted. Apart from this, we may venture to say that tight-lacing is by no means a modern evil, but was practised even earlier than the twelfth century; the figure in question shows a corset fastening up in front with a long lace depending from it.

FIG. 49.—The heraldic maunch.

Fig. 51, Pl., gives us no less than three varieties of the robe and its sleeves, also from Nero C iv.; the Virgin and Child, on their way to Egypt, being the first subject. She wears a sleeve which does not differ essentially from that of a monk's gown, while the second and third figures have sleeves of the period. To the uninitiated the peculiar figure of the heraldic maunch is quite unintelligible (Figs. 49 and 50), but a careful com-

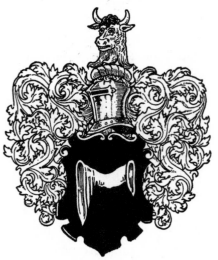

FIG. 50.—The heraldic maunch.

parison will at once simplify the difficulty. A further de-

velopment of the sleeve, called the pocketing variety, is
shown in Fig. 52, in which the terminations are very
largely distended.

The Mantle.—This
varied but very slightly
from those used in the
time of William I., as
will be seen on refer-
ring to the illustra-
tions.

The Head-dress.—
The head-gear lost its
primitive simplicity for
a time in consequence
of an extreme rise of

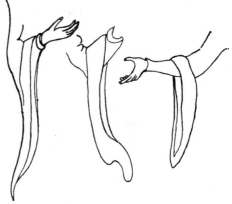

FIG. 52.—The maunch sleeve.

militarism among the ladies, engendered by the enthusiasm
then holding possession of the country consequent upon

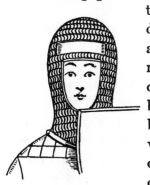

FIG. 54.—Knight in coif-de-
mailles.

the Crusades. Without actually
discarding this head-dress, they so
adapted it as to represent in a
marked degree the *coif-de-mailles*,
or head covering of chain mail worn
by their warrior lords. This will
be seen exemplified in Fig. 53, Pl.,
where the couvre-chef (in this case
of red material) is pulled tightly
down upon the head and kept in
place by a band of yellow embroidery round the forehead, thus
outlining the face similarly to that shown in Fig. 54, a
knight in coif-de-mailles.

This figure, which is an exact reproduction of one in an illuminated manuscript of the period, exhibits another trait of military feeling which is well worthy of notice. The super-tunic is purposely cut short, in order to show a garment which is a replica of that worn by the knights under their heavy mail, to prevent the latter chafing the skin.   It was termed the *Gambeson*, and was thickly quilted.   The dove-tail device of the hem is probably the lady's own design.

It is generally supposed that the *Tabard* was introduced as a garment for both sexes at this period, but as we have been able to find it represented only upon one female figure, we hesitate to state it as a certainty.   The tabard, however, undoubtedly came into use at a very early period, and was probably copied from the monastic habit, being identical in shape with the scapular.   Later the tabard took a very prominent place in civil, and especially in military, habits.

The method of dressing the hair at this period was very remarkable, and is plainly shown in a number of illustrations.   It was plaited into two tails, or otherwise divided, and each portion enclosed in a long tapering case, at times reaching nearly to the ground.   As a rule these were made of silk, and decorated in various ways, the ends bearing ornamental tassels.   There is a strong suspicion that this coiffure prevailed among the Saxon ladies before the Conquest, but it cannot be definitely stated as such. The two plaits preserved at Romsey, which were discovered in the Abbey Church in 1839, were taken from a coffin in which a woman of this early period had been buried.   They are eighteen inches in length.   The effigy of Matilda, Queen

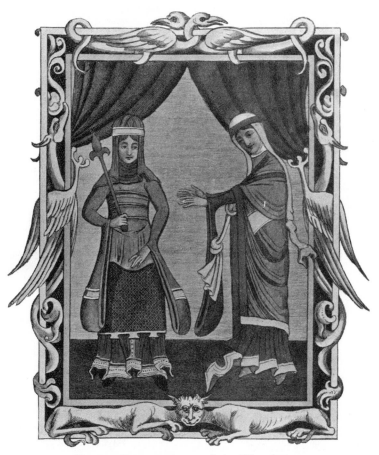

FIG. 53.—Norman costume, early twelfth century.

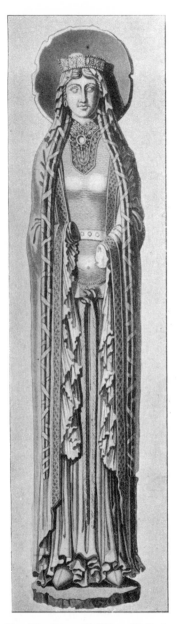

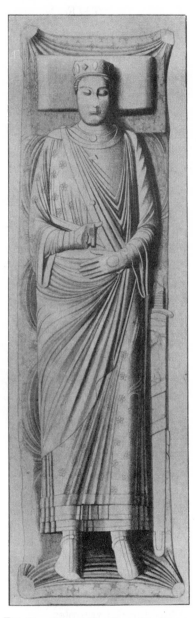

FIG. 56.—Queen Clotilda. Method
of arranging the hair.

FIG. 61.—Effigy of King Henry II., Abbey
of Fontevrault, Normandy.

of Henry I., at Rochester (Fig. 55), affords us an example
of this fashion; the two long plaits descend to the hips;
they are not encased, and the ends simply terminate in
small locks. Perhaps the finest example in existence is
that shown upon the effigy of Queen Clotilda, from Cor-
beil, which is here reproduced (Fig. 56, Pl.).
The plaits in this case reach below the knees;
they are two in number on either side, and
bound together by ribbons. That this style
of doing the hair was not confined wholly to
the upper classes is proved by a representation
in a Psalter in St. Swithin's Priory, Winchester, English twelfth century, where a
number of persons are shown in the place
of torment, and the women represented,
whether crowned or otherwise, have the two
long tails. This figure is not without interest
as exemplifying the cloak ornamented by
rich borders down the front. It is caught
up over both arms, and only partially exposes the long hanging sleeves of this period,
which are shown with an edging of pleated
silk. Upon referring back to Fig. 51, Pl., it
will be observed that the long encased plaits

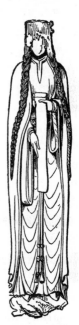

Fig. 55.—Matilda,
Queen of Henry I.

of the woman shown on the right exhibit the terminal
appendages; the uncovered hair shown in this example
is of the greatest rarity, and makes it a most remarkable
figure.

The shoes of Norman ladies are generally represented
black in manuscripts, but considering that the men wore
embroidered examples, sometimes elaborately ornamented

with jewels, it is only reasonable to suppose that the ladies did the same.

It must be carefully borne in mind that the distinctive civil costumes dealt with in these and succeeding chapters are essentially those of the wealthy and the well-to-do classes, and that they do not represent, except in a very remote degree, the general dress worn by the lower orders. In works upon costume it will be found, as a rule, that the dress of the masses is but briefly referred to, if at all, and we venture to think that this is a mistake. A mental picture of England in the past, so far as costume is concerned, cannot be accurately imagined without a knowledge of the dress of all persons connected. The general rule so far as it touches the mediæval period appears to be, that the costumes of the classes of one generation is to a certain extent the costume of the masses in the next, though, of course, there are exceptions. During the early Norman Period the dress of the Saxons preserved the same characteristics which had distinguished it for centuries (Fig. 57, Pl.), and many features pertaining to it survived even to the times of the Lancastrian monarchs.

Many illustrations of rustics have been handed down to us. In Cott. MS. Jul. A vi., the figures seen harvesting in the fields, felling trees, hunting, &c., are precisely similar to those shown three centuries earlier, and the same remarks may be made of artificers, gardeners, &c., in another eleventh century manuscript (Cott. MS. Claudius B iv.) slightly later in date, the only exception being the hair, which is rather longer. As a rule the rustics worked in the open air with the head uncovered, but in one illumination, dating from the time of William I., a figure is shown with a hood over the head, which may be taken as a very early form of the capuchon which subsequently prevailed for so many centuries. An exception also occurs in the case of the rustics appearing to Henry I. in his dream, where one holding the scythe is depicted wearing a hat of the form referred to previously. Another man grasping a pitchfork wears a cloak, which is very rarely shown among the lowest classes (Fig. 58).

The garment covering the body was usually of the

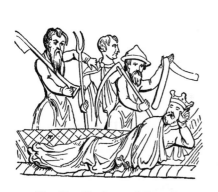

FIG. 58.—The dream of Henry I.

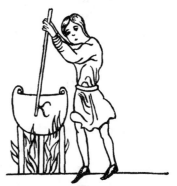

FIG. 59.—A cook.

simplest form that could be devised ; a close jacket reaching from the throat to the knees and furnished with sleeves generally too long for the arms, and rucked in Saxon fashion at the wrists (Fig. 59). It was invariably made of the tanned skin of some animal, upon which the hair had been left to be worn outside. This primitive garment, which was generally the only one worn amongst the lowest classes, was drawn in round the waist by a broad leather belt, which suspended a knife and other necessary articles. Shoes of a simple shape were always worn, and to this rugged simplicity, stockings of cloth and cross-gartering of leather were added by those in better circumstances.

The women of the lower classes were habited in as simple a manner as that which distinguished the men. A gown with sleeves, and reaching to the feet, with a piece

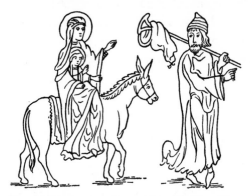

FIG. 60.—Norman travellers.   (Cott. MS. Nero C iv.)

of coarse linen swathed round the head after the manner of the rail or the couvre-chef, supplied a pattern which became almost stereotyped for three centuries. The hair was jealously guarded from exposure, as during the Saxon Period. The accompanying woodcut (Fig. 60), representing Norman travellers of the middle class, may afford interesting details to the student.

CHAPTER V

HENRY II., 1154-1189; RICHARD I., 1189-1199; AND JOHN, 1199-1216

THE MEN

THE sources of information for the costumes of the reigns of Henry II., Richard I., and John are somewhat enlarged when compared with the preceding period, inasmuch as we have more manuscripts, and those executed in a better style, and certain effigies of royalty. The latter are of extreme value in showing regal costume, which, somewhat modified in richness of ornament, and divested of attributes pertaining to royalty, also furnish us with the dress of the nobility. The coronation robes of these three monarchs, we glean from manuscripts, consisted essentially of a long tunic called a *Dalmatica*, with loose sleeves, covering an under garment with tight sleeves and being about equal in length. Over the dalmatica appeared the mantle. This dress, coupled with boots, gloves, and headgear, which will be subsequently described, furnishes us with the attire of the nobility. The earliest effigy of a King of England is that of Henry II., in the Abbey of Fontevrault in Normandy (Fig. 61, Pl.), a district which he much frequented with his Queen. It represents the monarch precisely as he appeared when lying in state. The dalmatica reaches to the ankles, and has the usual wide sleeves; it is crimson in colour, powdered with gold flowers. **A**

small portion only of the under tunic is visible at the
wrists, showing tight sleeves.   The mantle was originally
painted a deep red chocolate; it is fastened on the right
shoulder by a brooch, and falls to below the knees.   The
gloves have jewels upon the back of the hand, a token of
royal or high ecclesiastical rank; the boots are green, and
the gold spurs are affixed by bands of red leather.   The
shape of the crown may be discerned in Fig. 61, Pl., which
is reproduced from Stothard's "Monumental Effigies."   The
monuments of Richard I. at Fontevrault, and King John
at Worcester, are very similar to those of Henry II.; the
dalmatica of the latter is, however, much shorter, and
exposes a portion of the under tunic.   An illustration of
a contemporary king, which occurs in Roy. MS. 2 A xxii.,
circa 1190, is here reproduced (Fig. 62, Pl.).   The dalmatica
is ornamented with a rich design in which fleurs-de-lys
predominate; a heavily jewelled collar, with pendant and
a jewelled belt, are worn over it.   The sleeves in this
example are tight upon the forearm, and voluminous in
the upper part.   This peculiar shape of sleeve was prevalent
in this, and probably at an earlier period.   It will readily
be noticed that a marked peculiarity of this garment consists in its having one seam only on either side, which runs
from the under part of the wrist down to the hem.   The
mantle is white, richly lined with fur—the heraldic *vair*.
The high boots have an ornamental pattern which is very
common in manuscripts—a design upon a royal boot a
century later is precisely the same.

   A nobleman of the thirteenth century in Bod. Auct.
D iv. 17 (Fig. 63, Pl.) affords us a splendid example of the
costume.

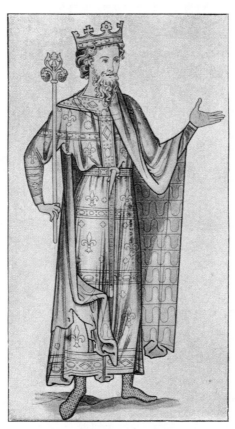

FIG. 62.—Regal costume, c. 1190.
(Roy. MS. 2 A xxii.)

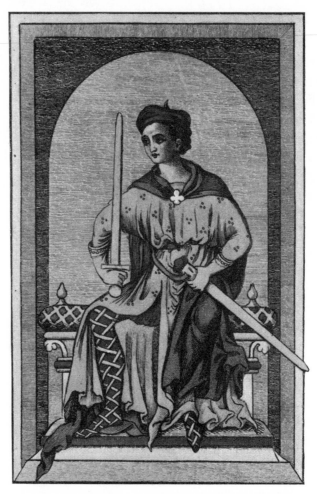

FIG. 63.—Nobleman, thirteenth century.   (Bod. Auct. D iv. 17.)

The dalmatica is clearly shown with a full sleeve previously described, and is open up the front. The colour of the original is red, and it is powdered with groups of three spots: the lining is white. The mantle of blue is fastened on the chest with a quadrilobed morse. The green gloves are a very distinctive feature; they have separate fingers, and reach half-way up the forearm, where they are elaborately embroidered. Upon the lower limbs red chausses are worn, covered with cross-gartering of gold, which, as will be seen, extends from the feet upwards. A garment, the *Braccæ*, similar to the knickers of the present day, is also shown. The blue hat appears to be of cloth, and is a departure from the Phrygian.

In Sloane MS. 1975 a doctor and his servant are shown (Fig. 64, Pl.); he wears a huge brown Phrygian cap, a red mantle fastening on the shoulder, a green dalmatica with an embroidered girdle and hem, from beneath which a brown tunic appears. The servant is clad in a single tunic, and wears green chausses. The boots in both cases are black.

Harl. MS. 4751 furnishes us with examples of hunting costume, in which the braccæ are very distinctly shown and no cloaks are worn (Fig. 65, Pl.). Upon the heads in two cases appear *Coifs*, almost universally used by hunters at this period. This is a very ancient head-dress, being worn at times by both men and women; subsequently it appears to have become a distinguishing attribute of the habit of the legal profession, and even at the present day has not fallen entirely into disuse. It is interesting to know that the bronze head of a Greek warrior has been found decked in a coif. During the twelfth and thirteenth centuries it appears

to have been common to nearly every class of society.
Thus, in Harl. MS. Roll Y vi., twelfth century, the "Life
of St. Guthlac," bricklayers and masons are represented with
it; a sailor wears it in a late twelfth century Harl. MS.
4751; it is seen upon the heads of the soldiery and a
number of spectators of different degrees in the "Vie de
St. Thomas," written *circa* 1230, &c.

Super-Totus.—This furnished the overcoat of the period
as a protection against cold and wet.   It was much used by
travellers and equestrians.   The shape of the garment varied
very much with individual taste, but the general pattern
adopted was one based upon the ecclesiastical chasuble.   A
circular piece of cloth had a hole made in the centre through
which the head was passed; in most cases a hood was
attached, and the wearing of this probably gave rise to the
capuchon, which came into use during the next period.

THE WOMEN

The Wimple and Peplum Head-dress, 1150–1280

Queen Eleanor, consort of Henry II., is buried at
Fontevrault, Normandy, and her effigy shows the regal dress
at the end of the twelfth century (Fig. 66, Pl.).   The under
tunic of white appears only at the throat, where it is fastened
by a circular brooch; a voluminous robe with sleeves tight
at the wrists and enlarging towards the upper arm is worn
over it, and is confined at the waist with a narrow girdle.
This robe is white, and a pattern is worked upon it consisting
of golden crescents in pairs, contained within the meshes
of an interlaced network, also of gold.   Over the robe a
blue mantle is shown, which, secured by a cord across the

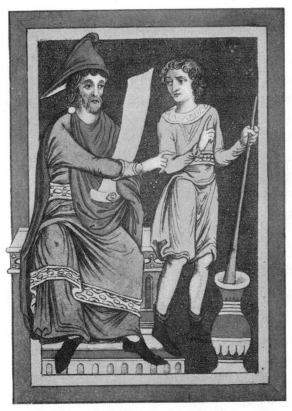

FIG. 64.—Doctor and servant, thirteenth century. (Sloane MS. 1975.)

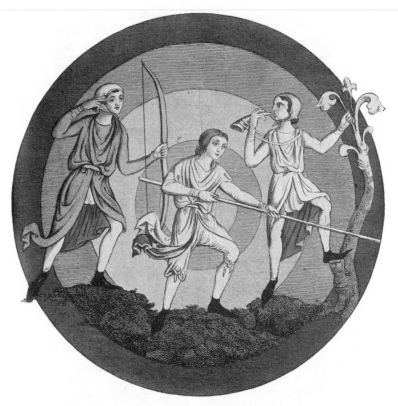

FIG. 65.—Hunting costumes, thirteenth century. (Harl. MS. 4751.)

chest, a fashion which subsequently prevailed for centuries, hangs down the back, but is brought forward over the lower part of the figure and held by the right hand.   It is studded with golden crescents.   The head is attired in a *Wimple* and *Peplum.*   This form of head-dress prevailed from the time of Henry II. to Edward I.   The wimple in its earliest form was a piece of white material, which was passed under the chin, and the two ends brought upwards towards the top of the head, where they were fastened together by a pin or brooch.   The peplum was only the couvre-chef masquerading under another name ; it was placed as usual upon the top of the head, and fell down symmetrically on either side of the face, and over the back of the head.   Originally of pure white material and without ornamentation, they subsequently became decorated, and of various colours, the wimple at times being of a different hue from the peplum.   As saffron is often mentioned by old writers in connection with the wimple and peplum, we must infer that yellow was the prevailing colour.   The term " wimple " includes the peplum, and will be used in this sense in the following chapters.   Long after it had been discarded as a head-dress by the upper classes, it remained in use by the middle and lower orders.

The same disinclination on the part of the ladies to show the hair was still manifested during this period, and practically in no illuminations is it apparent.   A curious exception to this unwritten law is that of the Queens.   On effigies of this and subsequent reigns, we find the hair fully exposed, sometimes in its natural condition and hanging down the back.   This was a special privilege of queenly rank ; upon their marriage the hair was worn flowing, and the same

fashion was represented upon their effigies; it is also natural
to assume that queens were above suspicion. The practice,
however, has led to much misconception, and persons not
representing royalty have appeared on the stage and elsewhere, in costume of the
period with flowing hair,
citing the queenly effigies as
authorities. There is no
doubt that an elaborate coiffure was invariably worn
under the wimple, for we can
distinctly discern the protuberance caused by it (Fig.
78, Pl.), but only under exceptional circumstances was

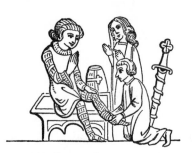

Fig. 67.—The hair exposed in the privacy
of home. (MS. 6956 Bibliothèque Nation-
ale, Paris.)

it ever seen. A rare example of the hair exposed in the
privacy of home is seen in Fig. 67. The dress of a lady of rank
at this time may be gathered from Fig. 68, Pl., which represents the Virgin and Child, and is taken from Roy. MS. 14
C vii., thirteenth century. So far as the head is concerned,
she is represented as a queen, with flowing hair and a crown.

The Robe.—This garment varies in no respect from the
preceding robes, except with regard to the sleeve, which
is now tight to the wrist. It lies in copious folds upon the
ground, and was evidently very voluminous. At times this
robe was termed the *Capa.*

The Cyclas played the same part in the lady's dress
that the dalmatica did in that of the man. It was not,
however, of the same form, being generally devoid of
sleeves; so far as length and appearance round the neck
is concerned, it is remarkably similar. The figure shows it

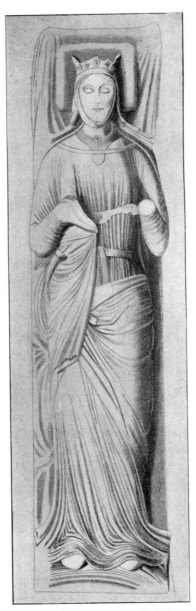

FIG. 66.—Queen Eleanor, consort of Henry II.

confined at the waist by a belt, while the ornamentation consists of small circles upon the yellow ground.

The Mantle in this case is shown very large, and, contrary to the usual custom, is not lined ; it is green in colour, ornamented with small circles with spots in the centre. Three young girls are delineated in Fig. 69, Pl. (Sloane MS. 3983), which exemplify the prevailing dress. The first wears a robe only, which spreads upon the ground; the sleeve is shown very clearly to be of large dimensions in the upper part, and was probably cut in the same method as that described in Fig. 62, Pl.; this, however, is not the case with regard to the robe upon the second figure, from which we must infer that the fashion was not universal. A peculiar feature is illustrated in these two figures, in looping up the robe in festoons to prevent it trailing upon the ground. The middle figure, in doing so, has exposed the hem of the under tunic, which appears to be fringed. She wears over the robe a cyclas with no decoration ; the shape, however, is very clearly seen, and leads us to conjecture that we have here the inception of the subsequent *Super côte-hardi* of a century later. In the case of the third figure the cyclas is so voluminous that a part of it trails upon the ground.

The Bliaut was a garment worn during inclement weather; it appears to have been of no particular shape or dimensions, and was common to both sexes. From descriptions of it, we infer that it must have been sometimes of expensive materials, but at the same time, as it is stated to have been occasionally made of canvas or fustian, we conclude that it was common among the middle and lower classes. Some writers trace the descent of the blouse of the French workman and the smock-frock of the English agricultural labourer from the bliaut.

CHAPTER VI

HENRY III., 1216-1272

THE civil costume prevailing during the long reign of King Henry III., embracing as it did the greater part of

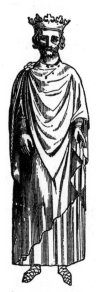

FIG. 70.—Effigy of Henry III., Westminster Abbey.

the century, was chiefly remarkable for the rich materials introduced, and not for any decisive alteration in style or the introduction of new garments. The great genius of the thirteenth century, Matthew Paris, was the historiographer of the kingdom, and not only did he write of the events passing before his eyes, but also drew a number of sketches which depict in a remarkable manner the costumes prevailing among all classes of people, and as such are particularly valuable. For the regal costume, however, the effigy of Henry III. at Westminster affords us an excellent example, and is chiefly notable for its extreme simplicity (Fig. 70). He is represented in a long tunic reaching to the ground, over which is a voluminous mantle, fastened upon the right shoulder by a morse of considerable proportions. There is no trace of a dalmatic having been worn. Nothing could possibly exceed the classic grace and kingly dignity of this effigy, which impresses by its very simplicity. Practically the

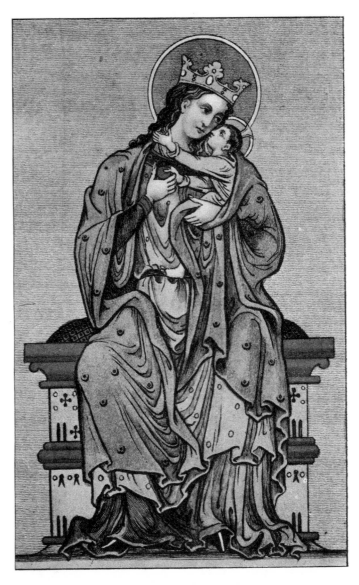

Fig. 68.—Virgin and Child, showing lady of rank, thirteenth century.
(Roy. MS. 14 C vii.)

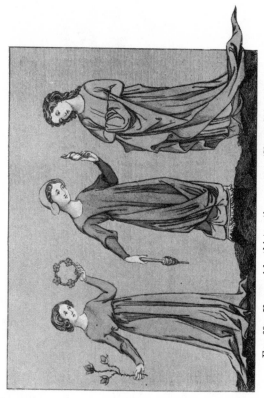

FIG. 69.—Young girls, thirteenth century. (Sloane MS. 3983.)

only trace of decoration, apart from the crown, appears
upon the boots (Fig. 71), which are of an extremely
ornamental character.   The usual reticulations characteristic of royalty appear upon them, but in each mesh a
leopard is shown worked in gold.   In Roy. MS. 14 C vii.,
a drawing by Matthew Paris of this king represents him
in a tunic having the peculiar sleeve of the time, a long
dalmatic which is sleeveless, and a
mantle, all being devoid of ornament.   In Cott. MS. Nero D i.,
his costume is the same.   Matthew
was no admirer of the pomps and
vanities affected by the Court.
Speaking of the marriage of the
King's sister Margaret with Alexander of Scotland, he says:
"There were crowds of knights so
pompously adorned with garments
of silk, so transformed with excess
of ornaments, that it would be impossible to describe their dresses.
Upwards of one thousand English

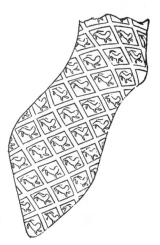

FIG. 71.—Design upon shoe.
Effigy of Henry III.

knights attended in vestments of silk, curiously wrought
in embroidery; they appeared on the morrow in new robes
of still more magnificent decoration.   Their breasts were
adorned with fibulæ, their shoulders with precious stones
of great magnitude.   The ladies had rings of gold set with
topaz stones and diamonds upon their fingers; their heads
were adorned with elegant crests or garlands; their wimples
were composed of the richest stuffs, embroidered with pure
gold, and embellished with the rarest jewellery."

THE MEN

The costume of the nobility and well-to-do classes
followed similar lines to that of the King, with the exception of the covering for the head.

The Capuchon or hood, which was adopted as a portion
of civil dress about this period, was evolved from the
monkish hood, and at first worn only as an attachment
to the *super-totus*. Its remarkable adaptability to all the
purposes which a head-dress could serve was soon recognised, and its adoption by all classes was only a matter of
time. Originating in the thirteenth century, the capuchon
eventually gained a remarkable popularity, and though after
a time it was partially discarded by the upper classes, it
did not finally disappear among the more humble people
until about the close of the fifteenth century, thus holding
its own for about three hundred years, an astonishing
example of persistence in an article of dress. It must not
be imagined that the same shape prevailed for these many
years, for various styles were evolved as time progressed,
some of which bordered upon the grotesque. In Henry

III.'s reign, however, the capuchon was in
its simplest form, and the general shape may
be gathered from the accompanying figures
(Fig. 73, Nos. 3 and 5). The shape when free
from the head may be gleaned from an interesting little sketch reproduced in Fig. 72,
which in the original represents a boy in pur-

FIG. 72.—The capu-
chon in its primi-
tive form.

suit of a butterfly about as large as a pigeon. He holds the
capuchon by its short *liripipe*, or point behind the head;
the back of the hood touches the boy's head; the neck is

in its proper position, and the opening for the face appears
upon the right.

The Hat seen in Fig. 73, No. 2, is represented in various
illustrations by Matthew Paris. Another style, only seen
upon persons of high rank, is No. 1, which appears to be of
soft material with the brim cut away in front. A variety is
indicated in a manuscript in Cambridge University Library,
dating from *c.* 1245, which
is only shown as a circular
pad upon the head, over
which is drawn the capu-
chon, No. 3. This circular
pad, furnished with a peak,
occurred on the walls of
the Painted Chamber,
Westminster, and has
been published in the
"Vetusta Monumenta."
It probably dated from the
early part of the thirteenth

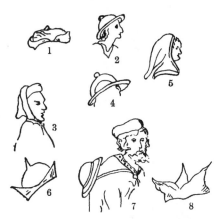

FIG. 73.—Capuchons and hats.

century. The hat, No. 7, is represented here suspended
over the shoulders by a silken cord which passes through
a ring upon the chest, and the evident use was to wear
both caps at the same time when circumstances required
it. We may say that for many years the custom prevailed
of wearing a hat over the capuchon, and this is evidently a
variety of the use.

The dress of the ordinary citizen partook essentially of
the character of that of the preceding period, the only variation being in the quality of the material, for the sumptuous
dresses and lavish display of the court percolated to the

middle classes, and induced them to dress far beyond their means, thus exciting uncomplimentary criticism from the national historian.

THE WOMEN

Berengaria of Navarre, the widow of King Richard I., died in 1235, and her effigy upon the tomb in the Abbey of l'Espau, near Mans, is full of interest (Fig. 74, Pl.). There is no indication whatever of her widowhood. In addition to her crown, she wears the peplum upon the head unaccompanied by the prevailing wimple, doubtless a concession to her position.

The Robe is of very ample proportions, and disposed in many graceful folds upon the figure; the sleeves, tight at the wrists, are somewhat enlarged at the upper arm. The mantle is but little seen, but the straps by which it is suspended pass across the chest. A narrow girdle decorated with gems is fastened round the waist by a buckle accommodating the long pendent tab. From this girdle is suspended a small aulmonière, or purse to contain alms, a fashion we shall find of great persistence until the Reformation. The brooch fastening the robe at the neck is of elaborate workmanship. A feature of this effigy is the book held in the hands, upon the cover of which appears a representation of the Queen lying in state with wax candles burning at her side in candlesticks. As an example of the head-

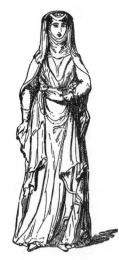

FIG. 75.—Aveline, Countess of Lancaster, 1269.

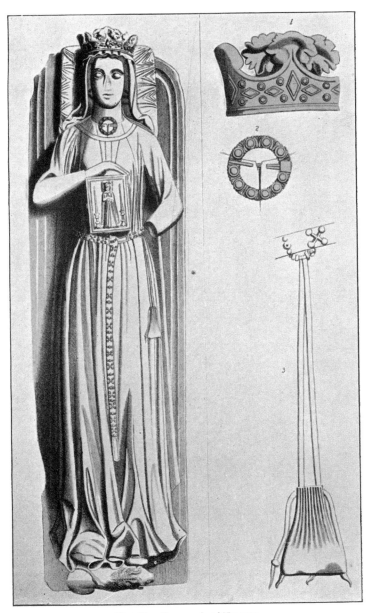

Fig. 74.—Berengaria of Navarre.

dress of the nobility, that of Aveline, first Countess of
Lancaster (1269), in Westminster Abbey, is an excellent
type (Fig. 75).   It should be remembered that at this period
the knights wore chain mail defences throughout, but underneath the coif-de-mailles an iron skull-cap had been
introduced, termed the pot-de-fer.   It caused a considerable protuberance over the ears, as seen in Fig. 76.   This

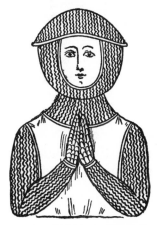

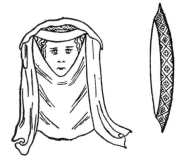

FIG. 76.—Knight, showing mail
over pot-de-fer, 1290.

FIG. 77.—Lady, showing imitation of
the knightly pot-de-fer.

feature was imitated by the ladies (Fig. 77), and the representation of these two figures of approximately the same
date are placed side by side for comparison.   The outlines
of the two faces are almost similar; the lady, however, as
will be perceived, has not erred on the side of modesty in
representing these lateral projections.   Although no decorative markings are discernible upon the wimple, no doubt
can be entertained but that it was made of the richest
materials, probably of two different colours.

The Hair during this reign was no longer done in two

plaits as formerly, but was gathered up into a network of gold or silver filigree, or in meshes of silken thread. The great difficulty is to obtain any illustration dating from this time of an exposed coiffure, so rigorously was the usual custom adhered to. The decorated cases enclosing the hair were of considerable proportions, as we may infer from the example given of the Countess of Lancaster (Fig. 75).

The ordinary dress of civilians may be judged from Fig. 78, Pl., which represents a simple robe sufficiently long to rest upon the ground, and confined at the waist. The sleeves are tight-fitting at the wrists. Over this is thrown a mantle, also reaching to the ground. It would be impossible to devise a dress more simple in aspect or more comfortable in use.

The shoes worn were of the short variety; they are generally represented black upon ordinary citizens, and with ornamental designs among the nobility—similar, in fact, to those of the men.

CHAPTER VII

EDWARD I., 1272-1307

It will have been perceived that in the preceding periods subsequent to the Conquest, the regal attire and also that of the nobility have been formed upon lines strangely monotonous as to contour and general shape. Robe, tunic and mantle—mantle, tunic, and robe, have succeeded with almost irritating regularity, and the student of costume experiences a feeling of relief to find some little deviation from the beaten track. The uniformity is broken to a small extent when we reach the reign of Edward I., by the introduction of the stole (Fig. 79). A manuscript of the thirteenth century exhibits regal costume, and affords us a good idea of the manner of adjustment, and also the dimensions

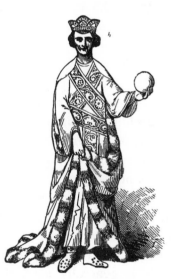

Fig. 79.—Regal costume, from a MS. of the thirteenth century.

of the stole. It is seen to be wider than the ecclesiastical article of dress, and to serve the purpose of a morse in fastening the mantle. Passing across the chest and round to the back, the two ends are again brought to the front, where they are probably fixed by a buckle, the longer portion forming a pendent tab.   In order to conceal the junction, and still further to confine the cloak, another piece of embroidery of a different design is fixed to the lining on either side.   This stole undoubtedly adds great dignity and richness to the attire.   Respecting the other garments, there is nothing of moment except perhaps the prominent part played by the fur upon the mantle.   Unfortunately no effigy of King Edward I. is in existence, but it is stated upon good authority that when the coffin of that monarch was opened in 1774, the body was found arrayed in a dalmatica or tunic of red silk damask and a mantle of crimson satin, fastened on the shoulder with a gilt buckle or clasp four inches in length, and decorated with imitation gems and pearls.   The sceptre was in his hand, and a stole of rich white tissue was crossed over his breast studded with gilt quatrefoils in filigree work, and embroidered with pearls in the shape of what are called true-lovers'-knots.   The gloves it is presumed had perished, for ornaments belonging to the backs of them were found lying on the hands.   The body from the knees downwards was wrapped in a piece of cloth of gold, which was not removed.   We may add that the whole of the jewellery found was imitation, an unusual thing at such an early period, though very common later. This is generally accounted for by the cupidity of the ecclesiastics.

THE MEN

Among the nobility this reign stands out in sharp contrast to that of the succeeding.   It must be borne in mind that Edward I. was essentially a military monarch, and that nearly the whole of his time was occupied in campaigns in different parts of his kingdom.   Under such a master, and remembering that the feudal system was still in force, the nobles had but little time to devote to the question of costume.   With the vitality almost crushed out of them by the terrible weight of the chain mail then worn, it was but natural that a loose and easy fitting garment would be the acme of luxury into which to change.   Not only this, but the King himself was never seen in what may be termed gorgeous robes, but was remarkably indifferent with regard to dress.   When expostulated with upon this point, he is said to have expressed the opinion that this subjects would not think any the more of him, or any the less, from the style of dress he affected.   Taking all these points into consideration, it is not to be wondered at that no striking changes were introduced.   The cyclas, tunic, and mantle of the form used in the previous reign still prevailed, but in place of the mantle the *Bliaut* was frequently seen.   This is represented as a long loose fitting coat, hanging straight from the shoulders and furnished with wide cylindrical sleeves, having holes cut a convenient distance down through which to pass the hands if required.   If, however, no new styles were introduced by the nobility, there was nothing to prevent them from using rich materials; and we consequently find that cloth of gold, cloth of Tars, silks, satins, and every kind

of rich cloth obtainable, together with ermine and other
costly furs for linings, were used in their garments.   One
peculiarity, however, should be mentioned, which is persistent
throughout the next three reigns, namely, the buttons upon
the forearm of the sleeve, which now appear for the first
time.   They extend from the elbow to the wrist, and were
common to both sexes.   In Roy. MS. 16 G vi., dating from

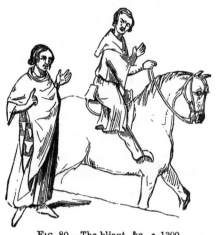

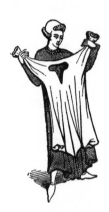

Fig. 80.—The bliaut, &c., c. 1300.   Fig. 81.—Man holding
(Roy. MS. 16 G vi.)   shirt.

c. 1300, are two figures (Fig. 80), and the man upon horseback
is represented with these buttons upon his sleeves; the bliaut
he wears is furnished with half sleeves, bell-shaped, while
his head is seen thrust through the opening of the capuchon
so that it lies upon his shoulders.   The peculiar pointing of
the toe downwards is a characteristic of mediæval equestrian-
ship, and will be more particularly seen upon representations of knights of that period.   The figure upon the left
wears a mantle lined with fur, under which we may perceive
the hanging half sleeve of the tunic.   The shape of this

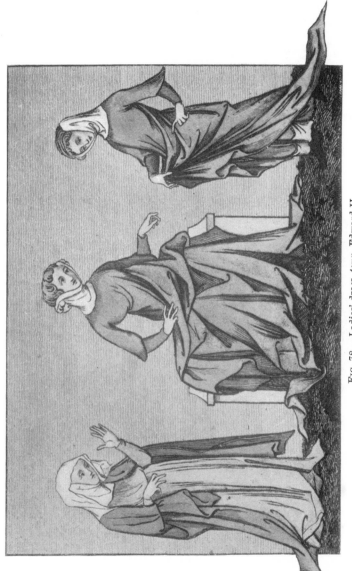

Fig. 78.—Ladies' dress, *temp.* Edward II.

sleeve should be carefully noted, inasmuch as it gradually developed from this primitive form.

For the simple dress of the peasantry of the time we may refer to Fig. 81, taken from a manuscript in the National Library, Paris (12,467). It is of great interest, inasmuch as very few representations of garments displayed in this form have been given. The person holding it is dressed in a longer tunic. An early thirteenth century MS. in the British Museum represents some hunters, from which we glean that the usual tunic of the citizens reached nearly to the ground, and frequently opened right down the front, being secured only to the waist. The loose knickers are consequently seen in one of the figures (Fig. 65, Pl.).

In Sloane MS. 2435 a small representation of the three classes of society is given—knight, ecclesiastic, and husbandman; the latter is clad in a short tunic reaching to the knees, and wears a white coif upon his head.

From Roy. MS. 2 B vii. we gather much useful information. The four figures (Fig. 82, Pl.) of minstrels represent the first in a wimple and a long robe with large sleeves. The boy is simply clad in a tunic. The third figure, that of a dancing girl, has the hair exposed, as usual with this class, and exhibits the low neck of the robe. The hood and the hats illustrated in the preceding chapter were persistent throughout this reign. The four figures shown in Fig. 83, Pl., represent the costume of one person at different seasons of the year.

Regal Costume.—The typical effigy illustrating English regal costume is that of Eleanor, consort of Edward I., in Westminster Abbey.   She is represented with the hair flowing and without the wimple.   The robe reaches to the feet, and the sleeves are tight at the wrist ; over it is the cyclas with its wide sleeves, but as a greater part of the figure is enveloped in a voluminous cloak, very few details are to be seen.

The statue representing the Queen upon the Eleanor Cross at Waltham is even simpler, only the robe and cloak being shown.   That the Spartan simplicity of the King affected the dress of his *chère reine* is undoubted.

The Robe.—This garment developed in length during this reign until it rested upon the ground probably a yard round the wearer, being extended in front almost as much as it was in the train.   This may be looked upon as characteristic of the end of the thirteenth and the early part of the fourteenth centuries.

Those taking an interest in the costume of the Middle Ages often express surprise at the beautiful draping of the mediæval dress as seen in contemporary illuminations, and the voluminous folds into which the dress naturally falls. At the same time they complain of the impossibility of obtaining the desired effect at the present day.   We venture to think that if similar material and the same design were used, the wished-for result would ensue.   The coloured plate is the photograph of a dress constructed upon the mediæval

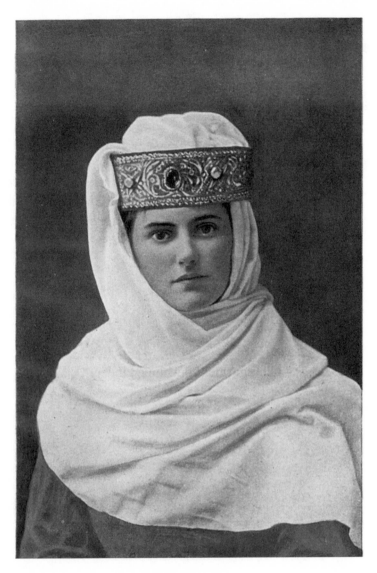

LADY, *circa* 1290

Head-dress.—Jewelled band, wimple and peplum showing modification in early part of reign of Edward I.

(Photographed direct from examples used in the Author's lecture upon "Mediæval Costume and Head-dresses.")

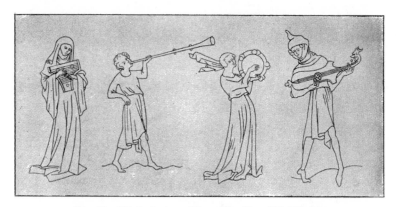

FIG. 82.—Minstrels, *temp.* Edward I.   (Roy. MS. 2 B vii.)

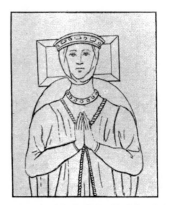

FIG. 84.—Countess of Oxford, Earl's Colne Priory, Essex.

principle, from which it will be gathered that the skirt of
the robe was a perfect circle when displayed. The material
used in the Middle Ages was invariably soft and clinging,
with none of the stiffness which characterised the Renais-
sance and subsequent periods. The sleeves seen in the
figure reach to the ground. The forearm is covered by the
sleeve of the under garment; it is tight-fitting, and shows
the buttons from the elbow to the wrist only.

The Cyclas, if worn, was a sleeveless dress of the same
length as the robe, and of a different colour. It is not
always represented, and the inconvenience of holding up
two long dresses when walking was probably the cause of
its omission. Like the nobles, the richest and most costly
materials were used by the ladies, but a striking feature of
the period appears to be the almost total absence of articles
of jewellery.

The Head-dress.—The wimple underwent a modification
towards the end of the thirteenth century. The peplum,
instead of being simply placed upon the top of the head
and falling on either side, was drawn up through a stiff
jewelled band made in the form of a crown, in the manner
shown in the coloured plate (p. 100); the wimple was put on
in the usual manner. One end of the peplum was fixed
to the inside of the crown upon the left side, and drawn
over the head to the right side; passing under the chin
it was carried round the shoulders, and the free end disposed in front. For this purpose the peplum was made
longer and more voluminous. A variety of this fashion
was shown upon the effigy, now destroyed by fire, of
one of the Countesses of Oxford in Earl's Colne Priory
Church, Essex (Fig. 84, Pl.). The above style of head-

dress (Fig. 85) was superseded in the last years of
Edward I. by the *Gorget and Couvre-chef.* These two
articles of female head-gear were merely

parodies upon the two preceding styles, but a distinct
advance was made towards the
fashion which subsequently prevailed of exposing the hair.
This did not actually occur to

FIG. 85.—Ordinary
head-dress of
linen.

FIG. 86.—Network
confining the
hair.

any great extent during the reign of Edward I., but
as it became usual to lay aside the couvre-chef when
indoors, the coiffure naturally had increased attention,

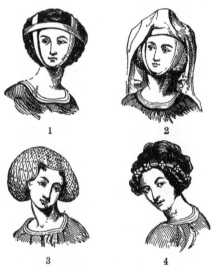

FIG. 87.—Hair-dressing, *temp.* Edward I.

and the ladies would be reluctant to hide it from view
more than was absolutely necessary. The method of
adjusting the gorget was simply to wind a piece of

material round the neck two or three times, and afterwards to raise portions of it at the sides and fix them
into the hair.   For this purpose the network for confining the hair (Fig. 86) was stiffened either by thickness
of material or by bands of linen, as in Fig. 87, No. 1,
from Roy. MS. 15 D ii. A similar method is shown in
the second figure, but this has the addition of the couvre-
chef. It will be noticed that this has precisely the same
appearance that the peplum presented.

CHAPTER VIII

EDWARD II., 1307–1327

THE reign of Edward II., the weak son of a warlike father, was given up to a wild debauch of costume and foppish eccentricities, strongly contrasting with the rigid conservatism of the previous reign. The rise of pampered favourites, each more extravagant than the last, produced a series of fashions which became the seeds of the true national costume under Edward III.

It may be admitted as an axiom that during the reign of a strong king, when the time bristles with stirring events, costume retires into the background, and makes little if any progress; whereas under a weak or effeminate monarch costume and all its accessories proceed by leaps and bounds. Probably the most eccentric and striking dresses ever evolved saw the light during the reigns of Edward II., Richard II., Henry VI., Charles II., and George IV.; and not only does the character of the monarch affect the civil dress, but the military equipment also reflects it. In this reign, for example, the knight of the Cyclas Period presents a more striking and picturesque appearance than he probably did at any other mediæval period (see " Arms and Armour "). With the advent of the reign of Edward II. we have a most valuable source of information introduced, which one might almost say exceeds in authentic and reliable information all the rest put together. We refer to brasses. The earliest in existence dates from 1277, and is of the military

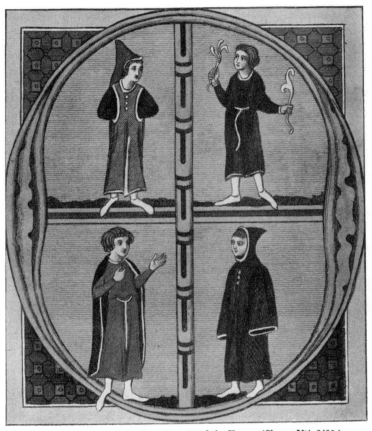

Fig. 83.—Costume of the Four Seasons of the Year.   (Sloane MS. 2435.)

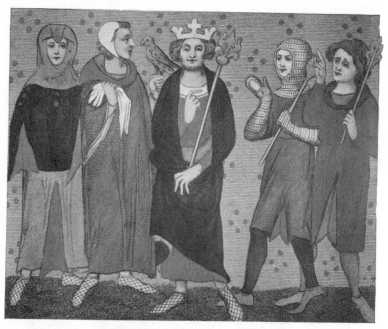

FIG. 90.—King and Court, *temp*. Edward II.

character ; the earliest of a lady is 1310, and that of a man
in civilian dress a few years later.   These sepulchral slabs
represent with the utmost fidelity every varying costume,
together with all minute details.   Of all the examples of
mediæval art yet remaining, none are of greater interest
or better known than these, and for the student of costume
they form rich storehouses of dress in its most comprehensive aspect.   They are as a rule much better preserved
than effigies of the same or even later dates, by reason of
the intense hardness and freedom from brittleness of the
material used.   It must not, however, be supposed that
every brass can be understood by the novice at the first
glance ; so far from this being the case, a certain amount
of education and practice in deciphering the salient points
are absolutely necessary.   Many features which escape the
beginner, and to him are of no moment, are invaluable to
the expert, and a knowledge of brasses, and of the artistic
delineation used by the old engravers, is a most valuable
accessory to the student.   Being represented upon a plane
surface, certain details which would be at right angles to
the spectator are swung back by the artist for display,
while others of a circular character are necessarily fore-
shortened.   One point concerning brasses should be borne
in mind,—the Continent is almost devoid of them, and
England is exceptionally favoured.   The destructive revo-
lutions and a long course of national disturbances in other
European countries have resulted in the almost total dis-
appearance of these works of art, and it is in England,
and England alone, that the study can be pursued.   The
Eastern counties, and the counties adjacent to them,
afford the richest fields for research.

THE MEN

The most drastic alteration which occurred in the men's dress affected the garment which had formerly been termed the dalmatica, its place being taken by

The Côte-hardi.—This consisted essentially of a very tight-fitting garment, closely following the lines of the body from the shoulders to the waist, where a skirt of much fuller proportions was added. The latter at first reached to the knees, and was of the same colour as the upper part. The junction of the upper and lower portions

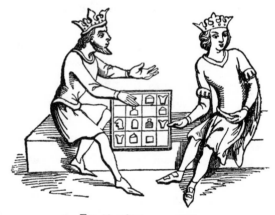

FIG. 88.—Costume, *c.* 1330.

gradually crept down the body, until by the middle of the reign it appeared below the hips. This feature is seen in illuminations of the early part of the fourteenth century in a most accentuated form, by giving the men a weasel-like length of body, which, combined with an extraordinary curve caused by bending the upper part of the trunk upon the hips, affords us an excellent clue to the chronology of a picture (Fig. 88). Even upon military brasses this peculiar feature is reproduced, as may be seen in Fig. 89. The côte-hardi was invariably fastened from the neck down to the waist by means of buttons, sometimes of great size, but no continuous fastenings are shown down the skirt. It is highly improbable, however, that no opening existed there, and as the skirt was made full, it was quite possible for it to overlap in front. A strong supposition exists that the opening was fastened under a flap down the front with a different kind of button from that used above, and that this feature survived for years afterwards, when the garment was much changed; for example, the côte-hardi shown upon the brass of Robert Braunche, Lynn Regis, 1364 (Fig. 114, Pl.), has buttons upon the lower part quite different from those above, although there is no apparent reason for it.

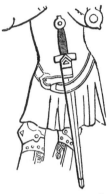

FIG. 89.—Knight, early fourteenth century, showing bending of the body.

The Tabard.—This article of clothing was of the simplest construction, and was really based upon the scapular worn by the monastic orders, precisely in the same manner as the dalmatica had been adapted from the dalmatic of the priestly order. It was merely an oblong piece of material, with a hole at or near the centre through which the head could be thrust, the shoulders being slightly shaped. The shorter portion as a rule hung down the front, thus presenting the general appearance of the knightly cyclas then prevailing. The courtiers, however, had their own particular tastes, and wore them long or short according to their fancies. This garment in its lengthy form reached to the ground; it was adopted by the members of the law, and was thus perpetuated for some considerable time. The bliaut, modified considerably in its proportions, was extremely fashionable, as will be seen in Fig. 90, Pl., which represents a king and his court.

The Court-pie was a short over garment for cold weather, and seldom exceeded three-quarters length; it was made upon the principle of the perfect circle, with a hole in the centre for the head to pass through, the sides being cut up for a short distance (Fig. 90, Pl., No. 1). It was always made in two or more colours, and therefore earned the term pie, or pied.

Balandrana.—This was merely another name for the super-totus, although its use was not entirely confined to cold weather, but, when made of rich material, formed a robe for parade (see Fig. 91, Pl.).

The Belt was in its incipient stage in this reign, but began to show signs of the splendour which distinguished it

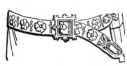

FIG. 92.—Belt of Humphrey de Bohun, Earl of Hereford, 1321.

in the reign of Edward III. (Fig. 92). It is generally shown hanging down more in front than behind, a little below the hips, and only upon the côte-hardi. The other garments worn over the côte-hardi, strange to say, are practically never represented as confined by a girdle. From this belt a gypcière was suspended on the left side or in front, more or less decorated in the case of the nobles.

Hats and Hoods.—The capuchon at this early stage of its inception began to undergo some of the metamorphoses which distinguished it during the long term of its existence. The point at the back gradually grew longer until it had reached to about the waist, and this develop-

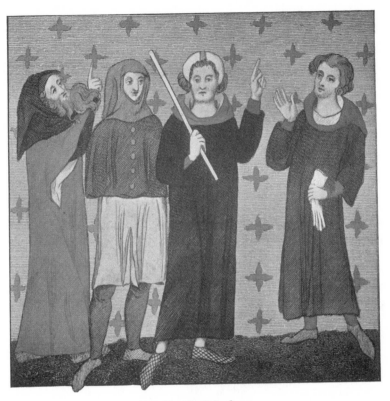

FIG. 91.—The Balandrana.

ment was dignified by a special name, the *liripipe;* at first it was useful, being passed round the neck when cold or wet weather occurred, but fantastic fashions prevailed, and it was seen in every conceivable position. At times a part of it was brought forward over the head, so as to reach almost between the eyes; others wore it in a short spiral, or passed it round under the chin and over the head, or wound it round the top of the head like a crown (Fig. 93, No. 3). The hat which prevailed during the

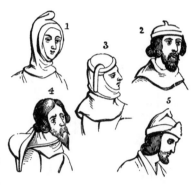

FIG. 93.—Head-gear, *temp.* Edward II.
From Sloane MS. 346.

reign of Edward I. was still in fashion, and a variety of it may be seen in No. 2, which is a flat cap with a narrow border covering the top of the head only; it sinks towards the centre, and then rises to a point. A

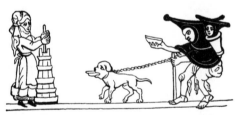

FIG. 94.—Milkmaid and beggar. From Add. MSS.
10,293, A.D. 1316.

very singular variety of hood is seen in Fig. 94, where it is sufficiently capacious to cover the shoulders like a cape, and is furnished upon the head with two projecting horns; this is taken from Add. MSS. 10,293.

The dress of the ordinary citizen of the period may be gleaned from Fig. 95, Roy. MS. 14 E iii., where one is represented enveloped in a bliaut with bell-shaped sleeves.

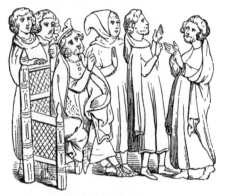

FIG. 95.—Edward II.
(Roy. MS. 14 E iii.)

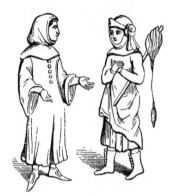

FIG. 97.—Costume of the commonalty, Edward II.

He wears an early capuchon not furnished with the liripipe. On again referring to Fig. 94, the blind beggar with the peculiar hood affords us an illustration, so far as his nether

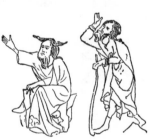

FIG. 96.—Boots and mittens of the lower classes, fourteenth century. (Arundel MS. 83.)

garments are concerned, of the tight-fitting cloth hose then worn by the men, and the loose knickers, although in this case both are in sad need of reparation. The method of carrying the child upon the back should be noted, as also the fact that it wears a similar hood to the man. The dog is apparently of a ferocious disposi-

tion, judging by the cable deemed necessary to restrain him. The general fashion prevailing among the upper classes at this time, of wearing or carrying gloves, was imitated by those in humbler circumstances, as will be seen in Fig. 96, which also illustrates the kind of boots they wore (Arundel MS. 83). Fig. 97 shows the pointed boot also in vogue at that period.

THE WOMEN

GORGET AND COUVRE-CHEF PERIOD, 1300–1350

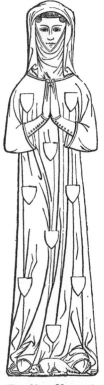

FIG. 98. — Margaret, Lady de Camoys, 1310.   Trotton Church, Sussex.

No effigy or brass of an English Queen at this period is to be found, but a statuette of Isabella of France, the most beautiful woman in Europe, occurs upon the well-known tomb of John of Eltham, in Westminster Abbey. Curiously enough the royal prerogative has been waived in this case, and she is represented in the gorget and couvre-chef, instead of the conventional loose-flowing hair and a crown. An example of the head of the Queen, shown without the disfiguring gorget, occurs in the nave of St. Albans Cathedral; she simply wears a couvre-chef, with a crown surmounting it. The costume is identical in pattern with the regal dress of the two previous periods. We know, however, from records and inventories of the royal wardrobe, that Isabella delighted in elaborate and splendid robes, made of the richest material procurable at the time, such as cloth of gold and silver, the most costly velvets and shot silks. The earliest known brass of a

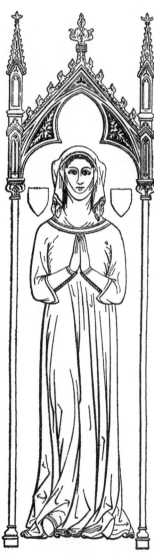

FIG. 99.—Joan, Lady de Cobham,
1320. Cobham Church, Kent.

lady dates from 1310, the reign of Edward II. It is that of Margaret, Lady de Camoys, in Trotton Church, Sussex, and is reproduced in Fig. 98. The adjustment of the gorget gives the well known V-shape identical with that of the knights of the period. Around the head is a narrow enriched fillet, below which on either side appears two small coquettish curls, an early example of the emergence of the hair. The couvre-chef falls gracefully upon the shoulders. An under garment has the usual tight sleeves buttoned to the wrist. A robe, unconfined at the waist, covers the entire person, and is of the simplest character; the sleeves are loose, and terminate below the elbow. This robe is powdered with small shields of arms, being the only sepulchral brass having this peculiar feature of ornament. Unfortunately they have been abstracted, and we are therefore unaware as to whether they bore her own arms or those of her first or second husband.

The emblazoning of arms upon the robes and mantles of ladies dates from the latter part of the thirteenth century, but as this is the first example which has been noticed in this work, a few explanatory notes are perhaps advisable. The custom prevailed in England for about two hundred and fifty years, and probably attained the zenith of its splendour during the fifteenth century. In all likelihood no more beautiful and effective method for the decoration of ladies' dresses has ever been devised; the rich tinctures imitated in the most costly material, with a contrasting hue

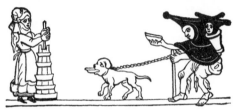

Fig. 100.—Milkmaid and beggar. From Add. MSS. 10,293, A.D. 1316.

of the garment, presented a scheme of ornamental wealth of colouring which has never been excelled. The knight in his jupon or tabard, blazing with his heraldic cognisances, stands out boldly in mediæval history; and the lady also, though in a less obtrusive form, is the appropriate complement to the perfect picture. The rule generally followed (although it must not be looked upon as hard and fast, in consequence of a few exceptions occurring) is for the lady to have her own family arms represented upon her robe, kirtle, or super côte-hardi, and those of her husband upon her mantle. If, however, they were shown impaled, they generally occurred upon the outer garment only.

At Cobham, in Kent, the brass of the first wife of Sir

John de Cobham is preserved; she died in 1320, and the

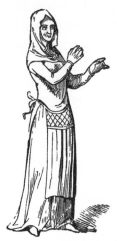

effigy differs but little from that of Lady de Camoys (Fig. 98). The fillet round the forehead is similar, and a small portion of hair is seen; the long robe is quite plain, but the termination of the sleeves are more of the lily shape. The buttons upon the right sleeve are touching each other (Fig. 99).

Among the well-to-do classes the general style of a loose-fitting gown prevailed, and the extraordinarily voluminous nature may be judged from the central figure of our illustration (Fig. 78, Pl.).

Fig. 101. — The barme-cloth or apron. (Sloane MS. 346.)

The same feature is also exemplified in the figure upon the right, which is also interesting in showing the *kirtle*, which would also sweep the ground were the hem not looped up in festoons.

The housewife of the period only copied to a partial extent the foibles of the aristocracy. In Fig. 100 she is represented churning in a dress which, like the kirtle above mentioned, is looped up; while the illustration gives us a very early example of the *barme-cloth*, subsequently termed the *apron* or *napron*. This protection for the dress had been in use for some considerable

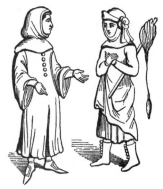

Fig. 102.—Costume of the commonalty, Edward II.

time, but rarely appears in an illustration; it was not always plain, as is seen in Fig. 101, taken from Sloane MS. 346, where the upper part is ornamented with reticulations. The barme-cloth was subsequently taken by the ladies, ornamented in a very rich manner, and became a favourite article of dress in the sixteenth century. The head-gear was the usual wimple, with the peplum tied in an ornamental knot at the side of the head (Fig. 102). A good illustration of boots worn by the women also occurs in these figures. The common name for these was *cockers* until about the time of the Commonwealth. They were generally made of crude materials, such as untanned leather. The term is not quite obsolete at the present day in the North of England.

CHAPTER IX

EDWARD III., 1327–1377

THE reign of "the King who taught the English people how to dress" should naturally be treated as a matter of paramount importance in a work of this nature. The King himself, warlike, and of strong common-sense, was not, however, the leader in the great movement which swept over England during his reign, and left the inhabitants with a characteristic national dress. There were many causes that led up to this consummation. The wealth which poured into the country from the wool trade with the Continent; the great war with France lasting so many years, with the victories of Creçy and Poictiers; the passing to and fro across the Channel of many thousands of men on trade or plunder bent—all these, and many others, were instrumental in building up a national character, and incidentally a national costume. Undoubtedly the garments evolved during the reign were hybrids between those prevailing at home and those in fashion on the Continent. The enthusiastic followers of an energetic king found themselves hampered by the long robes which had descended to them from their forefathers, and these were accordingly either relegated to the limbo of forgetfulness, or allowed to be perpetuated in the dress of those serving the law, medicine, or trade. The evolution of dress under an iron-willed king may perhaps be deemed a contradiction of the assertion made in a preceding chapter, but we may claim this as being the exception which is necessary to prove the rule. The great charm of the Edwardian dress, and that which stamps its superiority over the costumes of the majority of other reigns, is that, both with regard to the men and women, the garments follow the lines of natural beauty, namely, that of the body itself. There is nothing more exquisitely beautiful upon God's earth than the graceful outlines of the perfect human form with all its convolutions of marvellous symmetry; and the rational mode of dress, and that which is most pleasing to the eye, is to follow those lines as far as possible. All dress which tends to distort and disfigure the human form produces a bizarre result, displeasing to the eye, although the latter may become habituated to it; and a sigh of relief is unconsciously caused by the innate good taste, of which most of us are possessed, when the distortion is abandoned.

THE MEN: Early Period to c. 1350

The regal dress, as exemplified upon the effigy of Edward III., in Westminster Abbey, is notable for its noble simplicity. The chief garment is as usual the dalmatica, which reaches to the ground, and is open up the front, exposing the under tunic. The sleeves of the latter garment also show to a small extent upon the wrists, where they reach almost to the knuckles, embellished with the usual closely set row of buttons. The sleeves of the dalmatica are also somewhat tight, and curtailed at the wrist. A rich piece of embroidery borders the opening in front. The royal mantle resembles in a marked degree the ecclesiastical cope, both as to form and also in the morse which fastens it across the chest. The shoes are splendidly embroidered. The King's head is bare, and he is shown with long hair and beard. In Cott. MS. Nero E ii. (Fig. 103, Pl.), the King is represented in audience with Guy, Earl of Flanders. He wears a dalmatica of large dimensions, confined round the waist by a belt; it is provided with long hanging sleeves. This garment is purple lined with yellow; the sleeves of the tunic are identical with those of a Bishop at the present time. The Earl is habited in a long blue robe, having capacious sleeves lined with yellow. The curious pendants from the waist-belt should be noticed. It will thus be seen that with regard to the regal costume long flowing garments were still in favour, and considered inseparable from royal dignity.

The Nobles.—The characteristic garment of the whole reign of Edward III. is undoubtedly the côte-hardi, foreshadowed, and to a certain extent developed, in the preceding reign. At the termination of the reign the pendent sleeve was about a foot in length, and this continued to develop. A contemporary drawing (Fig. 104), representing a man and woman at dinner, shows this sleeve, but a better representation is seen in Fig. 105, where a scribe is seen seated upon a *huche*, and engaged apparently in writing a letter. About the year 1350 a marked innovation occurred, supplanting this feature. The sleeve became continuous to the wrist, hiding the buttons of the under tunic if any existed. To take the place of the pendent sleeve opening, bands of white material of various widths were affixed to the sleeve just above the elbow, which hung down to about the knees, as in Fig. 106, Pl. The first re-

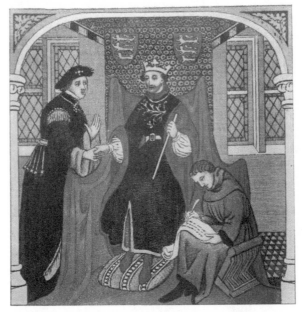

FIG. 103.—Edward III. and the Earl of Flanders.   (Cott. MS. Nero E ii.)

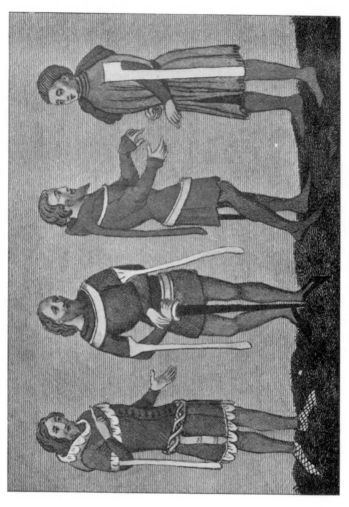

(Roy. MS. 20 D xiv.)　　(Roy. MS. 17 E vi.)　　(Roy. MS. 19 C iv.)　　(Roy. MS. 20 C vii.)

Fig. 106.—Early Edward III. costume.

presentation shows the côte-hardi buttoned tightly to the figure down to the hip-belt; the *tippets* are narrow, and a band of white material, dagged into pendent leaves,

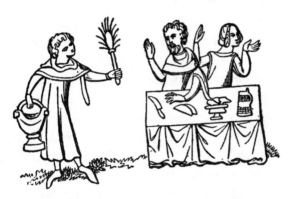

FIG. 104.—Illustration of pendent sleeve.   Early Edward III.

appears round the hem.   The côte-hardi is parti-coloured, half the garment with one sleeve being of one colour, and the remaining half of another contrasting colour.

Respecting the fashion of cutting into dagges, this decorative method was introduced about 1346, although some profess to find it earlier.   The term is applied to all ornamental edging, no matter how complex. The second figure shown deserves mention, inasmuch as it exemplifies a semi-military dress which often occurs at this period.   A

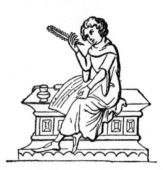

FIG. 105.—Pendent sleeve, illustrated. Early Edward III.

breastplate is hidden by the côte-hardi, which, like the military jupon of the time, buttons down under the left arm. The presence of the breastplate explains the reason for the small waist.

A late example of the *Côte-hardi* during the reign of Edward III. is shown in Fig. 107, Pl., by which time it had arrived at the height of its perfection. It accurately follows the outline of the figure, buttons down the front, has tight sleeves with no ornamentation, and is remarkably short. Omitting the sleeves, it is practically the counterpart of the military jupon, which did so much to render a knight of this period one of the most picturesque figures of mediæval times. The three persons represented in this plate are in black mourning habits. This question of colour for mourning is somewhat vague, but, speaking broadly, it may be said that until the fourteenth century practically all colours were used at different times for expressing signs of grief, but in the century mentioned black came more into use for this purpose than any other. At first it was customary to wear simply a black cloak or mantle over ordinary dress, but as time progressed other garments were also made of the same sombre hue. That the custom was occasionally broken through we may glean from the example of Henry VIII., who wore white mourning when Anne Boleyn was executed, and this unfortunate lady had in her turn worn yellow mourning for her predecessor. Probably black as a national hue for mourning was not finally established until the Commonwealth.

The materials used in making the côte-hardi were, so far as the aristocracy were concerned, of the most gorgeous and lavish description; cloth of gold or silver, velvet, silk, satin, baudekyn, &c., every rich and expensive material that money could procure, was used; while we read of gold

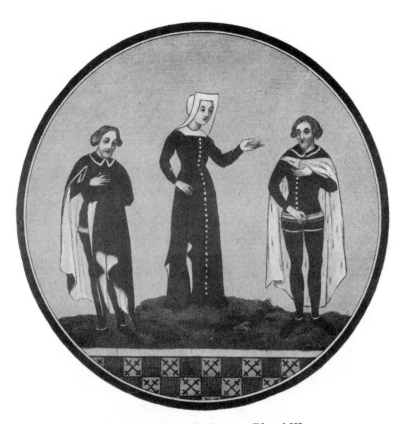

FIG. 107.—Mourning habits, *temp.* Edward III.

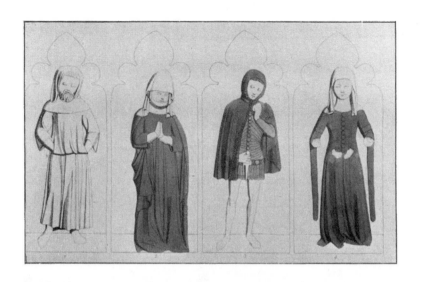

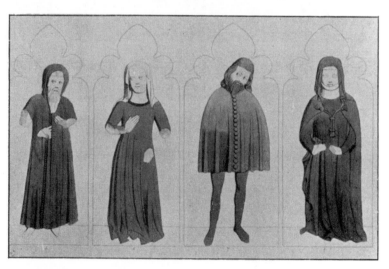

Stothard, Plate 54.

FIG. 110.—Figures of civilians round tomb of Sir Roger de Kerdeston.

embroidery, pearls and jewels being used in ornamentation. In its most perfect form the côte-hardi was in all probability padded, as creases are conspicuously absent.

A Mantle extremely characteristic of this period was one reaching to the ankles, and fastened on the right shoulder by three or more large buttons. It was ornamented by embroidery round the edge, the lower hem in

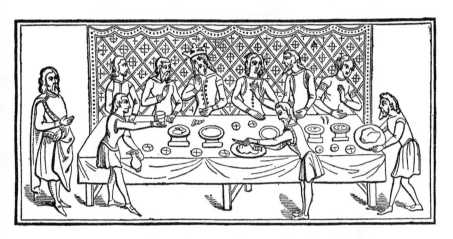

FIG. 108.—A king at dinner. Taken from Add. MSS. 12,228.

some cases being of the richest dagging from eight to ten inches deep. To the neck of this mantle the capuchon was affixed, which fell upon the chest and back when not in use. An adaptation of this mantle for use indoors is shown in Fig. 108, where the chief of the attendants is wearing one without a capuchon. The liripipe continued to grow both in length and width, often reaching to the ground.

The Chausses of the reign of Edward III. were a striking part of the general costume. They were made after the fashion of trunk hose, and fitted tightly to the person.

Pied chausses had been introduced during the reign of
Edward II., but are only occasionally seen during this
period; they did not become universal until the time of
Richard II.

The Shoes were strictly pointed, and the right and left
forms much accentuated, but we do not find the toes disproportionately long. They were made of very rich
material, and more of the shape of a half boot than a shoe.

The Belt.—This accessory to the dress vies with the
côte-hardi in being the most striking feature of the times.
It was always worn round the hips, and was universal.
The general construction was that of a number of square
brooches linked closely together by chains, each brooch
being as a rule a replica of its neighbours. The highest

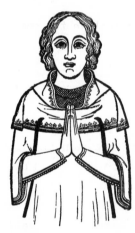

art of the goldsmith and jeweller
was brought into requisition, and the
costliness and magnificence were only
limited by the purse of the wearer.
It was, of course, merely the knightly
belt copied for the use of citizens.

The better class of civilian is well
depicted in the brass of Adam de
Walsokne at Lynn, 1349 (Fig. 109),
whose capuchon is ornamented with
a rich bordering. The tunic has
short pendent sleeves, from beneath
which the usual tight sleeves of the
under garment appear decorated with
thick rows of buttons (Fig. 110, Pl.).

FIG. 109.—Adam de Walsokne,
1349. Lynn Regis.

The costumes of the working classes were far more
striking in colour than they had hitherto been, and also

differed very essentially in style.   Upon the body the long
côte-hardi, reaching to the knees, appears to have been
almost universal; it was confined by a cord round the
hips in imitation of the knightly belt.   From this cord, as
a rule, a large square bag depended in front, which appears
to have served the functions of a purse, tool-holder, &c.,
so capacious were its dimensions.   In some illuminations it
is represented as large as a Highlander's sporran.   These
pouches were termed *gypcières*, a name which had previously been exclusively reserved for a pouch used in
hawking.   Others show this bag depending from the left
or right side, indiscriminately, and some, again, behind
the body.   The côte-hardi was in many cases pied, either
vertically, whereby the two sides show contrasting colours;
or horizontally, in which the upper portion differed from
the skirt.   The line of junction in this case was always
round the hips, the belt or cord serving to hide the seam.
This gave an opportunity for making the skirt of a thinner
material and of pleating it, whereby it hung in folds and
gave greater freedom in movement.   The attendants at
table, in the woodcut (Fig. 108), illustrate this feature,
which practically became disused about 1350.   The two
figures in the foreground also show the côte-hardi as
sleeveless, an under garment providing them.   In one case
a piece of embroidery is shown round the arm-hole.   There
are indications, in a few rare cases, of bands of different
coloured material bordering the lower hem.   The sleeves
were always of the same colour as the material on their
own side.

The *Capuchon* was by this time nearly universal; but
the lower part, which up to now had merely covered the

shoulders, was lengthened so as to reach to the elbows or even lower, thus fulfilling the purposes of a cape, and often buttoning down the front.   This capuchon was at times pied, but if so the côte-hardi was invariably made of a self colour.   Liripipes were of all sizes and dimensions, and

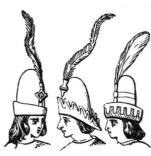

worn in a variety of ways, as in the preceding reign.   Although the capuchon was in use with the greater part of the nation, the nobles and those of high degree indulged in a fantastic hat, the style of which may be gleaned from Fig. 111.   These examples are taken from Add. MSS. 12,228, and are much more striking in the

FIG. 111.—From romance of King Meliadus, Edward III.

original colours than when reproduced in black and white. The brims are generally coloured, but the bodies of the hats appear to be of white felt.   The plumes waving from the front are in some cases disproportionately long—one, for instance, in the cap of a squire is probably a yard in length.   The ornamental sockets for holding these feathers often exhibit the art of the goldsmith.

The villeins and the lower class of labourers are well illustrated in the Loutrell Psalter, c. 1340, and they exhibit a strange medley of Edward III. costume combined with all the fashions of preceding reigns.   The ploughman, for example, is in a loose tunic girded round the waist; upon his head is seen an old-fashioned hat, which he wears underneath a capuchon with an incipient liripipe, but minus a cape; while upon his legs he has half stockings.   These socks, as we may term them, are discarded by the reapers, carters,

&c., who only wear boots.   In the case of threshers, the violent exercise necessitates the removal of every garment except those next to the skin, and they are represented in a short tunic only partially covering the universal loose knickers.   No protection whatever for the head is shown in many cases, and there are also examples of the feet being devoid of covering.

So far as the costumes for men have been described in the preceding pages, it should be distinctly understood that they are those of the earlier part of the reign of Edward III. to a very great extent, or, in other words, approximately before 1350.   After that time many innovations crept in owing to the increased traffic with the Continent.   We will treat of these in the usual order.

THE MEN: Later Period after 1350

The habiliments of a gentleman of approximately 1350 are portrayed in Fig. 112, where a close-fitting côte-hardi is shown with tight sleeves, encircled by a hip-belt with a large buckle.   To this is attached a gypcière having a dagger thrust through it.   His boots are long and pointed, and the garters are a prominent feature.   Over the left shoulder the capuchon is shown with ornamental bands round the neck and a short liripipe.   The parti-coloured dresses which came into fashion at this period were peculiarly objectionable to the ecclesiastic, and many caustic remarks were levelled at them by satirical contemporary writers; thus the red side of a gentleman is referred to as having been roasted by St. Anthony's Fire.

The effigy of William of Hatfield, in York Cathedral,

may be cited as an example of late Edward III. costume.
The cloak, which is still fastened on the right shoulder by

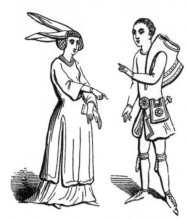

the usual buttons, is a very
graceful form, and has the
edge richly dagged into acan-
thus leaves. The côte-hardi
fits tightly to the form, and is
the regulation length for that
period; the sleeves are now
seen prolonged to the root of
the thumb, with the buttons
underneath. The greater part
of the côte-hardi bears a
pattern upon it of foliated
leaves and tendrils. The half

FIG. 112.—Edward III. costume, c. 1350.

boots are extremely ornate. A figure from the tomb of
Edward III., in Westminster Abbey, depicts a similar
costume, but plainer, the côte-hardi being unornamented
and the cloak being absent.

In the year 1363 a complaint was lodged in Parliament
of the excess to which the inhabitants of the realm generally
were in the habit of arraying themselves in costly materials
beyond their income or station; and in order to curb these
extravagances, a sumptuary law was passed which affords
us an insight into the dress of the period, so far as the
material, &c., is concerned. Thus :—

(1) Royalty, and nobles possessing upwards of one
thousand pounds per annum, were permitted furs of ermine
and lettice, and embellishments of pearls upon dresses, exception being made if the latter were required for a head-dress.

(2) Knights and ladies whose annual incomes exceeded

four hundred marks were permitted cloths of gold and silver, habits embroidered with jewels and lined with pure miniver and other expensive furs.

(3) Knights whose income exceeded two hundred marks, and squires with property valued at two hundred pounds, were allowed to wear cloth of silver, with ribbons and girdles reasonably ornamented with silver, also woollen cloth valued at six marks a piece.

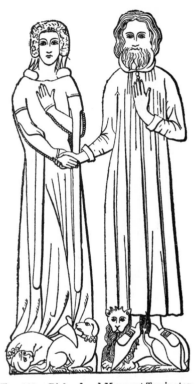

(4) Persons under the rank of knighthood were to wear cloth not exceeding four marks a piece, and were prohibited wearing silk or embroidered garments, or embellishments in their apparel with any ornaments of gold, silver, or jewellery, such as rings, buckles, girdles, ouches, ribbons, &c. The penalty in all cases was to be the confiscation of the offending articles.

FIG. 113.—Richard and Margaret Torrington, 1349–1356. Great Berkhampstead, Herts.

A civilian of the better class is depicted on the brass of Richard (d. 1349) and Margaret Torrington (d. 1356), in Great Berkhampstead Church, Herts, the singular simplicity of whose dress is very remarkable (Fig. 113). The only ornaments apparent are the buckles on the shoes.

Robert Braunche in St. Margaret's Church, King's Lynn, Norfolk (Fig. 114, Pl.), is portrayed upon a brass dating from

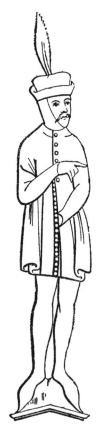

1364 in a long robe or gown with short sleeves, to which tippets are appended. The sleeves of his under tunic have buttons which reach from the wrist to beyond the elbow. The whole of the garments are finished with ornamental borders. The shoes in this case are laced.

In one of the compartments of this brass is shown a figure which is here introduced (Fig. 115). It is the plain costume of the period, but a hat is shown worn over the capuchon, which has a turned-up brim, from the back of which a feather springs. In Fig. 116, Pl., various figures representing the lower orders are introduced from Roy. MSS. 15 B iii.; 20 C vii.; 19 C i., &c., from which our readers will probably be able to glean a general idea of the dress of some of the working classes of England in the latter part of the reign of Edward III. Upon the first is seen a particularly large hood with no liripipe, covering a coif, which latter article of dress is very persistent throughout the period; while the second man is the agricultural labourer, pure and simple, his very action in wiping his brow being eminently suggestive of toil. The third upon the plate is an artificer of the better class, perhaps an armourer. The peculiar method of wearing the dagger is characteristic

FIG. 115.—Fig. from Brass of Robert Braunche, 1364. Lynn Regis, Norfolk.

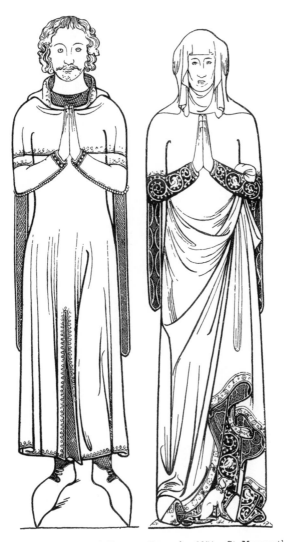

FIG. 114.—Robert and Margaret Braunche, 1354. St. Margaret's
Church, Lynn Regis, Norfolk.

of the next reign, as also are the pied chausses. The liripipe in this case is wide and bound round the head. No. 4 is seen in an old-fashioned tunic, bunched up at the waist, and illustrates the fashion of wearing an additional covering for the head, which is a marked feature of the whole of the fourteenth century. As another example of this double protection we reproduce a plate from a manuscript of the celebrated poem of Piers Plowman, preserved in the library of Trinity College, Cambridge, and written in the last years of Edward III. (Fig. 117, Pl.). Upon the head of the figure holding the plough is the universal capuchon, with the liripipe bound round the top, upon which is placed a very characteristic hat with a turned-up brim finishing in a knob. His tunic is pied, being mauve upon the right side, and white with red stripes upon the other; his chausses are red to match the capuchon, and the boots are black. His companion holding the goad is probably his helpmeet, though it is quite open to argument to assert that the figure it may represent is one of the sterner sex. Upon the head the old-fashioned wimple is seen, over which the capuchon, now lying upon the shoulders, can be drawn if required.

THE WOMEN: Early Period to c. 1350

Gorget and Couvre-chef Period, 1300-1350

We have now arrived at a very important part of the present work, in which it will be necessary to summarise to a certain extent that which has gone before, and to indicate the method of procedure with regard to the costume of the

next two or three centuries.   As this book is written with
the main object of affording the student certain characteristic
details and salient features which differentiate the dress of
one period from that of another, the simplification of such
a design is obvious.   In most books upon costume which
have hitherto appeared the dress of the lady has, to a
certain extent, been described in the vaguest terms as
having prevailed in such and such a style during, say, the
thirteenth century ; or else, that it was in evidence under
some particular king.   Now it is perfectly evident that a
costume did not change the minute a new king mounted
a throne, or that a garment was discarded immediately
upon the stroke of the last second of a century.   Fashions
do, and always will, overlap each other to a more or less
considerable extent, and the tendency to perpetuate an old
fashion was just as strong in the mediæval period as it is
among certain worthy ladies of our own.   There are probably few among our readers who do not know at least one
old lady who clings with affectionate regard to some early
Victorian fashion, and this trait was very marked in the
Middle Ages, when innovations were introduced at comparatively long intervals compared with the present age.   If
we make a careful survey of the dress of English ladies
from the Saxon Period to the Georgian, we find that, so far
as the gown and mantle (or the substitute for the mantle)
are concerned, the periods of change from one decided style
to another were extremely long, omitting certain eccentricities, like the maunch sleeve, for instance, which only
had an ephemeral existence.   A far better clue to the
chronology of the lady's dress is indicated by the sleeves,
which are at times decidedly characteristic of a certain

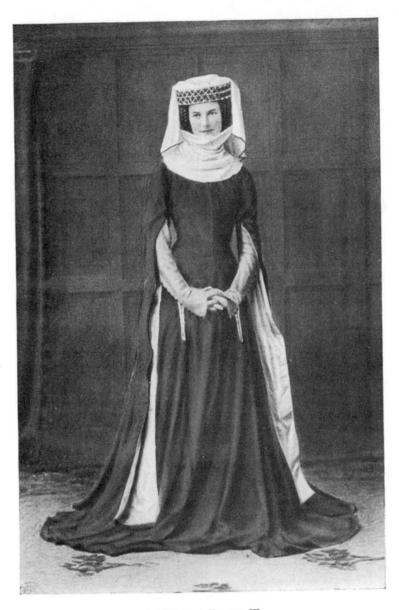

LADY, *temp.* EDWARD III.

Head-dress.—Gorget, couvre-chef and band.
Coiffure.—Thick plaits down either side of face.
Robe.—Of green thin cloth, sleeves lined cream silk.
Kirtle.—Sleeves only shown, with buttons.

(Photographed direct from examples used in the Author's lecture upon
    "Mediæval Costume and Head-dresses.")

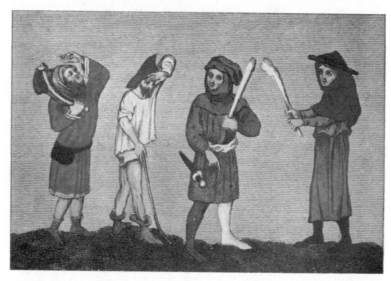

FIG. 116.—Artificers, &c., *temp.* Edward III.

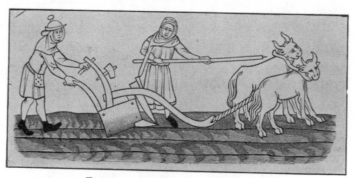

FIG. 117.—Ploughing, *temp.* Edward III.

epoch; but undoubtedly the best of all significant points is that afforded by the head-dress. This is almost as true at the present time as it was certainly true in the past. We would earnestly advise the student of costume to make this question of attire the memory-pegs upon which to hang the successive stages of development of female dress, and as a help we may adduce the following steps up to and including the present reign :—

1. The Saxon head-rail, closed during the greater part of the period, but worn open under the Danish and Norman influences, with the addition at times of a circle of gold.
2. 1066 to 1100. The Couvre-chef.
3. 1100 to 1150. The " Coif-de-mailles " head-dress.
4. 1150 to 1280. The Wimple and Peplum.
5. 1280 to 1300. Wimple and Peplum modification, with band.
6. 1300 to 1350. Gorget and Couvre-chef.
7. 1350 to 1380. The Nebule.

This method of differentiation has not to our knowledge been attempted prior to the issue of this work. It must not by any means be accepted as arbitrary—that is to say, the ladies did not in 1350 lay down the gorget and couvre-chef and take up the nebule; the date only approximates the period.

Undoubtedly examples may be found of the nebule before that date, and one of these will be given, while brass effigies showing the gorget and couvre-chef occur subsequently; but so far as can be ascertained, the nebule came into fashion somewhere about the year mentioned. These remarks also apply to each of the other dates. The

word "attire," it should be explained, always meant the
dressing of the head in the Middle Ages, and was used in
that sense in the translation of the Bible :

"She painted her face, and tired her hair, and looked out at a window."

The signification of the word since the Reformation has
completely altered; it now means the clothing of the
whole body.

In dealing with the costume of the men it was found
possible to divide the reign of Edward III. into early and
late periods, and it is just as advisable to do so with
regard to that of the ladies. Strange to say, the year 1350
is the same in both cases.

A well-known brass is that of Sir John and Lady de
Creke, in Westley Waterless Church, Cambridgeshire, which
dates from c. 1325 (Fig. 118). As will be noticed, the brass
should, to accord with dates, be placed in the preceding reign ;
but as the costume is so eminently characteristic of Edward
the Third's reign, it has been included in this chapter. The
head-dress of the Lady Alyne is the gorget and couvre-
chef, but the disposition of the couvre-chef is particularly
noticeable. It has a stiff band, with a serrated edge on
the forehead, and the two pendent sides are brought forward and pinned into the plaits of hair on either side of
the face. As the plaits show more clearly in the next
brass, it will be more satisfactory to describe them there.
The whole head-dress is an example of the many which can
be cited of the ladies imitating, in the material at their
disposal, the head-gear of the masculine sex. To facilitate
comparison the brass of Sir John has been introduced. Lady
Alyne wears a côte-hardi, as the robe began to be called, in

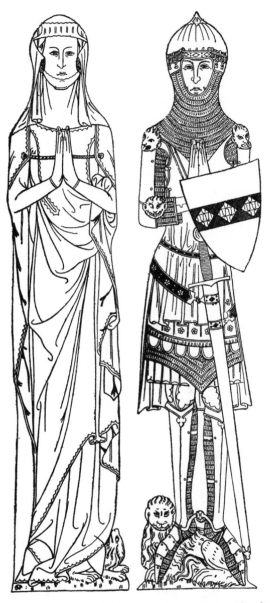

FIG. 118.—Sir John and Lady Creke, 1325. Westley Waterless
Church, Cambridgeshire.

imitation of the gentlemen's dress. It is long, with tightly fitting sleeves reaching to the wrist, and no buttons. Over this appears an extremely early example of the super côte-hardi, a garment which in various forms was to be a favourite among the English ladies for the next century and a half—an example of persistence in an article of European dress which it would be difficult to equal. To any one living in the twentieth century, the idea of a fashion lasting so long is to say the least appalling; but, on the other hand, we have to remember that the conservatism of the Middle Ages in this respect is as nothing when compared with some Oriental races, who still wear garments cut after the same fashion as their ancestors two or even three thousand years ago. The super côte-hardi as delineated is in an incipient form; the characteristic opening at the side reaches only as far as the waist, whereas before the reign ended it had assumed very much larger proportions. To facilitate walking, and also to show the richly decorated or emblazoned côte-hardi often worn underneath, it is drawn up on one side and passed through the arm opening. A cloak is worn lined with fur and fastened across the chest with a cord, which has no buckles, or ouches. The pointed shoes appear under the côte-hardi, and are quite plain. If the artist has represented this lady in proper proportions, she must have been exceptionally tall.

Another extremely interesting brass, dating from the year 1330, is that of Lady de Northwode, *née* Joan de Badlesmere, probably a daughter of Lord Badlesmere, of Leeds Castle, in Kent (Fig. 119). She married Sir John de Northwode, and the brass showing the effigies of both man and wife lies in Minster Church, Isle of Sheppey. The gorget is here shown in its fullest development, with a wire strengthening the upper edge; it passes round to the back of the head, and is secured as usual by pins into the hair. There is no couvre-chef. This year marks the approximate time when ladies dispensed with the couvre-chef when indoors or about their homes, or, to put it another way, the idea began to be recognised that it was possible for a lady to appear in public life with her head uncovered. This idea, once introduced, gradually developed until, after the lapse of twenty years, the ladies were able to lay aside not only the couvre-chef, but also the gorget. The method of arranging the coiffure should be noticed, inasmuch as it is characteristic of the first part of this reign. The hair at the back of the head is first dressed in two long plaits, which are brought round to the front and carried up on either side of the face, and fixed into the loose hair on the top of the head. She wears a fairly tight-fitting côte-hardi, of which only the sleeves and part of the skirt are visible.

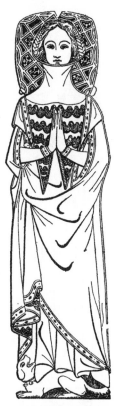

FIG. 119.—Lady de North-wode, 1330. Minster Church, Isle of Sheppey.

Strange to say, no buttons are shown upon the sleeves. The outer garment is a capacious cloak lined with the fur heraldically termed "vair," two pieces of which, in the form of lappets, are brought from either side and meet upon the chest, where they are buttoned down under the hands. The fastening may be continued if desired, as will be seen by the buttons which show upon the left side.

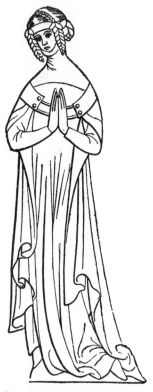

FIG. 120.—Lady, c. 1345. Wimbish Church, Essex.

This cloak is very gracefully caught up and draped into the opening for the hand upon one side, where it is kept in position by the arm.

As the question is often asked why a dog or some other animal appears at the feet of effigies, it may be as well to mention that this is merely a conventional style which prevailed from the earliest period, for giving a finish at the feet for precisely the same reason that we find a cushion under the head. That these animals were, however, sometimes the companions of the deceased is shown by the Stapleton brass in Ingham Church, where a small label is shown bearing the name of the dog lying at the feet of the knight, namely, "Jakke"; while a similar instance is that of Lady Cassy, who lies in Deerhurst Church, Gloucestershire, where the word "Terri" accompanies the dog.

The brass of a lady preserved at Wimbish Church, in Essex, and dating from c. 1345, affords us an example of the tiring of the hair, which is more complete than any yet given (Fig. 120). It can only be described as singularly quaint

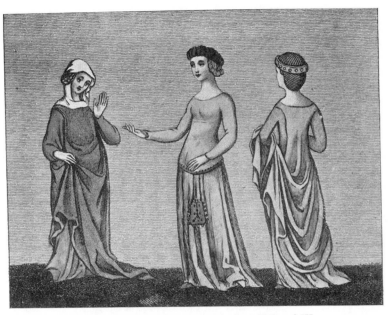

FIG. 122.—Costumes, first part of reign of Edward III.

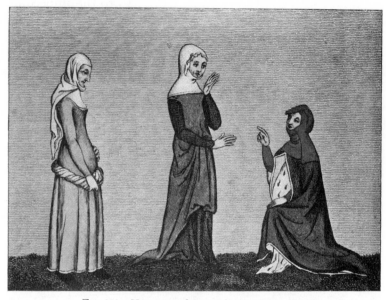

FIG. 123.—Matrons, early part of reign of Edward III.

and graceful, and in marked contradiction to the unbecoming style which succeeded it.   The method of doing the hair explains itself, but it should be mentioned that the plait passing over the head reached to a similar point on the right side of the head, although the mediæval artist has portrayed it somewhat out of place.   The gorget, as will be seen, is still the fashion, and remained so for approximately five more years.   Respecting the costume, which is singularly plain, there are no points of interest except the broad band encircling the upper part of the cloak.

The last brass we give of this early part of the reign of Edward III. is one of the most beautiful of the series—that of Margaret de Walsokne, 1349, the wife of Adam de Walsokne, a burgess of Lynn Regis (Fig. 121).   The head and shoulders only are given, as the characteristics of the dress are similar to those described before.

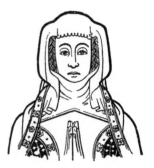

FIG. 121.—Margaret de Walsokne, 1349.   Lynn Regis.

The gorget and couvre-chef are here seen in their greatest perfection, the latter being ornamented with a scalloped edging across the forehead. On either side of the face the usual plaited hair is seen.   The côte-hardi, judging from the small portion showing, is of an extremely rich material with a decorated design ; the sleeves, which of course belong to the same garment, are furnished with the usual rows of small buttons reaching from the elbows to the wrists.   The super côte-hardi is plain, the only decoration being an ornamental border round the openings for the arms ; the skirt is raised according to the fashion of the time, and a portion of it held in position by the arm, similarly to that shown upon the brass of Lady de Northwode.

From a fifteenth century manuscript Bible, and also from Sloane MS. 2433, we give Fig. 122, Pl., which exhibit a few variations of style—for instance, the cincture round the hips of the middle figure is the forerunner of the jewelled belt of the latter part of the reign. No. 1 and No. 3 wear the super côte-hardi in its most primitive form, the length of which plainly demonstrates the reason for holding up the same under the arm.

Three matrons of the period, taken from Roy. MSS. 20 C v. and 19 D i., are here given (Fig. 123, Pl.), showing the ordinary costume of the well-to-do classes, the third figure being of higher rank, as it will be noticed that her cloak is lined with ermine.

THE WOMEN: LATER PERIOD AFTER 1350

The Nebule Head-dress, 1350 to 1380.—The period of the nebule head-dress trends somewhat upon the reign of the succeeding monarch, inasmuch as it lasted from 1350 to 1380 (Fig. 124, Pl.). During these thirty years, two features especially were prominent in ladies' dress—the nebule head-dress and the sleeve tippet. There are many brasses and effigies illustrating this period, whilst wealthy stores of illuminations and manuscripts are in existence; so much so is this the case, that the writer suffers from an *embarras de richesse* in selecting suitable types as examples. The earliest brass extant showing the distinguishing features we have mentioned is that of Richard and Margaret Torrington, 1349 and 1356, in Great Berkhampstead Church, Hertfordshire

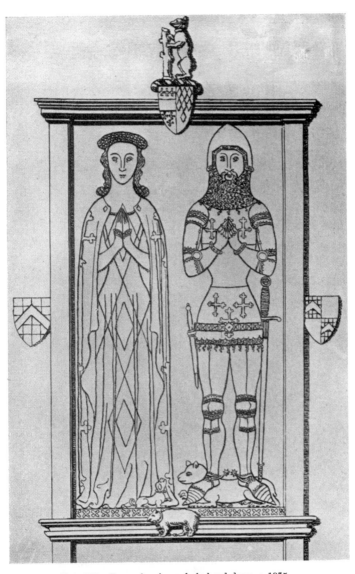

FIG. 124.—Brass showing nebule head-dress, c. 1375.

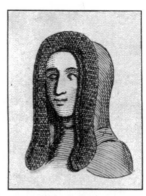

FIG. 126.—Catherine, Lady Berkeley, 1361. Berkeley
Church, Gloucestershire.

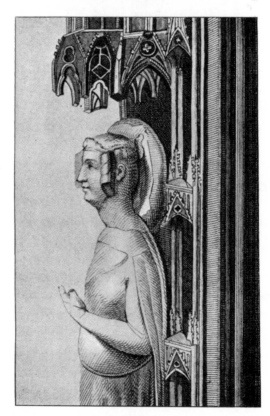

FIG. 127.—Queen Philippa, *d.* 1369. In Edward the Confessor's
Chapel, Westminster.

(Fig. 113), the two dates being respectively those of the two persons represented. The brass probably was not executed until the latter date. The lady shown in Fig. 125 wears a nebule head-dress, which is shown in its incipient stage. It consisted of a cylindrical case of woven wire, passing across the forehead and down each side of the face. The head of Catherine, Lady Berkeley, 1361, in Berkeley Church, is a valuable example, as affording us a side view of the head-dress (Fig. 126, Pl.). The effigy of Queen Philippa, consort of Edward III., in Westminster Abbey, exhibits this form of head attire (Fig. 127, Pl.).

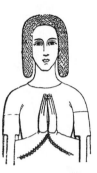

Fig. 125.—Ismayne de Winston, 1372. Necton Church, Norfolk.

The Tippet.—Margaret Torrington is habited in a côte-hardi having the tight sleeves and the usual buttons, which it will be noticed extend half the length of the upper arm. A special feature of this sleeve is the partial covering of the hand, which developed during the ensuing forty or fifty years until, by the commencement of the next century, more than half the hand was hidden. Round the upper part of the arm a band is fixed either temporarily or permanently, from which depends the long streamer called the tippet, which sometimes reached the ground. In all illuminated manuscripts these tippets are white. It should be noticed that they are fixed directly in front of the sleeves; a few years later, however, we find them occasionally fastened so as to hang down the side, and subsequently both styles prevailed until they went out of fashion. They are seldom if ever seen after about 1380.

The Vertical Front Pockets.—A figure from Roy. MS.

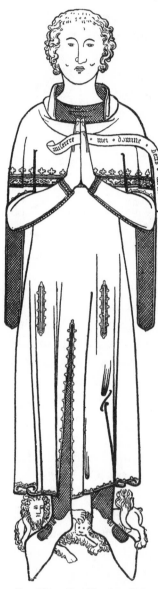

FIG. 129.—Alan Fleming, 1361.
Newark, Nottinghamshire.

19 D ii., and dating probably from about 1350 to 1360, exhibits these pockets, one on either side, and also affords an idea of the length of the tippet at that period (Fig. 128, Pl., No. 3). In order to show that these pockets were not strictly confined to ladies' costume, we give an example of their occurrence upon masculine dress in the case of the beautiful brass of Alan Fleming at Newark, in Nottinghamshire, 1361, which, in addition to illustrating this feature, also exhibits peculiarities which will doubtless be of interest to the reader (Fig. 129).

The tomb of King Edward III., in Westminster Abbey, is of bronze, as also is the effigy upon it; on the south side beautifully moulded statuettes, also in bronze, represent six of his children. These are to a very great extent in contemporary costume of the period of his death, 1377, but an attempt has been made to represent at least one of them

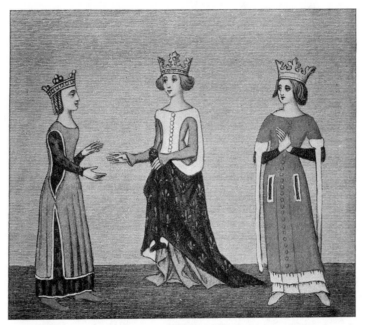

Fɪɢ. 128.—Ladies, second period of Edward III., showing vertical pockets, &c.

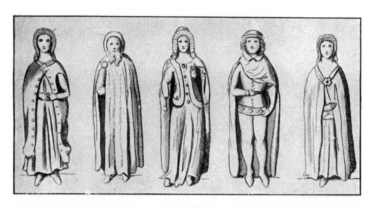

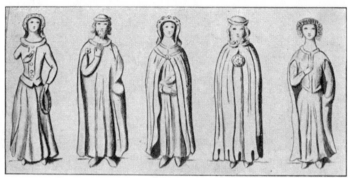

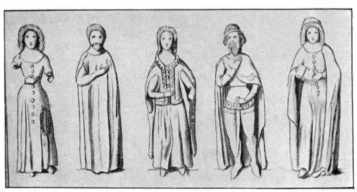

FIG. 131.—From the monumental tomb of Thomas Beauchamp, Earl of Warwick, 1370. In St. Mary's Church, Warwick.

in a dress which prevailed twenty years earlier, reproduced in Fig. 130. If this were intended to represent Blanche de la Tour as she actually appeared in life the costume is incorrect in several details, as she died in 1340, and vertical pockets are introduced—to mention but one feature.

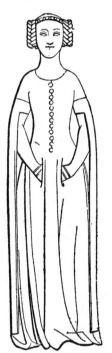

It will be seen by a study of the illustrations given that the unwritten rule which had prevailed for so many centuries against a woman showing her hair was broken through at the time of the advent of the nebule head-dress, although significant indications had appeared for years before. The emergence of the hair was also followed by the exposure of the neck, and during the later period we have just been discussing, both brasses and effigies afford examples of what may be termed low-necked dress, thus the Halsham, Bertlot, Stapleton, brasses, &c., may be compared. A noteworthy feature of this exposure is the absence of any embroidery, lace, or other decorative material to soften the hard line round the neck, which to our eyes is particularly unbecoming.

FIG. 130.—Blanche de la Tour. From tomb of Edward III., 1372.

In the monumental tomb of Thomas Beauchamp, Earl of Warwick, in the chancel of St. Mary's Church, Warwick, who died in 1370, a number of figures are inserted; they are very representative of the prevailing costume, and have been reproduced here for the benefit of the student (Fig. 131, Pl.).

CHAPTER X

RICHARD II., 1377-1399

THE assertion made concerning Richard II., that he was the greatest fop who has ever occupied the English throne, has not been promulgated without reason. The weak and effeminate character of this unworthy son of the Black Prince has been a theme for many historians, and practically none have risen to champion him. A king who could go so far in reckless extravagance as to possess at least one garment, among many others, which was valued at the equivalent of twenty thousand pounds of our money, must indeed have had dress upon the brain. For the first few years the style of costume introduced during the latter part of the reign of King Edward III. prevailed, and it was not until about 1389, when Richard had succeeded in throwing off the guiding hand of his uncle, the Duke of Gloucester, that the extraordinary and characteristic costume associated with his reign began to be evolved from the brains of the King and his sycophantic followers. Hence it is quite possible, if desired, to divide the reign into two distinct periods, but as a gradual leading up to the second period occurred during the earlier part, it is thought advisable to treat the reign as a whole. The last ten years may be aptly described as a wild debauch in all kinds of reckless extravagance in dress; not only among the King and courtiers did this madness prevail, but the middle classes also became obsessed of a reckless ambition to outdo their peers in sumptuary excesses, and, with the development of this craze, lavished money which they could ill afford in the wild riot of dissipation. It might be imagined that at least the heroes of the period, the hardy veterans of Chevy Chase, might have risen superior to this effeminate weakness; but so far from this being the case, we find the garments prevailing in civil life adopted by the military with ludicrous effect, and illustrations of the same will be given in the course of this chapter.

The method previously adopted in this work of distinguishing the regal dress from that of the nobility, and the nobility from that of the commoner, is rendered impossible, inasmuch as, to quote the words of Knighton, "the vanity of the common people in their dress was so great, that it was impossible to distinguish the rich from the poor, the high from the low, the clergy from the laity, by their appearance," and it would be obviously futile to attempt to differentiate in this matter at the present day, when it was found too difficult in the past. The satirists and reformers of the time were loud in their outcries against the national extravagance. Geoffrey Chaucer, the great English poet of this period, who died in 1400, declaimed vehemently against the "superfluitee of clothing" which he saw prevailing around him. He animadverts upon "the coste of enbrouding, disguising, endenting, or barring, ounding, paling, winding, or bending, and semblable waste of cloth in vanitee; but ther is also the costlewe furring in hir gounes, so moche pounsoning of chesel to maken holes, moche dagging of sheres, with the superfluitee in length of the foresaide gounes, trailing in the myre, on

hors and eke a foot, as wel of man as of woman, that all
thilke trailing is veraily wasted, consumed, thred-bare,
and rotten, rather than it is geven to the poure, to gret
damage of the foresayd poure folk." His " Canterbury
Tales " furnish descriptions of some very characteristic
dresses.

THE MEN

A representation of the King in his childhood is contained in a Psalter preserved in the British Museum; it
depicts him with his father, the Black Prince, and was
formerly in his possession (Fig. 132, Pl.). The effigy of the
King and also of his Queen, Anne of Bohemia, lie in
Westminster Abbey; they are of bronze, and evidently
authentic portraits. The most striking feature of both
figures is the extreme richness of the material of their
garments. They are ornamented all over with devices
and decorations, being the royal badges, namely: The hart
crowned and chained, the sun emerging in splendour from
behind a cloud, and the *Planta genista*, or broom plant,
from which the Plantagenets derived their name. Alternating with these devices are the letters R and A.

The Houppelande.—This extraordinary garment, which
was in fashion altogether for more than twenty years, may
be seen in its earlier form in the accompanying Fig. 133, Pl.,
of Richard II. at his devotions. It is from a small painting
preserved at Wilton House, and the figures of his patron
saints accompany him in the original. The collar of
the garment is of ordinary dimensions, and the sleeves,
although reaching the ground, are comparatively short
when the King is standing. Both collar and sleeves, to-

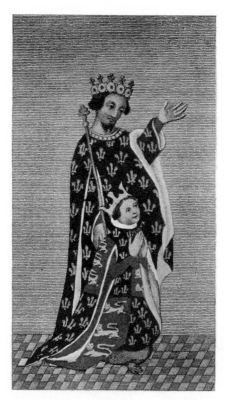

FIG. 132.—Richard II. and his father, the Black
Prince. (Cott. MS. Domit. A xvii.)

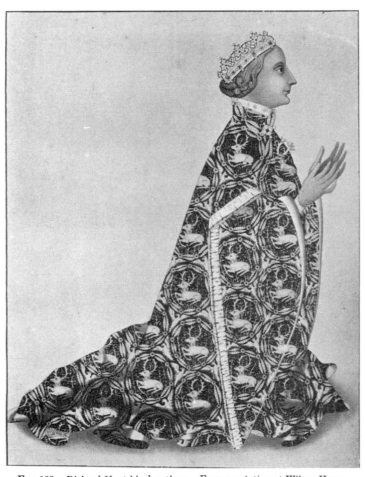

Fig. 133.—Richard II. at his devotions.   From a painting at Wilton House.

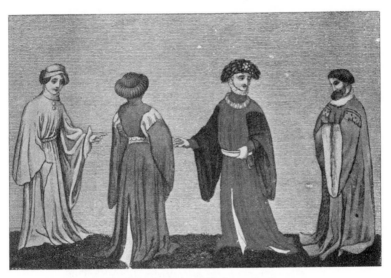

FIG. 134.—Varieties of the houppelande.

(Sloane MS. 2433 and Roy. MSS. 20 C vii. and 15 D iii.)

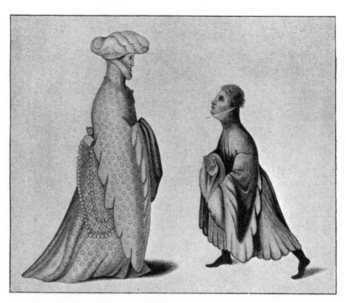

FIG. 135.—Examples of the houppelande. (Harl. MS. 1319.)

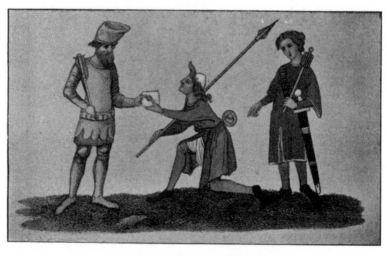

FIG. 138.—Costume, *temp.* Richard II.
(Sloane MS. 2433 and Roy. MS. 16 G vii.)

gether with the youthful appearance of the King, point to the year of its execution as being *c.* 1380. There is one great feature in all the subsequent houppelandes which is entirely absent in this, namely, the dagging. The badge of the white hart is sown all over the garment and enclosed in ornamental circles, while the small figure in relief of the same, with jewelled antlers, performs the office of a morse. In Fig. 134, Pl., taken from Sloane MS. 2433 and Roy. MSS. 20 C vii. and 15 D iii., four separate styles of the houppelande at this early period are given, in which it will be distinctly seen that the collar had attained to large dimensions, reaching as high as the chin and the back of the ears. Ornamental work in the shape of dagged embroidery has begun to show itself upon the shoulders, while the sleeves of one costume are of a different colour from the body. In all cases these garments are lined, that of the King in Fig. 133, Pl., being of ermine. For the fullest development of this dress we reproduce examples from Harl. MS. 1319, probably one of the most valuable illuminated manuscripts in our national collection. It is a history in verse of the closing years of the life of Richard II., written by a French gentleman who took a share in the events, and is illuminated with a fidelity which is simply extraordinary. Both figures are habited in houppelandes (Fig. 135, Pl.), but that upon the left is the more highly developed. The height of the collar, the fur edging round the face, the embroidery depending from the middle of the back, the circles with which the whole dress is powdered, and the rich dagging of the sleeves, are all points for observation, while other distinctive features of the period may be gleaned from the figure upon the right.

The Chaperon.—This remarkable head attire for men sprang into existence during the period under discussion. It is really a head covering with which the reader is quite familiar, being in fact nothing more than the capuchon and liripipe, but so utterly transformed as to be completely unrecognisable in its new condition.   Some inventive genius was bent upon the development of a new head-gear, and, candidly speaking, we think that any innovation in this direction was pardonable, seeing that the capuchon, having been in vogue for a matter of three centuries, was getting a trifle old-fashioned.   He accordingly thrust the top of his head into the aperture through which his face had erstwhile protruded, and, passing the part which had previously covered his neck and shoulders over the top of his head, the ornamental dagging of necessity fell down on the left side of the face ; then, boldly seizing the liripipe, he wound part of it round his head, and after fastening it allowed the end to fall down upon the right side.   Delighted with the novelty, the exquisites at once adopted it, and, although it under-

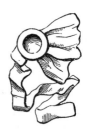

went many transformations, the chaperon was in evidence for nearly one hundred years.   Even at the present time we have reminiscences of its former favour, for it is perpetuated in the shoulder knots upon the Order of the Garter (Fig. 136), while the head covering, with its attendant dag-

FIG. 136.—Shoulder-knot : Order of the Garter.

ging, is readily discernible in the metal cock-ades of our coachmen.   It must not by any means be considered that the chaperon described above was a stereotyped fashion; it soon began to show chameleon-like changes, some of which we reproduce

(Fig. 137). In one example the whole of the drapery is brought boldly to the front; in another, exactly the opposite style is shown; while in a third, we find a part of it hanging down the nape of the neck, and the liripipe twisted round

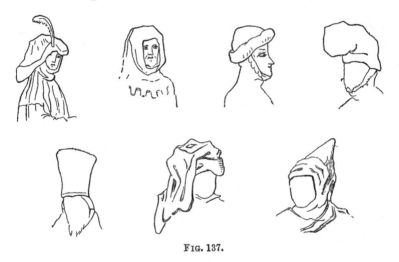

FIG. 137.

the crown of the head like a turban. A hat which is occasionally represented in this reign is depicted upon the head of the knight in Fig. 138, Pl. The same type may also be recognised in the large selection of hats in use during this reign, and appended for the benefit of the student (Fig. 139, Pl.).

The Paltock.—So many different garments were introduced at this time, each bearing a different name, and probably changing that name before they became obsolete, that there is great difficulty in understanding precisely the written description concerning them. There is one, however, which is so frequently represented, that it may be the paltock of Piers Plowman. "They have a weed of silk called a

Paltock, to which their hosen are fastened with white latchets "
(author of "Eulogium," *temp.* Richard II.). The garment
shown in Fig. 140, Pl., is undoubtedly a paltock. It was
worn with tightly-fitting chausses, which reached to the
waist, and were then fastened by points tied to corresponding points fixed to the lining of the paltock. This garment,
which may be looked upon as a short jacket, was at times
so scanty that only a short frill appeared below the waist.
Probably Chaucer was referring to these when he speaks of
"the horrible disordinate scantiness of clothing as be these
cut slops or hanselines." This short jacket was undoubtedly
of German origin, and, as will eventually be seen, was by no
means peculiar to this reign. The sleeves were, as a rule,
highly ornamented and dagged, and the usual high collar
encircled the neck. From Fig. 141, Pl., it may readily be
perceived that the paltock was simply the houppelande with
the skirt cut away.

The Court-pie.—This was an outer garment or mantle,
and is merely mentioned by the chroniclers without being
described. As a short kind of cloak, somewhat resembling
a tabard by reason of its being split up at the sides, was in
vogue during this reign, it is more than likely that this may
have been the court-pie. In Fig. 142, Pl., the personage on
the right is habited in a garment of this description. It will
be seen that it is split up at the sides and richly dagged, and
also that a high houppelande collar is provided ; the sleeve,
however, belongs to an under garment, probably a paltock.
The chaperon is shown very large, the hanging portion
falling down the back. This figure also serves to illustrate
a very common method for combining the wallet or gypcière
with the dagger. As will be noticed, the belt is put round

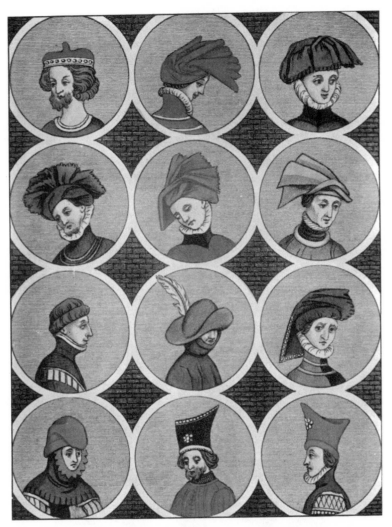

FIG. 139.

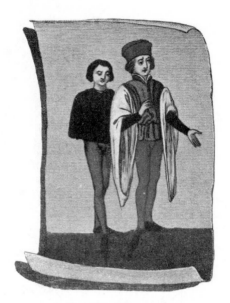

FIG. 140.—The paltock.

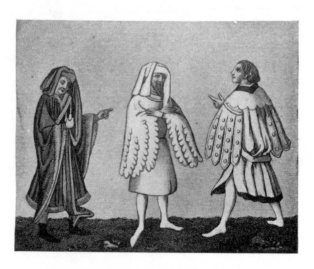

FIG. 141.—Costume, Richard II.

the hips in this case, but as a rule all cinctures round outer garments passed round the waist. The wallet is occasionally shown hanging down the back from a strap which passed round the neck; in fact, there was no general rule for its position. The dagger did not pass through the centre of the wallet, but two straps were provided upon the outside which served to secure it in position; at times the weapon was suspended down the back (Fig. 143, Pl.).

Boots.—The reign of Richard II. is noted for its extravagance respecting foot coverings of all descriptions, and probably the longest pointed shoes of any age were then in evidence. The three personages shown in Fig. 144 exemplify this feature; they represent the Dukes of Lancaster, York, and Gloucester, and are reproduced from Roy. MS. 20 B vi. It is probable that the length of the boot is more than twice that of the foot. These long-toed shoes were termed *cracowes*, and first came into England in 1384; it is highly probable that they derive their name from Cracow, then in the domains of the father of Anne of Bohemia, the Queen. Another term for them was *poleyns*. These toes were at times stuffed with

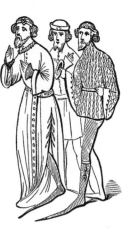

Fig. 144.—Costume, late Richard II. (Roy. MS. 20 B vi.)

wadding, and wired so as to assume fantastic shapes, such as ram's horns, &c.; as locomotion was obviously impossible if the lengths were inordinate, we understand from the chroniclers that the toes were fastened up by chains to the knees, and in some instances even to the waist.

But very few illuminated examples of this fashion have been handed down to us; we reproduce the following from

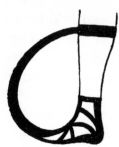

FIG. 145.—Poleyn. From
Harl. MS. 1319.

Harl. MS. 1319 (Fig. 145), where the method is plainly shown, and which also furnishes us with an example of an ornamental shoe. It is quite possible that the small chain depending from the garter, seen in Fig. 144, may be for this purpose, but it is also open to supposition that it is intended to represent the Order of the Garter. The knights of the period also affected this extraordinary style in their steel sollerets, but the long toes in their case were removable by merely severing a strap. A variety of cracowe is shown in Fig. 146. The general method for fastening poleyns was either by straps or by means of a buckle; an example of the latter, from the brass of Robert Attelath at Lynn, 1376, is given here (Fig. 147).

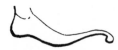

FIG. 146.—Shoe, Richard II. (Sloane MS. 335.)

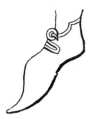

FIG. 147. — Shoe buckle, Robert Attelath, 1376, at Lynn.

The uncles of Richard II., shown in Fig. 144, well illustrate the multiplicity of the prevailing dress, and also indicate some special points. Two of them have the sleeves of their under garments developed so as to cover the knuckles, a point alluded to in dealing with the last reign. The houppelande has remarkably small sleeves, and is only dagged at the sides, while the figure upon the right, clad in a paltock, well exemplifies the shape of that garment, although the skirts would be too long for the exquisite of the time. The jewelled circlets round the head should be noticed, and also the peculiar hat worn by the central figure (Fig. 144). Brasses of civilians of this period are rather uncommon, and as they are generally of merchants, they show, as a rule, only the long robe affected by that class of the community and the capuchon. That of Thomas de Topcliffe, 1391 (Fig. 148), is an example of the case in point,

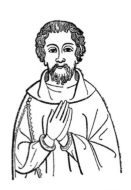

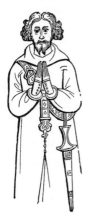

FIG. 148.—Thomas de Topcliffe, 1391.
Topcliffe Church, Yorkshire.

FIG. 149.—John Corp, 1361.   Stoke
Fleming Church, Devonshire.

where, however, one feature is shown in its incipient stage which became very prominent in the succeeding century, namely, the sleeves, which, though tight at the wrist, show signs of enlargement at the elbow. As was customary at this period, he wears an *anelace*, not shown in the figure; but in order to represent this feature, which was common among civilians of this period, a copy of the brass of John Corp, 1361, in Stoke Fleming Church, Devonshire, is given here, which shows the weapon depending from a very elegant baldrick (Fig. 149). It had a very broad blade, narrowing from hilt to point, and was sharp on both edges (*vide* Cinquedea, " Arms and Armour ").

In Fig. 150, Pl., we have an example of costume dating from the last years of King Richard II., which were distinguished by the peculiar horizontal position in which the dagger was worn, both by civilians and the military. The boot upon the right leg is red to match the tabard, and upon the left, white.

THE WOMEN

THE RETICULATED HEAD-DRESS, 1380–1400

Although for a great number of years—probably two or three hundred—the ladies had dressed their hair more or less by the aid of a wire decoration or shape, the full development of the system did not appear until the advent of the reticulated style proper, which prevailed approximately between the years 1380 and 1400. The nebule design undoubtedly paved the way for this consummation.

The *Reticulated Head-dress*, considered as a whole, was the most beautiful style which had hitherto been evolved, although to modern eyes it may appear stiff, hard, and incongruous. It cannot be denied that any head-dress which in any way hides the hair, the most beautiful adornment of woman, is to be deprecated; and the above remarks are only to be taken as a comparison between the different mediæval styles in which the hair was covered. Its chief features were its costliness and its beauty as a work of art. In building up this remarkable coiffure, gold wire, woven into a net-like mesh or reticulation, played the prominent part, being held in position by a rigid framework of the

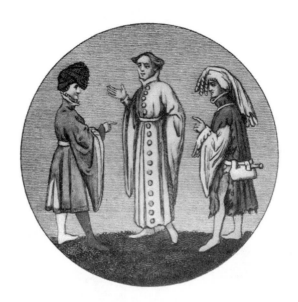

Fig. 142.—The court-pie.

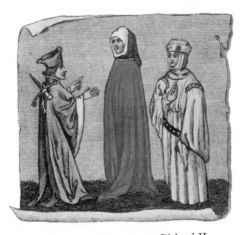

Fig. 143.—Costume, *temp.* Richard II.

1. Chron. S. Denis.   2. Roy. MS. 20 C vii.   3. Sloane MS. 2433.

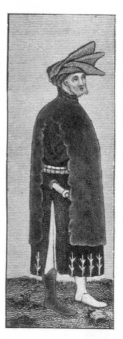

FIG. 150.—Costume, late Richard II.
(Harl. MS. 2897.)

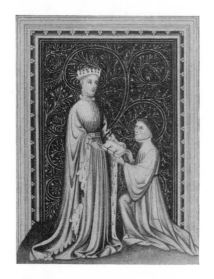

FIG. 167.—Occleve the poet and King
Henry V. (Arundel MS. 38.)

goldsmith's art.   An early example is that of Lady Burton, 1382, in Little Casterton Church, Rutlandshire (Fig. 151).   The rigid piece crossing the forehead, and extending on both sides, is called the *crespine*, while the portions appearing on either side of the face are termed the *cauls*.   The whole head-dress is, however, generally referred to as the crespine.   The general construction of these head-dresses is for the crespine to be made after the fashion of a coronet, but having a semicircular projection on either side forming the tops of the cauls. The latter in the case of Lady Burton are two half cylinders fitting over the ears, and enclosing the hair ; at the back of the head, which is seldom or never seen in brasses, a network, fastened to the coronet at the top and hanging down, is carried tightly round and fixed to either caul.   The coronet was, as a rule, a stiff gold band ornamented with jewels ; the cauls were of narrower bands of gold strengthening the wire nets.   At the inter-sections of the reticulations, jewels

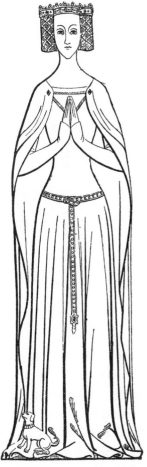

FIG. 151.—Lady Burton, 1382. Little Casterton Church, Rutlandshire.

were used to fasten the bands together.   Within these cauls the hair was carefully plaited, as seen upon the

brass of Lady Harsick (Fig. 152). The reticulated head-
dress was from its very nature extremely costly, and
no expense was spared in its lavish decoration; as a
consequence, we find these head-dresses dignified as heir-
looms, and frequently mentioned in the wills of the
period. A later example, that of Eleanor Corp, 1381,
Stoke Fleming, Devonshire (Fig. 153), affords us an
example of another variety of this style, in which the ears
are not enclosed, but the whole head is enveloped in what

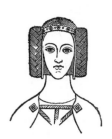

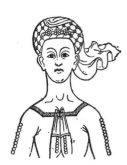

Fig. 152.—Lady Harsick, 1384.
South Acre, Norfolk.

Fig. 153.—Eleanor Corp, 1391.
Stoke Fleming, Devonshire.

may be termed a hemispherical cage. The veil should be
noticed, as it is an early example of the style prevailing
after 1400. A quaint little figure from Harl. MS. 4425 is
reproduced here, which shows a head-dress somewhat similar
to that of Eleanor Corp, but encloses the ears. The white
portion of the super côte-hardi should be noted (Fig. 154,
Pl.). A splendid example of the pure style of this head-
dress is afforded us by an effigy of the first wife of Ralph
Neville, Earl of Westmoreland, who died about 1397. The
massive goldsmith's work and generally elaborate character
of the whole coiffure are very striking, and certainly one

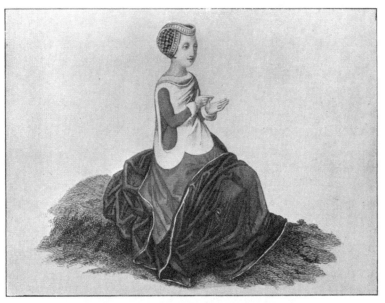

Fig. 154.—Lady, *temp*. Richard II. (Harl. MS. 4425.)

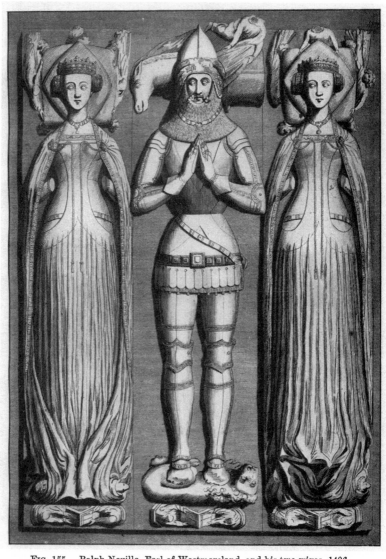

FIG. 155.—Ralph Neville, Earl of Westmoreland, and his two wives, 1426.
Staindrop Church, Durham.

of the handsomest we have preserved upon an effigy (Fig. 155, Pl.).

There are many readers who may be tempted to criticise this mediæval mode of arranging the coiffure, but, as we have before intimated, the bizarre fashions of old-world times constantly repeat themselves. For example, if this head-dress delineated upon the accompanying coloured plate

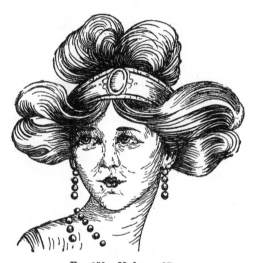

FIG. 156.—Modern coiffure.

(p. 128), which is a reproduction to measurement of an ancient example, is compared with the above sketch (Fig. 156) of an up-to-date method of doing the hair, the amount of projection at the sides of the face, and also upon the head, bear a strange resemblance to each other, the only difference practically being, that in one example the hair is free, and in the other confined.

It is interesting to note, in connection with other fashions of this extraordinary period, that the appearance of any hair outside the head-dress was deemed indecorous, and that ladies habitually kept a small pair of tweezers in the *aulmonière* or gypcière depending from their hip-belts with which to remove the short hair at the back of the neck. To such an extent did this fashion ultimately prevail that ultra-fashionable ladies were also furnished with a small mirror, by the aid of which, and the tweezers aforesaid, they were enabled to remove the eyebrows, even performing this ceremony when in their carriages or at public functions. Upon no brass, however, have we been able to detect the eyebrows removed.

The Côte-hardi and Super Côte-hardi.—During this reign the côte-hardi maintained its general tight-fitting form, but as the years progressed it became customary at times to wear it without the super côte-hardi. The reason for this was undoubtedly the extremely rich material of which it was made, very costly cloths of gold and silver being used. Consequently many effigies and brasses represent the ladies attired in the côte-hardi and a mantle, as in the case of Lady Burton (Fig. 151). In the brass mentioned the jewelled hip-belt is seen, fastened with a buckle and an Order of the Garter knot, with a long pendant. This fashion of belt is almost the same as that worn by the knights twenty years previously. Very soon, however, the lady's belt became nearly as wide as that of the knight, and fastened in the same manner, namely, by a buckle in front. The openings at the sides of the super côte-hardi were cut low to enable the belt to be seen, and that part of the garment hanging down the front was considerably narrowed, while the back was correspondingly widened. The French ladies carried this fashion to such an extreme,

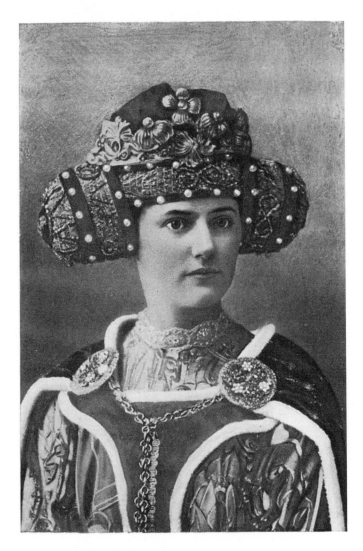

LADY, *temp.* RICHARD II.

Head-dress.—The reticulated, richly jewelled.
Côte-hardi.—Purple silk.
Super Côte-hardi.—Rich embossed velvet, lined white fur.
Cloak.—Green velvet, edged with ermine; fastened by morse across
the chest.

(Photographed direct from examples used in the Author's lecture upon
"Mediæval Costume and Head-dresses.")

that the body part of the dress hanging down the front at times resolved itself into a simple chain.   The coloured plate (p. 132) is a costume modelled upon the lines of the dresses prevailing during the last decade of the century.   The head-dress in some respects resembles that of Lady Burton, but attains to somewhat greater dimensions.   The jewels largely consist of pearls.   The côte-hardi is better seen in the coloured plate, p. 166, where it has a rich design wrought in green and gold.   The wearing of corsets under this costume is perfectly justifiable, for the ladies of the period were in the habit of confining their waists, as may be seen upon brasses and effigies.   The côte-hardi reaches to the ground.   The massive jewelled belt round the hips is unfortunately hidden, but is made of what may be termed the regulation square brooches; from the belt upon the right side is suspended the aulmonière, with the *baselard* fixed upon the outside in the usual manner.   It should be explained that ladies were in the habit of carrying this small dagger, partly on account of the lawless times then prevailing, and which sometimes justified its use, and also to a certain extent in imitation of the misericorde worn by the knight, and the anelace carried by the civilian.   Upon the left side, as seen in the figure, a small chain suspends the mirror and pincers before referred to.   The super côte-hardi illustrates the fashion prevailing throughout the period of emblazoning and quartering armorial insignia upon garments, concerning which we have written when dealing with the early part of the reign of Edward III.   The left side is of black velvet (which also extends down the back), and upon it a lion rampant appears worked in gold.   Upon the upper half of the right side fleurs-de-lys occur upon green velvet, and below a chevron upon a scarlet ground. The seams are finished with gold braid. Around the arm openings appears a white fur with which the garment is lined. The cloak, of a rich brocade in black and gold, has shields of arms worked on either side. The lining of blue silk is edged with fur.

The fashion prevailing for ornamental jewellery is very aptly seen upon the brasses and effigies of the period; both represent jewelled examples which pass round the neck or shoulders and have a pendant in front of a very highly ornate character. The embroidery upon the arms and also upon the super côte-hardi should be noted. It will be readily evident upon inspection that the super côte-hardi was made at times in two separate pieces joining below the hips. There can be no doubt that during this period the wearing of a piece of soft material down the

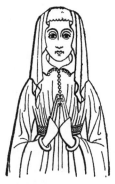

FIG. 157.—Lady, c. 1400. St. Lawrence Church, Norwich.

back of the head was coming into fashion; it is shown upon the brass of Eleanor Corp (Fig. 153), and also in a few other examples. Towards the end of the century ladies appear habited in houppelandes which reached to the ground and are very voluminous. Upon a brass in St. Lawrence Church, Norwich, c. 1400, a lady is represented (Fig. 157) in one, the high collar of which is turned over; the buttons and loops for fastening it are shown. It may be a source of wonder to some readers how ladies could indulge in such sports as hunting when attired in the prevailing fashionable head-dress. So far as the

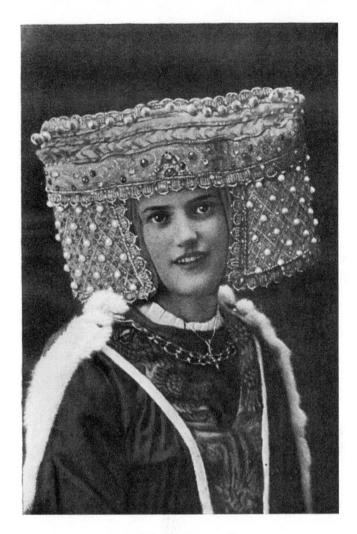

LADY, *temp.* RICHARD II.

Head-dress.—Reticulated, variety of, ornamented with goldsmith's work and jewels.

Cloak.—Of green velvet with design in gold, lined ermine.

Morse.—Of goldsmith's work and jewels, connected by gold chain from which hangs a pendant.

Super Côte-hardi.—Of red velvet, edged with fur.

Côte-hardi.—Of rich baudekyn.

Hip Belt (not seen).—Of square brooches and jewels, from which depends the aulmonière with baselard thrust through it; also the mirror and pincers on left side.

(Photographed direct from examples used in the Author's lecture upon "Mediæval Costume and Head-dresses.")

nebule was concerned no great difficulty was experienced, and in Fig. 158, dating probably from *c.* 1370, as indicated by the tippet sleeves, a lady is shown engaged in

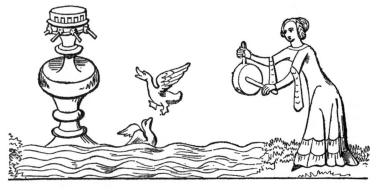

FIG. 158.—Lady rousing game with a tabor.   Taken from Roy. MS. 10 E iv., *c.* 1370.

the occupation of rousing game, with no other head covering; while Fig. 159, approximately of the same period, represents a lady possibly still farther afield.   Rabbits appear

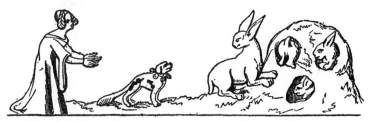

FIG. 159.—Lady at the rabbit warren.   From Leland's "Collectanea,"
vol. iv. p. 279.

to have deteriorated somewhat in size since the mediæval period.   When, however, upon horseback and engaged in the violent exertion of the chase some other head covering was necessary, and from numerous illustrations we glean that something after the nature of a wimple and peplum was worn. The illustration given here (Fig. 160) represents a lady in a super côte-hardi hunting the stag,

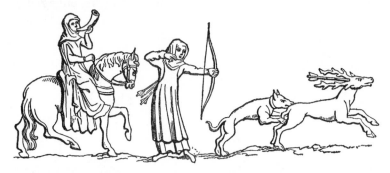

FIG. 160.—Ladies hunting the stag. Taken from MS. Reg. 2 B vii.

accompanied by an attendant on foot, and wearing a head covering of this nature. The lady is seen riding astride,

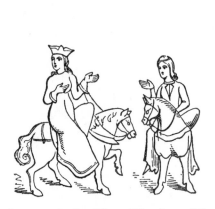

FIG. 161.—Ladies riding. Taken from a MS. in the French National Library, No. 7178.

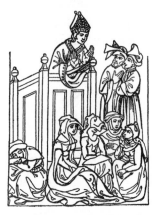

FIG. 162.—In church. Taken from a MS. of the fourteenth century.

and, as at the present time a tendency towards this method is being exhibited, it may not be out of place to mention that it has never been fashionable in England in the true

sense of the word. Anne of Bohemia is credited with
having introduced the side-saddle into England, but there
is abundant evidence to show that this is incorrect. It is
probable that she merely brought in an improvement upon
the existing saddle, conjecturally the pommel. The lowest
classes, undoubtedly, rode astride always; the nobility only
adopted it when hunting, or when they were engaged in
a journey which necessitated speed. The general arrange-

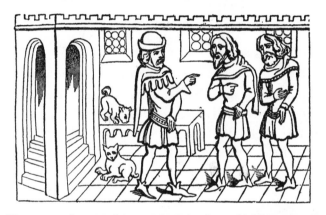

Fig. 163.—Two serving men of the period.   Taken from Add. MSS. 12,228, fol. 310.

ment for ordinary riding is shown in Fig. 161, taken from
a manuscript of the fourteenth century. Examples of ladies
riding side-saddle may be found in the British Museum
and other manuscripts as far back as the early Saxon
period (*vide* Cott. MS. Claudius B iv.; Cott. MS. Nero
C iv., &c.).

The Lower Orders.—The dress of the people varied
little from that of the time of Edward III., the long plain
dress and capuchon prevailing. In Fig. 162 a portion of the
congregation, sitting, as was customary, upon the ground,

or upon low stools, exemplifies this. Two men standing are wearing the chaperon, and are probably of a better class. This is taken from a manuscript of the fourteenth

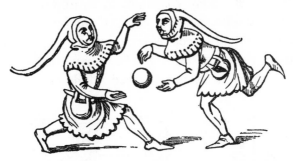

FIG. 164.—Taken from one of the carvings of the miserere seats in Gloucester Cathedral.

century. Two serving men are shown in Fig. 163 belonging to the later half of the fourteenth century, while two ordinary citizens playing ball are seen in Fig. 164.

CHAPTER XI

With the accession of Henry IV. we find a totally different feeling or sentiment towards costume from that prevailing in the preceding reign. The King and his chosen councillors had something better with which to occupy themselves than devising new foibles, in consolidating the tenure by which the monarch held his throne. Not only was there no sympathy in high quarters with the fantastical extravagance of the reign of Richard, but practical demonstrations antagonistic to it in the form of drastic sumptuary laws were successively passed by the Government. To make a law, however, and to enforce it are two totally different things, and the regulation of a people's dress by Act of Parliament has never been a satisfactory procedure. This was especially the case at the present time, when the people had become so imbued with the love of dress, and so steeped in the passion for ostentation and display, that we find the reigns of both Henry IV. and of his son but little varied from that which had previously prevailed. In fact, this period may be looked upon as a transition one, in which the chief extravagances and riotous excesses underwent modifications, and were practically the seeds of that severe style —comparatively speaking, of course—which was called forth in the reign of Henry VI. The diatribes of ecclesiastics and denunciations of contemporary satirists were especially

137

directed against all garments of the dagged or slashed variety, and "those possessing such fanciful devices as edges cut in the form of letters, rose-leaves, and posies of various kinds." The reference to letters is explained by the fact that short sentences, mottoes, and initials were very commonly worked upon the borders of garments.

THE MEN

Although the effigies of King Henry IV. and his Queen, Joan of Navarre, in Canterbury Cathedral, are rightly classified as being among the most beautiful of our regal monuments, they possess but very little interest for the student of costume in the way of novelties. The chief point of interest is undoubtedly centred in the crowns, which are of magnificent proportions and workmanship (Fig. 165, Pl.). The King is habited in the style affected by monarchs of that and preceding periods, the only innovation discernible being the cape of ermine, which is shown reaching to the girdle. This cape became a regulation dress for royalty and superior officers of state, and will be met with in succeeding reigns, although in a more modified form, being considerably curtailed in length. Thus in Harl. MS. 2278 an illumination occurs representing Lydgate presenting his poem to the King (Henry V.); the regal costume shows the cape of ermine furnished with a collar of the same material; the cape, however, does not reach so far as the waist. The cloak, or mantle in this case, is also of ermine, and of such large proportions that it spreads upon the ground around his feet. The cape in the illustration is worn over the mantle, which certainly appears to be a much more natural position than

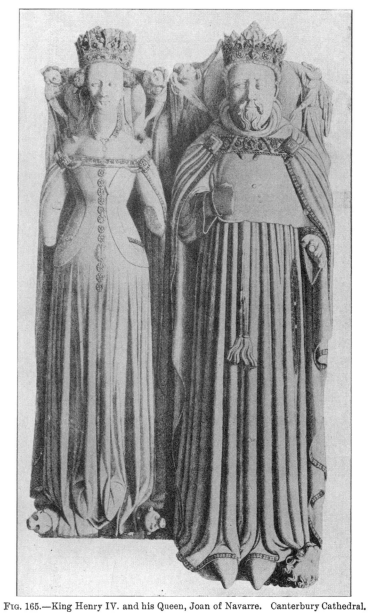

Fig. 165.—King Henry IV. and his Queen, Joan of Navarre. Canterbury Cathedral.

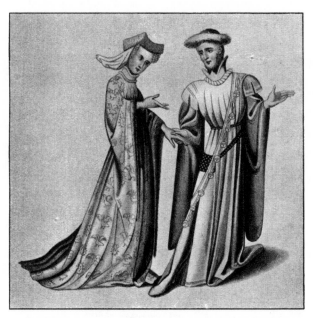

FIG. 166.—Costume, *temp.* Henry IV. (Roy. MS. 15 D iii.)

under the mantle, as seen in the Canterbury effigy. It may perhaps be mentioned that another peculiarity of the latter figure lies in the vertical openings for pockets, similar to those used in the reign of Edward III.; these occur in the dalmatica, and are ornamented with a richly-wrought border. The morse confining the cloak is also of exceptional beauty.

The dress of the nobles during the reigns of Henry IV. and Henry V. is well illustrated in the accompanying sketch, Fig. 166, Pl., taken from Roy. MS. 15 D iii., early fifteenth century. It will be at once perceived that the houppelande differs in no essential respect from that prevailing in the reign of Richard II., except that it has lost the dagging of the sleeves, &c. Upon the shoulders, however, some epaulettes are shown which manifest tracings of dagging. The high collar and gypcière are preserved. The belt round the waist, instead of round the hips, is a feature which prevailed at this time amongst the military and civilians. Undoubtedly the greatest innovation, and one which came in c. 1400, is the bag sleeve, which remained in fashion for about seventy or eighty years. It was tight at the wrists and also at the arm-hole, and the dandy of the period had them made as long and as voluminous as possible. The universal colour for these houppelandes was scarlet. One pronounced feature in the sketch is the baldrick hung with bells, a fashion which was introduced from Germany, where it had been prevalent for many years.

We are able now to understand a passage from Roy. MS. 17 B xliii., an extract from "Visions of Purgatory," by William Staunton, c. 1409 : "I saw some there with collars of gold about their necks, and some of silver, and some men I saw with gay girdles of silver and gold, and harneist horns

about their necks, some with more jagges on their clothes
than whole cloth, some had their clothes full of gingles and
belles of silver all overset, and some with long pokes (bags)
on their sleeves, the women with gowns trayling behind
them a great space, and some others with gay chaplets on
their heads of gold and pearls, and other precious stones."
It must not be supposed that the houppelande as seen in
the previous reign had died out altogether; on the contrary,
we find an illuminated manuscript (Arundel, No. 38) in the
British Museum depicting Occleve the poet presenting his
book to Henry, Prince of Wales (afterwards Henry V.), in
which the Prince is clad in a decided houppelande of the
old fashion, with dagging upon the fur-lined sleeves
(Fig. 167, Pl.). The poet wears a scarlet houppelande

of the prevalent fashion, which exemplifies
the shape of the sleeve to a marked degree.
Incidentally we may refer to the hideous
method of wearing the hair then coming
into vogue, and which, although so extremely unprepossessing, remained in fashion
until the time of Edward IV. In order to
show the style in its most exaggerated form,
we append Fig. 168, taken from a portrait of the Duke of
Bedford (*temp.* Henry VI.).

Fig. 168.—Duke of Bedford, *temp.* Henry VI.

With regard to the civilians, a brass executed in 1400,
and lying in Tilbrook Church, Bedfordshire, well illustrates
the style then coming into vogue. The man, who exhibits
the bifid beard affected by Richard II., wears a paltock,
which is only visible at the neck, and has the sleeves reaching
to the knuckles. Over this is a houppelande, the high neck
being shown unbuttoned and falling upon the shoulders.

The bag sleeves are very clearly indicated, together with the method for fastening them by buttons at the wrists. An ornamental belt is worn round the waist (not the hips, as in the previous reign), and from it depends the anelace of very large dimensions (Fig. 169). This brass may be taken as a general type of the brasses of civilians for the next fifty years at least, only slight variations occurring in the height of the collar, the lining of the dress with fur or otherwise, the cloak sometimes worn over the houppelande, &c. One of the most valuable manuscripts in the British Museum is Cott. MS. Nero D vii., the Catalogue of Benefactors to St. Albans Monastery. It was written and illuminated by Alan Strayler, and covers a period from c. 1390 to c. 1445. This artist has limned the faces and dresses of the persons who presented gifts to the Abbey, and affords us one of the best and most reliable sources for contemporary costume. Nigel Lorringe (Fig. 170, Pl.), for instance, is shown in a houppelande, the collar of which apparently reaches over his head, and is ornamented with one of the startling patterns which prevailed shortly before the demise of Richard II., in this case conjecturally the Order of the Garter. The hat we have seen in various illustrations with but slight alterations during the past two centuries (vide Fig. 139, Pl., and Fig. 37). He wears long poleyns, and has an anelace suspended by a baldrick. His gift to the monastery was evidently worth receiving, judging from the size of the bag. William de Albeneis presented a goblet, and is shown in the usual baldrick and anelace (Fig. 171, Pl.). His bifid beard shows him to be contemporary with Nigel Lorringe. The lady and gentleman in Fig. 172, Pl., are Johannes Gyniford and wife, and we have here an example of the profusion of ornament which characterised the men about the year 1400.

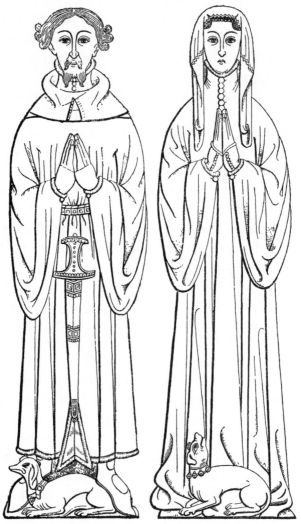

FIG. 169.—Civilian and lady, *c.* 1400.   Tilbrook Church, Bedfordshire.

The imitation of the SS collar, the large roses upon the

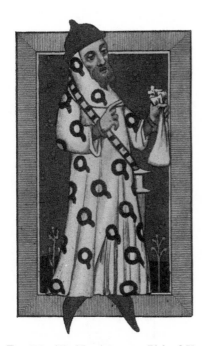

Fig. 170.—Nigel Lorringe, *temp.* Richard II.
(Book of Benefactors of St. Albans Abbey.)

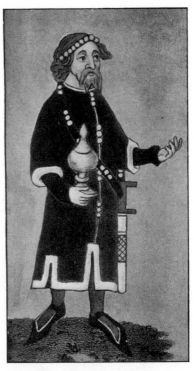

Fig. 171. — William de Albeneis, *temp.*
Richard II. (Book of Benefactors of
St. Albans Abbey.)

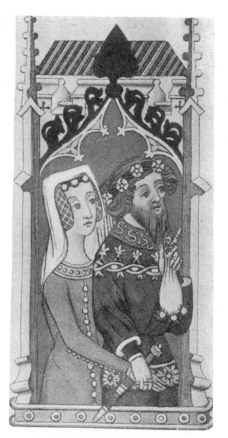

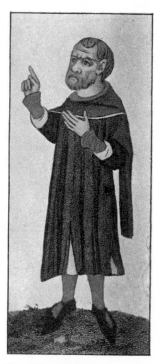

Fig. 172.—Johannes Gyniford and wife, *temp.*
Richard II. (Book of Benefactors of St.
Albans Abbey.)

Fig. 173.—Alan Strayler, artist.
(Book of Benefactors of St.
Albans Abbey.)

chaplet, the highly decorated hip-belt of large dimensions, and
the ornamental design round the shoulders, all tend to give
us the feeling in costume prevailing at that time even among
the middle classes.   It should be noticed that he wears no
less than six rings upon his fingers.   The painter himself,
Alan Strayler, is shown in Fig. 173, Pl., and the modesty
of his costume is commend-
able when compared with
those he depicts.   Thomas
Bedel, of Redbourne (Fig.
174, Pl.), is shown in an extraordinary hood, which is
evidently padded to give the
appearance it presents.   The
enormous buttons on his
houppelande are decidedly
obtrusive.   An interesting
little sketch (Fig. 175) represents Walter de Hamuntesham attacked and seriously
wounded by the rabble of St.
Albans while standing up

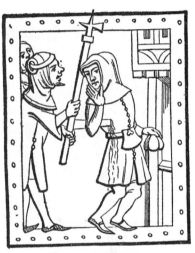

FIG. 175.—Walter de Hamuntesham
attacked by a mob.

for the rights and liberties of the Church.   Like most of
the illuminations, there is no date attached to it, and
the only clue to chronology lies in the costumes depicted.
The hood of the sufferer is remarkably like that of the
Thomas Bedel above; the townsman wielding a pole-
axe has the liripipe of his hood twisted round the crown
of his head and knotted at the back, in one of the
approved fashions of the lower orders, while his outer
garment is singular from the fact that it is split up at

the side like a tabard, and buttoned. The dresses worn
by Law officials did not, generally speaking, undergo many
alterations, but remained very constant, innovations only
occurring at long intervals. As an example, at the present
time we may cite the fact that the dresses of our Judges,
Corporation officials, &c., are based upon those used at
the time of Queen Elizabeth.

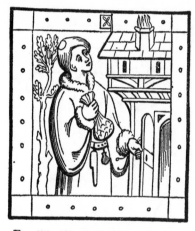

We append illustrations of
law costumes prevailing
generally in the fourteenth
and fifteenth centuries (Figs.
176, 177, Pls.).

The woodcut of Alan
Middleton (Fig. 178) is of
later date, and represents
him with the bag sleeves of
the fifteenth century; a
penner and ink-horn depend
from his girdle. He was a
collector of rents for the
monastery. These series of
sketches are valuable, not only on account of the costume,
but also as affording authentic portraits of personages who
lived five centuries ago.

FIG. 178.—Alan Middleton, collector of
rents. St. Albans Abbey.

THE WOMEN

THE CRESPINE AND VEIL PERIOD, 1400–1420

The period from c. 1400 to 1420 may be memorised
as the "Crespine and Veil" Period with great advantage;
although the dress changed somewhat during this time,

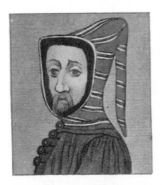

Fig. 174.—Thomas Bedel, of Redbourne, *temp.* Richard II.
(Book of Benefactors of St. Albans Abbey.)

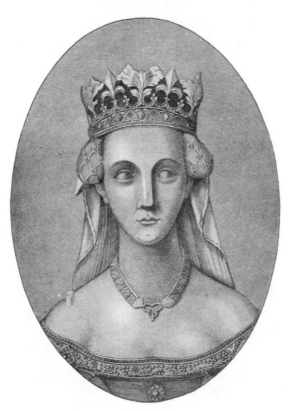

Fig. 179.—Joan of Navarre, consort of Henry IV.   In Canterbury Cathedral.

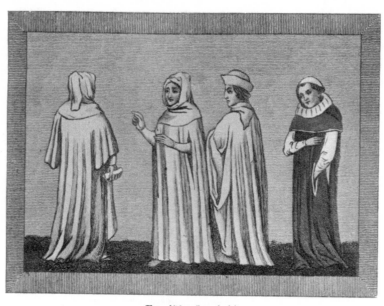

FIG. 176.—Law habits.

(Nos. 1, 2, and 3, Sloane MS. 2432.   No. 4, Roy. MS. 20 C vii.)

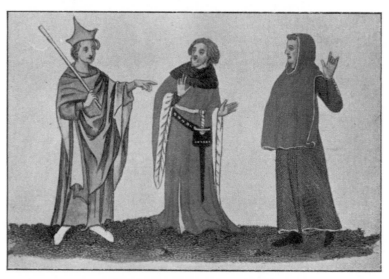

FIG. 177.—Habits of officers of the law.

(Roy. MSS. 2 B vii. ; 20 C vii. ; 16 G vi.)

the head-dress underwent but little, if any, modification. It is a strange but noteworthy fact that, although the costumes of the men, from the reign of Richard II. to that of Richard III., passed through a series of kaleidoscopic changes, both in cut and colour, the dress of the ladies altered but slightly. This remark, however, does not apply to head-dresses, for during this period of one hundred years more startling and grotesque varieties of head-gear appeared before an astonished world than during any other century of English history.

The effigy of Joan of Navarre, the consort of Henry IV., lies in the Chapel of St. Thomas à Becket, in Canterbury Cathedral, by the side of that of her husband. She is the first queen to exhibit reticulations in the head-dress upon a regal effigy (Fig. 179, Pl.). She wears a côte-hardi and a super côte-hardi, both remarkably low-necked. As nothing whatever appears upon the shoulders, the two garments have perforce to terminate in the ornamental band which passes round the chest. The cloak also depends from this band, which has jewelled morses fixed into it. So far as the rest of the costume is concerned, it is precisely similar to the super côte-hardi costumes already described.

The Houppelande.—Many ladies affected this style of outer garment, one of the earliest of this period being shown in Fig. 169, dating from 1400. It will be seen that it is high-necked, and fastens down the front for a short distance with very large buttons. Both sleeves are of the bag pattern, buttoning tightly round the wrists, where an edging of fur is seen. The hands are partly covered by the sleeves of the côte-hardi underneath, which are ornamented with the usual buttons.

Upon a brass in St. Lawrence Church, Norwich, *c.* 1400 (Fig. 157), a lady is shown similarly attired, but having a belt confining the houppelande; the high collar is here thrown back, showing the buttons and loops.   An earlier form still of the houppelande, but without the bag sleeves, is shown upon the brass of Lady Lora de St. Quintin, *c.* 1397, Brandsburton Church, Yorkshire (Fig. 180), where the extraordinary development of the sleeves of the côte-hardi over the hands is a very marked feature.

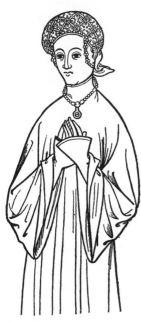

FIG. 180.—Lady Lora de St. Quintin, 1397. Brandsburton Church, Yorkshire.

A similar garment to that of Lady Lora may be seen in Fig. 166, Pl., taken from Roy. MS. 15 D iii., and is probably ten or fifteen years later.   In the original it is shown most beautifully ornamented with small golden cygnets upon a white ground.

A brass dating from 1410 lies in Spilsby Church, Lincolnshire (Fig. 181), and depicts a knight and lady of the eccentric d'Eresby family.   We say eccentric advisedly, for not only does the knight present peculiar features in his armour, but the lady, as will be seen, has some distinct touches essentially her own.   The display of the collar of the houppelande, and also the dark material with which the sleeves are lined, should be noticed; but the manner in which

the palms of the hands are
shown to the front, instead
of being placed as in prayer,
together with the pendent
lawn cuffs, form very striking peculiarities. From the
foregoing examples, it will
be seen that not only was
the houppelande a favourite
with the men during the
reigns of Henry IV. and
Henry V., but also with the
ladies, the remarkable absence of dagging and the
grotesque fantasies of Richard II. being a noteworthy
feature.

The Short-waisted Gown.
—Fig. 182, Pl., is an interesting group, depicting
Christine de Pisan presenting her book to the Queen
of France. All the ladies
(except the poetess, who is
upon her knees) are habited
in houppelandes having long
open sleeves, and with the
collars turned down. It
should be noticed that the
cincture round the waist is
in all cases high, and in this

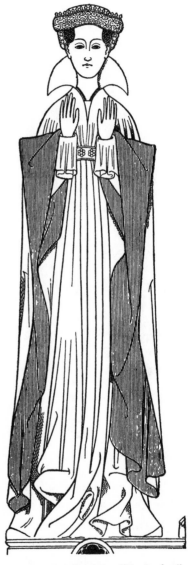

FIG. 181.—A lady of the d'Eresby family
o. 1410. Spilsby Church, Lincolnshire.

feature we have an early form of the well-known short-waisted gown of the fifteenth century.   In future chapters we shall trace the development of this gown, and show how, when fully evolved, it ran side by side with the super c\^ote-hardi costume until about the reign of Richard III.   It is curious to notice how the fantastic dresses of Richard II. left their traces upon subsequent costume.

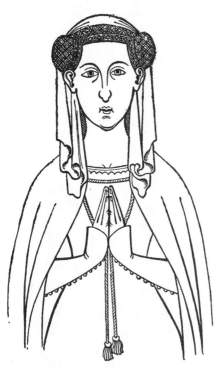

FIG. 183.—A lady at Sawtrey, Hampshire, 1404.

The Crespine and Veil.—In dealing with the reign of Richard II. we pointed out that the reticulated head-dress was often accompanied by a small veil hanging down the back.   This custom, once introduced, gradually developed, until about the year 1400 the veil became a prominent feature, covering not only the back part of the head, but also at times hanging down on either side of the face, after the fashion of the peplum of a century earlier.   In fact, the head-dress between 1400 and 1420 merely consisted of the reticulated crespine partially covered by the veil. One of the earliest forms may be seen in Fig. 169, where a small crespine, suitable to the lady's position, appears to be

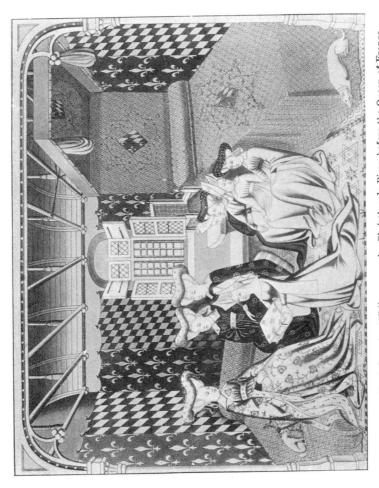

Fig. 182.—Head-dress in stiff linen worn by Christine de Pisan before the Queen of France.

almost entirely covered by the veil, while in Fig. 157 the head-dress is completely covered by this feature. A form of attire which came in later was the square crespine, the cauls of which alone were permitted to emerge. If the crespine had been allowed to appear, it would most probably have been of the shape shown in Fig. 181. Here the elaborate attire may be seen in one of its fullest developments, and unquestionably in one of its

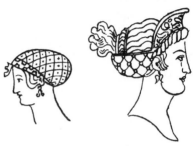

FIG. 184.—Greek heads.

most pleasing forms. The veil is not visible, but it probably covers the crown of the head and hangs down the back. The general and most popular form of the crespine may be noticed in Fig. 183, which shows the general arrangement very clearly. If the face depicted here is a correct portrait, the lady probably died an unappropriated blessing. It is curious to note how fashion repeats itself, and a comparison of the crespines of this period with that of the Greeks shows similarities which can only be described as remarkable coincidences (*vide* Fig. 184).

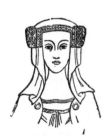

FIG. 185.—Lady Felbrigg, 1413. Felbrigg Church, Norfolk.

The brass of Lady Felbrigg, 1413, in Felbrigg Church, Norfolk, shows a graceful arrangement of the veil, and the whole front of the crespine is visible (Fig. 185). A brass dated 1420, in Herne Church, Kent (Fig. 186), shows the fullest development of this style, from which it will be at once perceived that the cauls were quite as large as they had been forty years previously. This remark also applies to Lady Shelton, who died in 1423, and lies in Great Snoring Church, Norfolk (Fig. 187). A feature of the veil shown here is the goffering along the front, being probably the earliest example of a fashion which lasted for over twenty years. That the cauls of Lady Hallé were not out of proportion for the period, we may cite the crespine of Lady

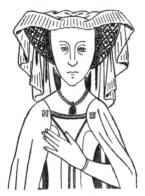

Peryent five years previously (Fig. 188), who wears a much larger head-dress, with the strange

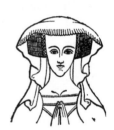

FIG. 186.—Lady Hallé, c. 1420.
Herne Church, Kent.

FIG. 187.—Lady Shelton,
1423. Great Snoring
Church, Norfolk.

feature of the veil appearing draped upon the top only. There is one significant peculiarity in Fig. 186 ; the cauls are beginning to show an upward tendency, and we may trace the subsequent horned head-dress from this inception. The same peculiarity may be noticed in all the crespine and veil head-dresses depicted in Fig. 182, Pl. A late example of the crespine and veil head-dress, with the goffering distinctly shown, is seen upon the brass of a lady in Horley Church, Sussex, dated 1430, some ten years after the fashion had been generally discarded (Fig. 189).

Among the many charms attendant upon the study of costume, it may with confidence be asserted that the gradual

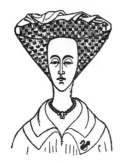

FIG. 188.—Lady Peryent, 1415. Digs-well Church, Hertfordshire.

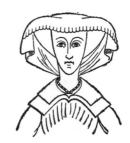

FIG. 189.—Lady, c. 1430. Horley Church, Sussex.

development of some insignificant detail into a subsequent prominent feature, and the dying out of the same, is not the least interesting point to those who follow it minutely.

CHAPTER XII

It is with a considerable amount of diffidence that we commence this chapter upon the costume prevailing during the reign of Henry VI., for an uneasy consciousness prevails that, however earnestly it may be attempted, it will assuredly fall short in fully coping with the subject. The material to hand is so vast, and the varieties so complex, so confusing, and, worst of all, so overlapping, that it is impossible to make any hard and fast rules, and to a certain extent any definite statements, concerning the dress of the period. So far as costume is concerned the reign presents itself to one's mind as a fantastical phantasmagoria of all the odds and ends of the garments prevailing during the preceding centuries, with no prominent salient features that may be definitely grasped. The boundless disorder, civil dissensions, and internal struggles of the reign could in no way have been more vividly portrayed than in the heterogeneous agglomeration of jumbled fashions with which the unhappy subjects of a weak and, at times, mad king attempted to clothe themselves.

THE MEN

During his long reign of thirty-nine years, Henry VI. would naturally be depicted a considerable number of times by the illuminators of contemporary manuscripts. One of

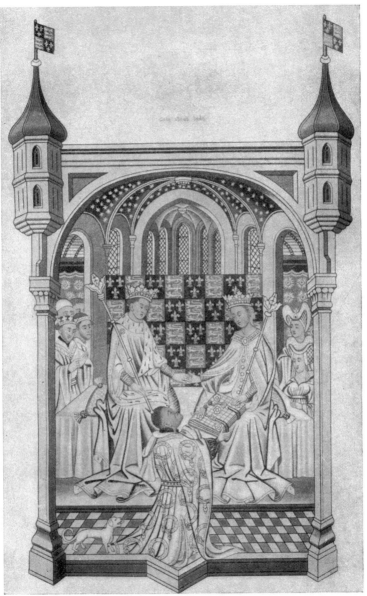

Fɪɢ. 190.—John Talbot, Earl of Shrewsbury, presenting a book to
Margaret of Anjou, c. 1445. (Roy. MS. 15 E vi.)

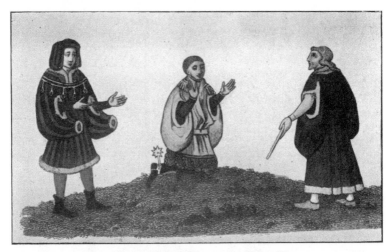

Fig. 192.—Bag sleeves, *temp.* Henry VI.
(Roy. MS. 15 E vi. and Harl. MS. 2278.)

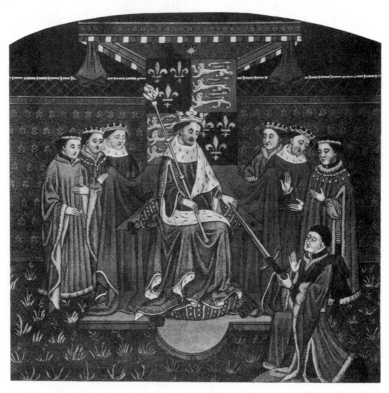

Fig. 196.—Henry VI. presenting a sword to John Talbot, Earl of Shrewsbury.
(Roy. MS. 15 E vi.)

the best known is that in which the warlike Talbot, Earl of Shrewsbury, is presenting a book, composed expressly for her at the cost of the Earl, to Margaret of Anjou (Fig. 190, Pl.). This figure, reproduced from the actual book in the British Museum, Roy. MS. 15 E vi., shows the King in a short tippet of ermine, a most voluminous mantle open at the side and lined with ermine, covering a houppelande with open sleeves, from which appear the tight sleeves of an under garment. As usual the houppelande is red. In Cott. MS. Julius E iv. there is a representation of Henry VI. attired in a long flowered blue houppelande, over which is draped a capacious mantle. This manuscript is most remarkable for containing a series of full-length figures of English kings from the time of the Conqueror to that of Henry VI., who is shown as a young man, and underneath each illumination are descriptive verses written by Lydgate. The artist has exercised his powers of personal recollection only, and has not availed himself of any opportunities of research. Thus his representations of English kings is essentially the costume prevailing in his own period, together with a few suggestive reminiscences of the three previous reigns. The figure of Richard II. has the berretino, with its pendent becca and the dagged appendage upon the top, which the student will at once recognise as being derived directly from the chaperon. A peculiar variety of côte-hardi covers the figure, upon which is the hip-belt, effectually denoting the period. The hose is white, as also are the shoes, which have turned-up cracowes. If we divest these figures of their crowns, there can be no doubt that we have representations of the costumes of the nobility of the period. In that portraying King John we are introduced to the short mantle, which was very prevalent in the last reign and the commencement of this. It was termed the *heuke*, and in the example is composed of a mixture of colours, red, blue, and purple, probably indicating variegated silk. The lining is purple and the outer border is of gold embroidery. It is fastened upon the right shoulder by a rich jewelled brooch. The côte-hardi with its hip-belt is significant of the reign of King Richard II.; the sleeves, covering the hands and furnished with rows of buttons, recall the reigns

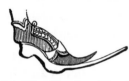

FIG. 191.—Clog, *temp.* Edward IV. (Roy. MS. 15 E iv.)

of Henry IV. and V.; while the clogs bring us back abruptly to that of Henry VI. These clogs (Fig. 191) were worn by gentlemen throughout this reign, and there are even examples to be found in the time of Richard III. The fashion is a remarkably singular one, and quite in accordance with the time of Henry VI.; the enormously long toes, exceeding the length of the shoe by some inches, must have proved most inconvenient for walking. In this gallery of kings, Henry II. wears a paltock, having extremely long and wide sleeves lined with ermine which hang to the knees. Edward II. is represented in a purple houppelande edged with fur and reaching to the ground; it is secured round the waist by a jewelled girdle. The great majority of kings are shown in armour, which is treated of in another volume in this series.

Among the upper classes the characteristic bag sleeve of the reigns of Henry IV. and V. became peculiarly the sport of circumstances. In Fig. 192, Pl., No. 1 is taken from Roy. MS. 15 E vi., and exhibits the modification of the sleeves by the addition of two other exits for the arms.

In order to assume this shape we may infer that the sleeves
were stiffened.   No. 2, taken from Harl. MS. 2278, represents a gentleman who is endeavouring apparently to sit
upon his spur.   Only one opening appears in his sleeve,
and the same may be said of the third figure adapted from
the same manuscript.

Among the multitudinous hats of this reign, that depicted in Fig. 193, Pl., is fairly common, and its exceeding
grotesqueness is only excelled by the specimen shown in
Fig. 194, Pl.   This represents a small group taken from Harl.
MS. 2278, and clearly shows the enormous extent to which
the becca depending from the head-gear became developed.
The childish figure to the left illustrates the mode of
carrying the capuchon or berretino when not in use,
and many examples of this feature occur in illuminated
manuscripts and also upon brasses.   To emphasize this
statement we append Fig. 195, taken from an incised slab
in the Church of St. Ouen, at Rouen, and representing
the architects of the church.   In both cases the berretino
(also at times called the *roundlet*) is shown thrown over the
right shoulder; the end of the becca shows quite clearly
on the second figure a little above the head upon the right
side.   Upon the first figure the head portion is very distinct.
Before leaving this figure, we should like to draw the
attention of the reader to the fact that the bag sleeve in
its primitive form was still prevailing in 1440 amongst
certain classes, and that the hair was cropped in the same
ungainly manner upon the Continent as prevailed in England.
Reverting to Fig. 194, Pl., we notice that the third personage represented affords us another example of what may be
termed the " mandarin " hat, and in fact the whole figure is

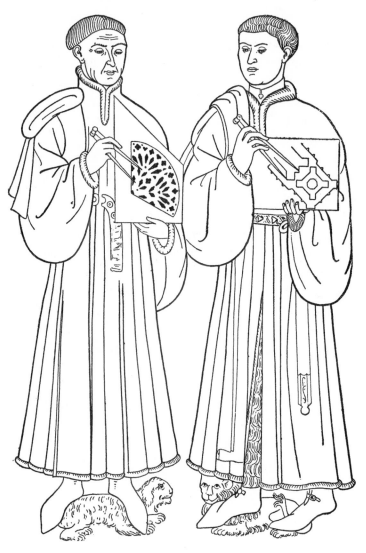

FIG. 195.—Incised slab, *c.* 1440. The architects of the Church of St. Ouen, at Rouen.

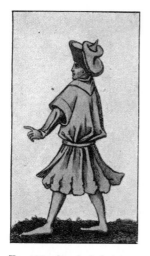

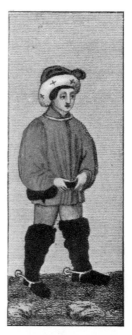

FIG. 193.—Mandarin hat, *temp.*
Henry VI.

FIG. 197.—Riding habit, King Henry
VI.   (Harl. MS. 4379.)

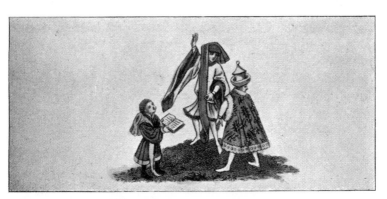

FIG. 194.—Development of the becca.

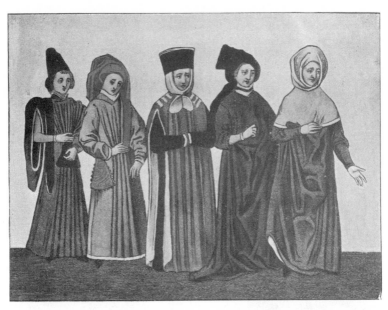

FIG. 198.—Costumes illustrating Transition Period, Henry VI.–Edward IV.
(Harl. MS. 4379, &c.)

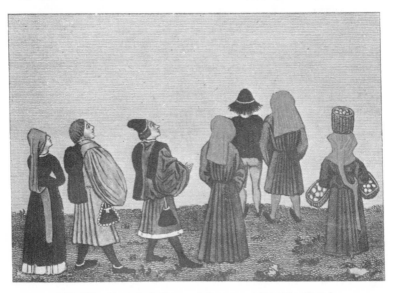

FIG. 199.—Group including market women. Transition Period.

extremely suggestive of the Celestial. In Fig. 196, Pl., three varieties of apparel are illustrated, taken from Roy. MS. 15 E vi. The figure kneeling upon the ground is habited in a capacious houppelande edged with fur, and has his berretino thrown over his shoulder in the approved fashion. Immediately behind him is a personage wearing a cloak, the side opening of which is so extensive that it presents a tabard-like appearance. Next to him we see a man in a long houppelande fitted with bag sleeves.

Towards the end of the reign of Henry VI. the dresses insensibly began to trend in the direction of the style prevailing in the reign of the succeeding sovereign, and the following figures are selected to illustrate this tendency. Fig. 197, Pl., which we may aptly dub a caricature in spurs, is wearing a turban lined with white fur; his pied jacket has one side green and the other red; while so much of his nether limbs as are not hidden by boots are shown dark in the manuscript. Fig. 198, Pl., is taken from the Harl. MS. 4379, which is an edition of Froissart's Chronicles written during this reign. It will be of interest to the reader to differentiate between the styles of the two reigns, as illustrated in these transition figures.

In Fig. 199, Pl., a group of persons including a market woman is shown, as also Fig. 200, Pl., to illustrate the ordinary dress of the ordinary working people.

THE WOMEN

The extravagances to which we have alluded at the commencement of this chapter as prevailing during the reign of Henry VI. were not intended to apply exclusively to the members of the sterner sex. We find a remarkable exemplification also in the case of the ladies, though strange to say they exhibited it in a most marked degree in fantastical head-dresses, and showed but little variation in the fashions of their robes. There is therefore a possibility of classification in their case, which is utterly wanting, and has not been attempted, in dealing with the men.

The Robe.—Throughout the whole of this reign a robe was in fashion which was perhaps more generally prevalent than the super côte-hardi costume, although the latter remained a great favourite with many, and is constantly seen in illuminations. As an example of this assertion we may refer to Fig. 196, Pl., where it will be seen that Queen Margaret is vested in the latter costume. Her côte-hardi is of cloth of gold, with a black hip-belt encircling it; over it appears a white super côte-hardi, part of which, *i.e.* round the arm openings, is probably fur. Upon this is draped a simple red cloak, lined with ermine.

The robe alluded to above had one or two distinguishing characteristics, by means of which it may be readily recognised from that of all other periods. It is always represented as being extremely short-waisted, and at one period was encircled by a very broad cincture. The skirt was very long, and not only had a train of great length, but the front was cut almost equally long, which, if required, could be spread out to a considerable distance in front. The bodice was tight-fitting, and at a later period was cut very low, almost invariably to a V-shape in front, and often the same behind.

At the commencement of the reign, when the influence of the houppelande was still felt, the sleeves of the robe

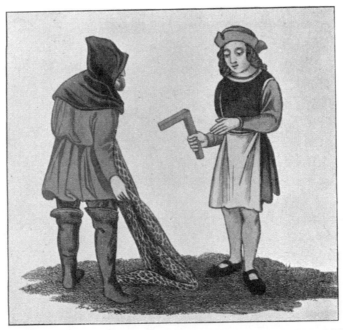

FIG. 200.—Carpenter and fisherman, Transition Period, Henry VI.–Edward IV.
(Harl. MS. 4379.)

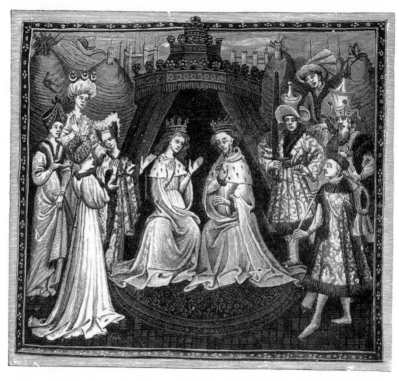

FIG. 201.—King, Queen, and Court, *c.* 1450. (Harl. MS. 2278.)

were cut somewhat loose, but they became smaller as the reign progressed.

The Head-dress.—Undoubtedly the first of the startling series of head-dresses was the Turban Head-dress. This fashion was in vogue for a considerable period, and instances may be found of its use throughout the reign, and even afterwards. It was undoubtedly based upon an Oriental model, as during the early part of its use a very common ornament for its decoration was the crescent (Fig. 201, Pl.), which appears to point to a Turkish origin, and no doubt became fashionable in consequence of the Moslem looming large in European affairs, by reason of the persistent attacks upon, and subsequent capture of, Constantinople. That it was not of Indian origin is proved by the shape, and also by the fact that it was not commonly of white material. This medi-

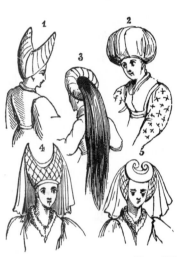

FIG. 202.—Head-dresses, *temp.* Henry VI.

æval turban was of very light construction in spite of its bulk, being simply composed of a wire framework, over which was stretched a covering of silk or other material, often of the richest description. In Fig. 202 two turbans are depicted, one being of a very voluminous form, and another in the centre of the picture exhibiting a smaller variety; it differs from the other in having the hair flowing through the centre and down the back. One thing may certainly be said in favour of the turban—it was the least aggressive of the many head-dresses which sprang into existence at this period. That it was a favourite is shown by its persistence. For example, the annexed figure (Fig. 203) represents a card party in the early part of the sixteenth century, where one of the ladies appears in a turban of no small dimensions.

The Horned Head-dress.—Of all the head-dresses which

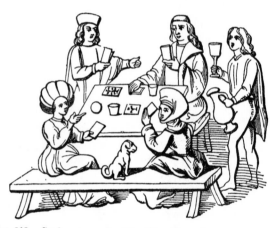

FIG. 203.—Card party, early sixteenth century, showing persistence of turban head-dress.

came into fashion during this extraordinary reign, the horned variety was *par excellence* undoubtedly the most grotesque and bizarre. It neither fitted the head nor adorned it—it was merely an uncouth excrescence. We find it pursuing its mad course upon the Continent for some time before its introduction into England; the invasion of our own country occurred about 1420. On referring back to Fig. 186, the cauls shown upon the head of Lady Hallé are seen to have an upward tendency, and here we doubtless

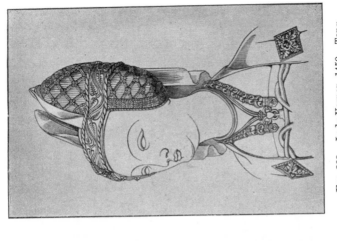

FIG. 208.—Lady Vernon, 1450. Tong
Church, Shropshire.

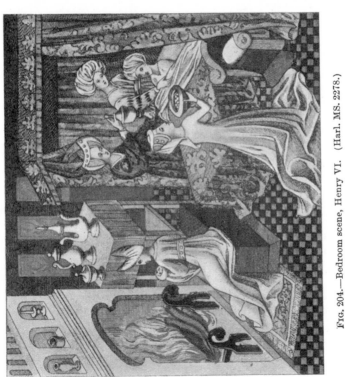

FIG. 204.—Bedroom scene, Henry VI. (Harl. MS. 2278.)

witness the origin of this species of attire. During the next forty years we find it of all shapes and dimensions; it does not seem to have gradually developed as one would imagine, finally attaining its maximum size at the end of this period; on the contrary, some of the largest coiffures are noticed much earlier, as, for example, the magnificent specimen in Arundel Church, Sussex, upon the effigy of Beatrice, Countess of Arundel, 1439, which is considered to be the finest and most perfect illustration of the horned head-dress in existence, either in the British Isles or upon the Continent. A reproduction of this is shown in the *Frontispiece*, which has been made according to original measurements. If a comparison of this figure is made with that of Lady Burton (Fig. 151), it will be seen that so far as the width of the cauls are concerned they are almost identical in size, and it is only the addition of the huge horns which make it of such gigantic proportions. With the advent of these inflated specimens of attire, the coronets of noble ladies underwent a corresponding increase in size.

In Fig. 204, Pl., taken from a MS. of Lydgate's Metrical Life of St. Edmund (Harl. MS. 2278), a bedroom scene is depicted, and the nurse seated upon the huche before the fire wears a very common form of the horned head-dress, such as was affected for many years by the middle and lower classes. The voluminous dress upon two figures in this engraving should be noted, also the fact that two examples of the turban head-dress are illustrated. The lady holding the hanap in her hands wears a species of horned attire which is often met with, and which subsequently developed into the heart shape. The figure kneeling shows the caul upon the right side and the two horns from which depends the veil, although the mediæval artist in this case has not been very happy in his perspective.   The kneeling figure of Christine de Pisan in Fig. 182, Pl., illustrates the method of imitating the horned head-dress in stiff linen; we have referred to this figure as illustrating the beginning of this style. The wearing of horns upon the head naturally suggested the father of all evil to the irrepressible satirists of the time, and many ungallant allusions were made respecting them. Probably no attire excited more uncomplimentary and sarcastic remarks from writers, and even the greatest poet of the day, Lydgate, the Monk of Bury, appears to have been untiring in his condemnation, and even concocted a ballad upon the subject, " A Ditty of Women's Horns," in which he mentions that horns were given to beasts for defence, a thing contrary to femininity, and beseeches them to cast their horns away, inasmuch as the Virgin Mary never wore them.   At the same time he appears to have had a shrewd eye for beauty, as he acknowledges that the latter *would* show in spite of the horns.   A writer, who compiled a work for the use of his three young daughters about this time, describes the horned head-dress.   He introduces a holy bishop declaiming from the pulpit against the fashionable follies of the fair sex, whom he accuses of being marvellously arrayed in diverse and quaint manners, and particularly with high horns.   He compares them to horned snails, to harts, and to unicorns, and tells a story of a gentlewoman who went to a feast with the head so strangely attired with long pins, that her head-dress resembled a gallows—and she was consequently scorned by the whole company, who said she carried a gibbet upon her head.

However, these diatribes and animadversions had about as little effect in discouraging this fashion as the proverbial water upon the duck's back. In fact it seemed rather to add to the growth than otherwise, for we read that " it was judged necessary to enlarge the doors of the apartments of the Château de Vincennes," and also that the ladies " wore

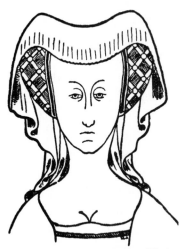

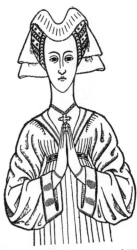

FIG. 205.—Joyce Halsham. West Grinstead Church, Sussex, 1441.

FIG. 206.—Lady Staunton, 1458. Castle Donington Church, Leicestershire.

horns wonderfully high and large, having on each side, instead of pads, ears so large that when they would pass through the door of a room, it was necessary for them to turn aside and stoop." That all ladies did not, however, exceed the ordinary bounds is proved by many figures upon brasses. Lady Halsham, for instance, 1441, in West Grinstead Church, Sussex (Fig. 205), wears a modified example; and seventeen years later Lady Staunton, 1458, in Castle Donington Church, Leicestershire, shows one of similar dimensions

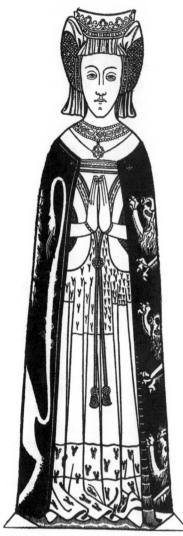

FIG. 207.—Lady Tiptoft, 1446. Enfield Church, Middlesex.

(Fig. 206). Joice, Lady Tiptoft, 1446, in Enfield Church, Middlesex (Fig. 207), wears an extremely elaborate headdress which falls under this category, although the coronet has the effect of dwarfing the horns. This magnificent brass is given full length in order to illustrate the armorial bearings upon the cloak and super côte-hardi—it is one of the finest examples we possess delineating this feature. The effigy of Lady Vernon, wife of Sir Richard Vernon, 1450, in Tong Church, Shropshire, affords us an exceptionally fine example of the horned head-dress in an unexaggerated form which is well worth attention (Fig. 208, Pl.). The method of fixing the cord upon the cloak between the two morses is distinctly shown, while the collar of "esses" is very elaborate. In order to exemplify the ridicule with which the horned head-dress was greeted by

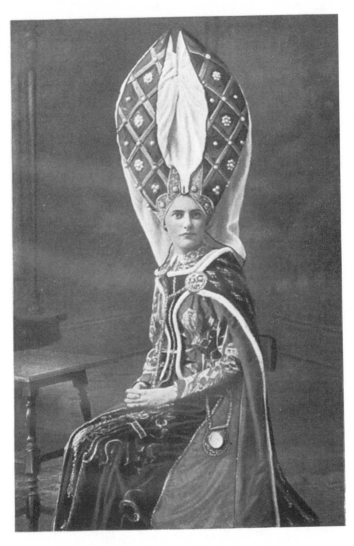

LADY, 1450–1470 (Henry VI., Edward IV.)

Head-dress.—Forked. Adapted from a representation on a contemporary misericorde.

Cloak.—Ermine; black velvet powdered with golden fleurs-de-lis; lined blue satin.

Jewelled Morse.—With pendant chain.

Super Côte-hardi.—Parti-coloured; black velvet stamped with heraldic lion rampant, collared; panel right side, red and green with heraldic quarterings in gold.

Côte-hardi.—Of rich baudekyn with strong pattern.

(Photographed direct from examples used in the Author's lecture upon "Mediæval Costume and Head-dresses.")

some, we append Fig. 209, taken from a *miserere* in Ludlow Church, Shropshire.

The Heart-shaped Head-dress was a direct development of the style seen in Fig. 182, Pl., for as the cauls grew higher and higher, the pad resting upon them was gradually pushed upwards, until it finally developed into the heart-shape.

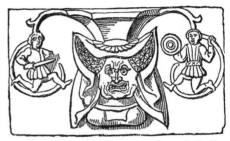

FIG. 209.—Horned head-dress. *Miserere* in Ludlow Church, Shropshire.

Two heart-shaped head-dresses of a later date, taken from Roy. MS. 15 E vi., are illustrated in Fig. 210, Pl.; one of them has a very peculiar imitation of a fashion prevailing among the gentlemen of the time of Edward IV., in the streamers hanging from the right side.

The Forked Head-dress.—This was undoubtedly a variety of the horned, which was formed by the horns standing up perpendicularly upon the head, instead of curving outwards, and having drapery depending from the points. The reproduction shown in the coloured plate (p. 166) has been made from a design upon the blade of a misericorde now preserved in the Wallace Collection. As will be readily seen, it is of very large proportions, but it corresponds exactly with the dimensions of the original. The forked head-dress had varieties, as may be seen in Fig. 211, Pl., representing Isabella of Bavaria, Queen of France, who died in 1435. She is depicted in a forked head-dress surmounted by a crown; one attendant has a similar attire, while the third is a peculiar variety often represented at this period, but probably more in fashion on the Continent. The extreme richness and voluminous character of the super côte-hardi is worthy of notice. We find that certain classes of the lower orders were in the habit of imitating their betters in the Middle Ages as they are in our own, and the ale-wife in Fig. 212 appears to have been an example;

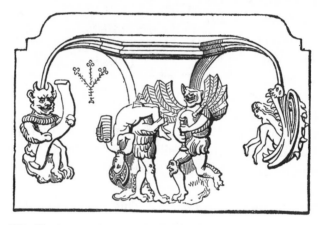

FIG. 212.—The doom of the ale-wife. Taken from a *miserere* in Ludlow Church.

any attempt to curtail the amount of liquor due to customers was deemed by them as a most heinous offence, and worthy of the punishment which has befallen the lady in question. It will be noticed that she still holds the token of her office while being carried to the place of punishment which looms on the right. The head-dress she wears is of the forked variety.

The Crescent Head-dress was a variety of the horned style, which very seldom appears of unwieldy proportions. An example of it is given in Fig. 202, No. 5, and another

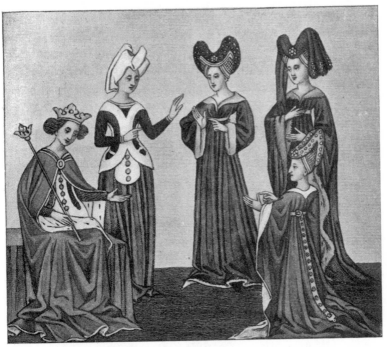

FIG. 210.—Heart-shaped head-dresses, &c.   (Roy. MS. 15 E vi.)

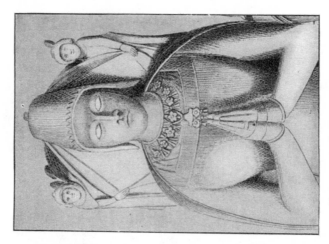

Fig. 216.—Lady Crosby, 1466. Great St. Helen's Church, London.

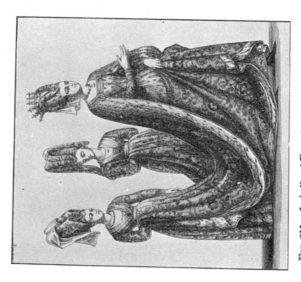

Fig. 211.—Isabella of Bavaria, Queen of France, 1435. The forked head-dress.

in a somewhat modified form upon the brass of an unknown
lady at Ash, in Kent, *c.* 1460 (Fig. 213).

As an example of the overlapping of styles, and of the
strict conservatism in head-dress which prevailed then as
now among certain individuals, we give here
a representation of the effigy of the second
wife of Ralph Nevill, Earl of Westmoreland,
dating from 1426 (Fig. 214, Pl.), which may
be looked upon as a magnificent example of
the reticulated head-dress, pure and simple,
in use twenty-six years after becoming obsolete. This lady, however, is by no means
the last, for, as will be seen in Fig. 215, Pl.,
Margaret Holland, who lies buried in Canter-
bury Cathedral, and died in 1440, is two-score years behind
the times.

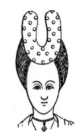

Fig. 213.—Brass of
unknown lady, *c.*
1460. Ash, Kent.

In Great St. Helen's Church, London, is the monument
of Sir John Crosby, and the appended illustration (Fig. 216,
Pl.) represents Lady Crosby, who died in 1466, although
the monument was not erected until 1475, when Sir John
died. The head-gear, as shown, is an exact copy of that
prevailing in Flanders at the time, as may be seen in
Raoul de Presle's French translation of St. Augustine's
"Civitas Dei," and, so far as we know, was never accepted
as an English head-dress.

CHAPTER XIII

EDWARD IV., 1461–1483. EDWARD V., 1483.
RICHARD III., 1483–1485

THE student of costume need be under no apprehension respecting his ability to recognise the dress prevailing in this period, and to differentiate it from that of all others. So marked and apparent are its characteristics, both as regards men and women, that it stands out pre-eminently distinct from all other ages. He will find a mass of material ready to hand in the form of brasses, effigies, paintings, and illuminated MSS., that afford rich stores with which to satiate his thirst for knowledge, and to these must be added a new and ultra-important source which cannot be over-estimated. The art of printing had been introduced upon the Continent about the middle of the century, but did not find its way into England until 1477, when Caxton produced his first book. Wood blocks had appeared not very long after movable type, and although they were at first executed in a barbarous manner, yet improvement came fairly rapidly, and towards the end of the fifteenth century we begin to recognise that valuable attention to minute detail which is so eminently a feature of the other authorities enumerated.

A great division occurs in the costume prevalent during this period as compared with that which antedated it, namely, the introduction of that accuracy and quality of

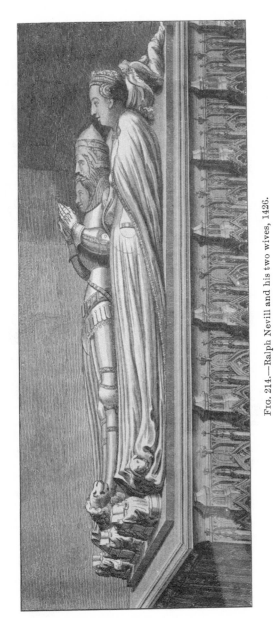

Fig. 214.—Ralph Nevill and his two wives, 1426.

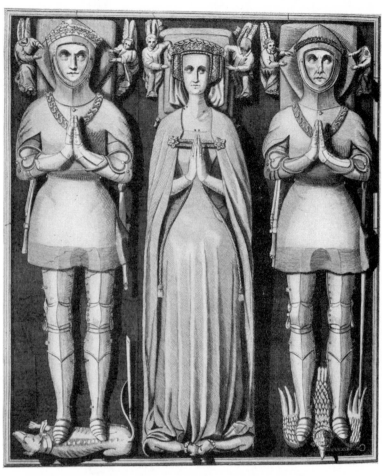

FIG. 215.—Margaret Holland, 1440, in Canterbury Cathedral, with her two husbands, John, Earl of Somerset, and Thomas, Duke of Clarence.

perfect fit into the garments of the men which had not hitherto distinguished them. Putting it in another way, we may say that, broadly speaking, it had been perfectly possible for a dressmaker to cut out and complete any garment worn by men up to that period; after the reign of Edward IV. the era of the tailor began.

The period under consideration is essentially that of the short garment, practically all the long robes and gowns of preceding reigns being rigorously discarded, and only a few retained to serve purposes of state for officers of the law and a few court functionaries. These short garments undoubtedly had a German origin, which filtered through France and found their way across the Channel. They appear to have been adopted and worn with a total disregard to feelings of decency, which it is the pride, object, and aim of all civilised nations to instil into the minds of their subjects, and we are compelled to believe that the vehement diatribes of the preachers of the day were fully justified when we behold some of the representations of fashions which have descended to us.

THE MEN

No effigies are extant of the three kings whose names head this chapter, and it is only from MSS. that we can glean any particulars of regal apparel. Edward IV., as depicted in a MS. (No. 265) preserved at Lambeth Palace, wears the imperial arched diadem which first made its appearance upon his seal (Fig. 217). He wears a cape of ermine, with a cloak having a wide border of the same fur. The cloak is so very voluminous, that it hides the shape of the robe beneath. By the King's side is the young prince, for three short months Edward V.; his robes are practically the same as his father's. Of the coronation robes of Richard III. we have a detailed description; there appears to have been two complete sets, one of crimson velvet edged with miniver and richly embroidered with gold,

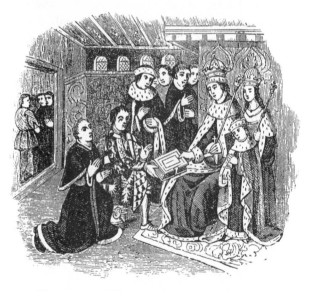

Fig. 217.—Lord Rivers and Caxton before Edward IV.

while the second was of purple velvet with an edging of ermine. The chausses worn were of crimson satin, as were also the mantle and hood, the coat, surcoat, and shirt. The sabbatons were covered with crimson cloth of gold. Towards the end of the ceremony he wore a tabard of white sarcenet, and a coif of lawn. Two hats were also provided, with rolls behind and peaks before.

The dress of the nobility was extremely varied, and

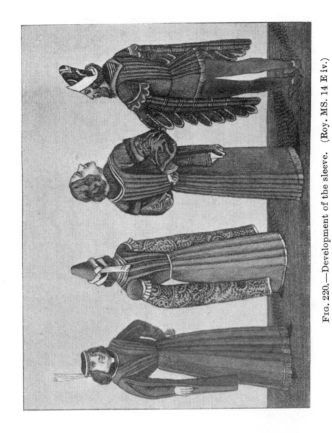

Fig. 220.—Development of the sleeve. (Roy. MS. 14 E iv.)

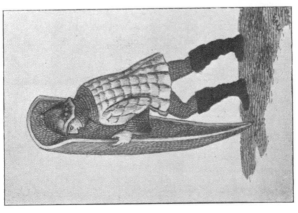

Fig. 219.—The military pourpoint.

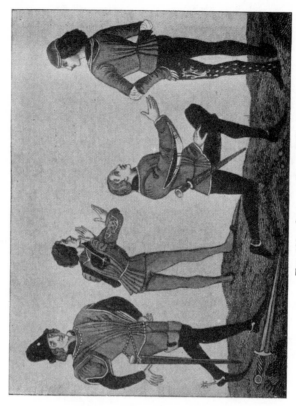

FIG. 223.—Costume, Edward IV.

1. Cott. MS. Nero D ix.   2, 3, and 4. Roy. MSS. 15 E iv. and 15 E ii.

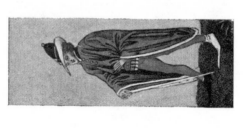

FIG. 221.—An exquisite, early Edward IV. (Harl. MS. 4380).

no definite style can be adduced. In Roy. MS. 15 E iv., representing a book presentation to King Edward IV., two courtiers are seen standing by the side of the King, which are generally considered to depict Clarence and Gloucester, his brothers (Fig. 218). Gloucester, afterwards Richard III., wears the fashionable *pourpoint*, or short jacket of the period. The term "pourpoint," strictly speaking, signifies any garment, no matter the shape, which is made by sewing or quilting two layers of material together with a padding between. It had been used as a defensive equipment for the military for many generations as the gambeson or haqueton, and now came into general vogue as a style for civil dress. There can be little doubt that the idea for the pourpoint originated in this knightly gambeson, a garment worn under the armour to prevent chafing, and thickly quilted in parallel rows; its initiation in this reign was followed

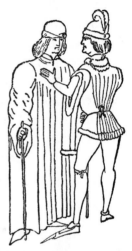

FIG. 218.—Costume, *temp.* Edward IV. (Roy. MS. 15 E iv.)

by a general use of the system for the next half century. A soldier habited in a pourpoint is inserted here for illustration (Fig. 219, Pl.). The method adopted for making a pourpoint consisted in having a perfect-fitting garment of the shape required to serve as a lining; upon this was laid the proper dress material, which was sewn down to the lining to form the desired flutings, the latter being kept in position by a padding of moss, flock, wool, or any light substance. The radiations seen upon the back of the

pourpoint worn by Gloucester indicate these quiltings; the
colour is red, and the edges have a border of fur. The
sleeve is extremely characteristic of this reign, being formed
like a cylinder, and having a hole in the upper part for the
arms to pass through (Fig. 220, Pl.). The chausses are blue
in colour, and around the left leg is the Order of the
Garter. The clogs or pattens upon the feet have been
referred to before. Clarence has a long green gown with
loose sleeves; a close red hat peaked in front and rolled
behind covers his long bushy hair. Gloucester's hat is red,
but of a different pattern; a jewelled brooch fastens the
feathers which droop over the top of it.

In Fig. 221, Pl., is indicated a dandy of the early part
of Edward's reign, in which the peaked cap with a black

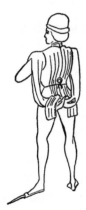

FIG. 222.—Costume,
Edward IV. (Roy.
MS. 15 E iv.)

crown and a white brim, the *Bycocket*, is
plainly shown; his green pourpoint has long
hanging sleeves edged with ermine; the
chausses are red, while the long-toed poleyns
are black and white respectively. He carries
a walking-stick, now coming into fashion.
An example of this short jacket may be
seen in Fig. 222. A strange style began
to come into vogue during this period,
whereby the shoulders were rendered disproportionately broad and the waist correspondingly small. This is well shown in
Fig. 223, Pl., No. 1, where an extra piece
of material is given to the sleeve to heighten
the effect which has been already produced by the *mahoitres*. These were pads of moss or flock sewn within the
shoulders. In the third year of the reign of Edward this

style of padding was prohibited to be worn by any yeoman or person under that degree, under a penalty of six and eightpence, and twenty shillings fine for the tailor who manufactured them. The chausses are red, and nearly encased in long tight-fitting black boots with yellow tops. He wears the usual peaked cap. No. 2 should be noticed for the enormous length of the poleyns. During this time no one under the estate of a lord was allowed to wear them more than two inches in length.

The third figure has the arm within the cylinder sleeve, and affords us an example of its double use. The fourth figure illustrates a peculiarity of this period, the sleeves being in two pieces and joined together at the elbow by *points*. As this is the first occasion where this term is used, we may say that this method for fixing garments together became very common during the sixteenth and seventeenth centuries, and this example may be looked upon as an early one. The points were simply ties furnished at the end with pointed aiglets, which were sometimes made ornamental. Many references to points may be found in

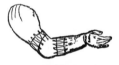

FIG. 224.—Sleeve showing method of pointing.

Shakespeare and other early plays. A further illustration of the pointing or lacing of sleeves is given in Fig. 224.

Fig. 225, Pl., No. 1, shows the method of carrying the berretino with its hanging becca, while the second exhibits the development of the poleyn, which is being demonstrated for our special edification. These long toes were rendered flexible to a certain extent by a judicious system of padding and stiffening, as otherwise they would double up under the feet in the act of walking. An interesting cut (Fig. 226) shows us the effect of the mahoitres upon the pourpoint, and also informs us that even the serving men and minstrels affected the long poleyns of the period.

Hats.—One of the most prominent coverings for the head which came into vogue approximately at the beginning

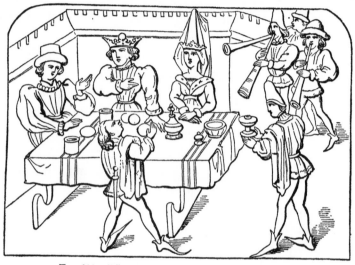

FIG. 226.—Effect of the mahoitres upon the pourpoint.

of the reign of Edward IV. is one which had been in use for some time upon the Continent; it was termed the *Bycocket,* and in all its varieties appears to have possessed two essential features connected with the brim which may generally be recognised, namely, a peak standing out well in front, and another mounting upwards to the crown at the back. These two points gave it the name of bycocket (Fig. 227). A magnificent example shown upon a king is given in Fig. 228, Pl., where a gold crown encircles it, and

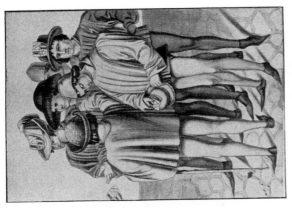

Fig. 234.—Proclamation of a tournament :
crowd affixing favours in their hats.

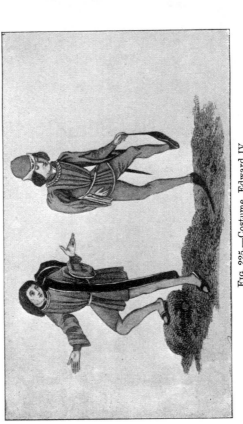

Fig. 225.—Costume, Edward IV.

1. Roy. MS. 15 D i.   2. Roy. MS. 14 E iv.

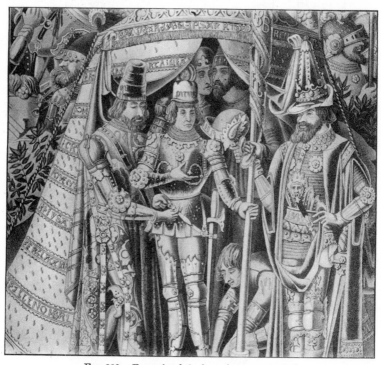

Fig. 228.—Example of the bycocket, ornamented.

the summit is finished with an ornamental boss of gold. The brim of the hat is of white material, but the remainder is of the most brilliant scarlet decorated with metal studs. Divested of its crown, the by-cocket proper appears as in the illustration. In Fig. 221, Pl., the usual form of bycocket is seen which prevailed in England, the domed top being of rare occurrence; but in Fig. 229, a bycocket is seen upon one of the cloaked characters, where the domed top is shown, but in a much modified form. In Fig. 230 Clarence is represented in the same style of hat,

FIG. 227.—The bycocket.

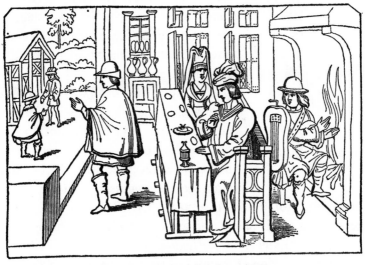

FIG. 229.—The bycocket, &c., c. 1470.

but with a very small peak in front. The usual form in use among ordinary persons is illustrated in Fig. 231, No. 2.

About the same time that the bycocket appeared another style of hat, the sugar-loaf, was introduced, which most

probably had its origin in a feeble attempt to copy the
steeple head-dress of the ladies. We will state the case
in this fashion, though it is quite open to question whether
the ladies did not introduce the steeple in imitation of
the sugar-loaf. In Fig. 232, No. 1, the sugar-loaf is seen
in its early form before being stiffened, but in No. 2

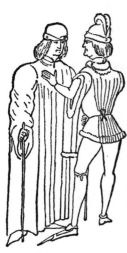

this omission is remedied. These two
figures give in an extremely exaggerated
form the general appearance of the
costume of the period. The addition
of a rolled brim to this sugar-loaf produced an almost infinite variety of
shapes; for example, in Fig. 233, representing a mediæval dance, we find
four of these hats based upon the sugar-
loaf-and-brim principle, and a bycocket
appears upon the head of one of the
minstrels. These by no means exhaust
the styles of hats worn during this
time; a few more may be seen upon
the heads of an interesting little group
taken from a manuscript in the Biblio-

FIG. 230.—Costume, *temp.*
Edward IV. (Roy MS.
15 E iv.)

thèque du Roi, Paris (Fig. 234, Pl.). The characters here
are placing small shields of arms in their hats, being those
of their partisans in a forthcoming tournament. We also
give an illustration (Fig. 231) of twelve examples of varieties
of head-gear prevailing at this period which will probably
be of interest to the reader.

Shoes.—At this period the long pointed toes of the
shoes are a very remarkable feature, as they probably
exceeded those of any other reign. A writer of the

period describing the poleyns states, "That the men wore
shoes with a point before, half a foot long; the richer
and more eminent personages wore them a foot long, and
princes two feet; which was the most ridiculous thing that
ever was seen."   The sumptuary law of the third year of the

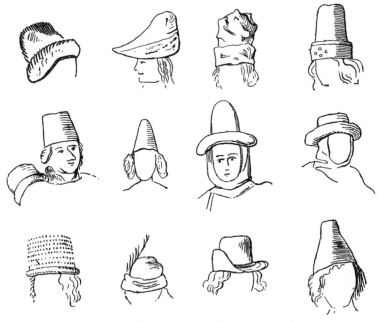

Fɪɢ. 231.—Varieties of hats, *temp.* Edward IV.

reign of Edward IV. prohibited a person wearing poleyns
having cracrowes more than two inches in length if he
were under the estate of a lord, but this apparently had
but very little effect.   In the British Museum are preserved
specimens of these shoes, excavated in the neighbourhood
of Whitefriars, and in all probability dated from that period.
They were found in an old rubbish heap, and the general

shape may be gleaned from Fig. 235. In many mediæval illustrations the extraordinary appearance of the boots is

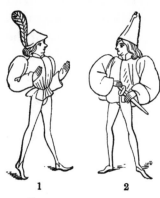

FIG. 232.—Costume, *temp.* Edward IV.

generally ascribed to inaccurate drawing on the part of the artist; but a brief inspection of the shape of the sole of these examples leads to the conclusion that they were faithfully represented, and that the suspected distortion does not exist. The toes were tightly stuffed with moss or hay, and a curious confirmation of this custom is preserved to the present day in a proverb current among the French peasantry, who describe a wealthy person by saying, "He has hay in his shoes." The method of constructing this strange foot-

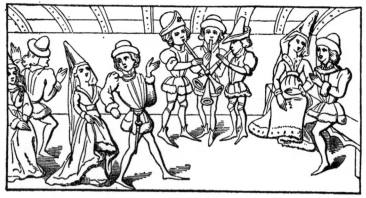

FIG. 233.—A mediæval dance, *c.* 1470.

wear is well shown in the accompanying diagrams of an example preserved in a Continental museum (Fig. 236,

Pl.). It will be seen that they open down the sides as in the previous figure, and this forms a peculiarity distinct from preceding periods. The strengthening of the sole by cross pieces, shown in the central diagram, is ingenious. Boots of the period are but rarely shown, but one example, from Roy. MS. 15 E vi., has a long-pointed, turned-up toe, and the top is shown of a lighter leather than the lower part in the original. The pattens

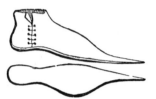

FIG. 235.—Shoes, Edward IV.

worn by the gentry during this reign were made of aspen-wood, and necessarily became much lengthened to accommodate the long toes ; an example is given in Fig. 237. There was no arbitrary rule respecting the fashion for the tops of these shoes, as may be seen by comparison with the illustration previously given. The shape of the foot-wear during the last part of the reign of Edward IV. was entirely

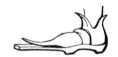

FIG. 237.—Shoe and clog, Edward IV.

different from that which has just been described. When the change took place in England it is somewhat difficult to decide, but it probably occurred between 1477 and 1480 —these years may be termed a transition period. The beaux of the day had apparently become satiated with long-toe vagaries, which had certainly been in vogue for an astonishing number of years under more or less aggravated conditions. Now, however, they were swept relentlessly away, never again to appear as an English fashion. In their place we find a foot-gear substituted which was broad instead of long at the toes, and at first partook somewhat of the nature of the old fashion, as shown in Fig. 238, where a point may still be seen; it is in Roy. MS. 15 E

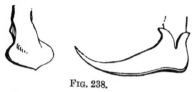

FIG. 238.

From Roy. MS. 15   From a painting in Salis-
E ii., 1482.   bury Cathedral.

ii., and dates from 1482. The toes, however, soon showed a tendency to broaden out to such a width as to almost rival their predecessors in distortion of the human foot.

Many examples of this feature will be given in succeeding reigns.

THE WOMEN

THE HENNIN HEAD-DRESSES, 1420–1490

In the introduction it was stated that the reigns of Edward IV. and his immediate successors were essentially the age for short garments. That remark applied exclusively to the men, and one is almost tempted to say that, so far as the women are concerned, it was the age of long garments. Of novelties introduced during the reign there are but few; all changes which occurred appear to have been made upon the basis of the old costumes of the reign of Henry VI.

Respecting regal habits, they may be judged from the plate already shown on page 172, where the Queen is represented liberally ornamented with ermine which covers the dress, of which nothing can be said except that it is low-necked, and is probably of the short-waisted variety.

The Gown.—Only two kinds of dress were prevalent, the super côte-hardi, and the short-waisted. The former appears to have undergone only slight modifications, which

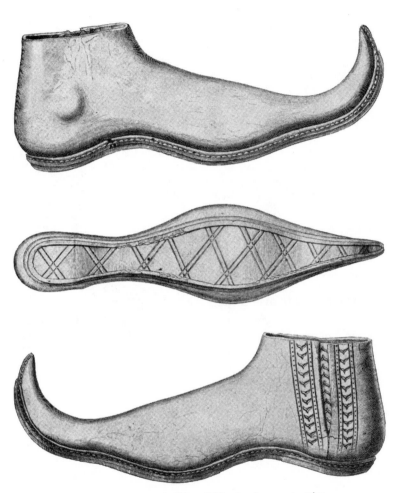

Fig. 236.—Poleyns, *temp.* Edward IV., showing construction.

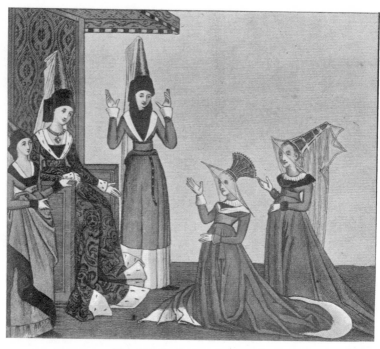

FIG. 242.—Ladies, *temp.* Edward IV.

Nos. 1, 2, 3. Cott. MS. Nero D ix.   4 and 5. Roy. MS. 19 E v.

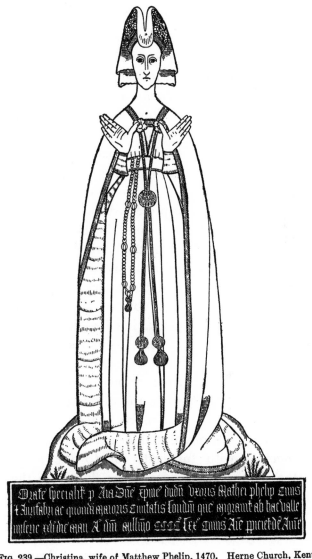

FIG. 239.—Christina, wife of Matthew Phelip, 1470. Herne Church, Kent.

did not in any way affect the general characteristics of the
costume as a whole. The short-waisted, on the other hand,
became extremely short-waisted, and the effect of this was
accentuated by the exceedingly low neck which became
the fashion. The broad cincture round the waist dwindled
into a comparatively narrow band
having generally a long pendent
tab.

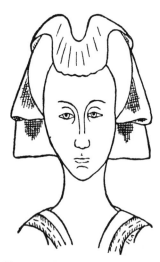

FIG. 240.—Petronilla Bertlot, 1490.
Stopham Church, Sussex.

In Herne Church, Kent, there
is preserved the brass of Christina,
wife of Matthew Phelip, 1470
(Fig. 239), which shows the lady
in a short-waisted gown undoubtedly very long in the skirt,
but covered by the capacious
cloak, lined with fur, which lies
in folds upon the ground. Her
waist is encircled by a cincture
from which depends a rosary,
while the tassels of her cloak are
a noteworthy feature. About this
time a fur collar was often an addition to the short-waisted
gown, together with fur cuffs cut to the shape of a
gauntlet, and the figure under notice illustrates the latter.
The head-dress of Petronilla Bertlot, 1490, in Stopham
Church, Sussex, is remarkably like that of Christina
Phelip, although it is twenty years later (Fig. 240). The
fur collar is well seen upon the brass of Isabella, wife
of William Cheyne, in Blickling Church, Norfolk, 1482
(Fig. 241), where cuffs are also apparent, and a long pendent
tab to the girdle. Incidentally we may call attention to

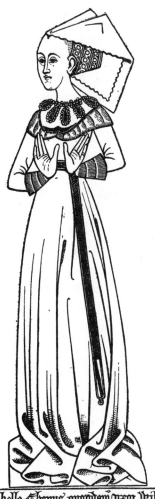

hic iacet Isabella Cheyne quondam vxor Willi Cheyne
armigeri de Insula de Thypen in com cantie q obijt xxiiii die
mens Aprilis ao dni mo cccc lxxxo cui aie pruciet deus amen

FIG. 241.—Isabella, wife of William Cheyne, 1482. Blickling Church, Norfolk.

the extremely awkward form of holding the hands which appears upon brasses about this time, and is shown upon these two examples. Even if seen in the attitude of prayer, they are almost as awkwardly rendered as in the foregoing examples.

The richer furs were forbidden to any persons who were not in the enjoyment of forty pounds yearly income; and girdles of gold, silver, or silver gilt, or any way ornamented with such material, were also forbidden to them. In Fig. 242, Pl., five representations of ladies in the gowns of the period are given, where the fur collar and cuffs, narrow cinctures, and general short-waistedness, together with other features, form a very interesting group for study.

The Head-dress.—Although the period under discussion was not quite so prolific in startling head attire as the reign of Henry VI., yet the four varieties evolved are sufficiently striking to compensate for the lack of numbers. Undoubtedly the chief form distinguishing the years from 1460 to 1480 was—

The Steeple Head-dress—sometimes irreverently called the " chimney-pot." This grotesque style was in favour on the Continent at a much earlier period, and is generally attributed to the Queen of Charles VI. of France, Anne of Bavaria, who introduced it from her native land into that country, and it naturally after a time appeared in England. The French style, however, differed somewhat from the English, as may be seen in Fig. 243, where a distinct bending forward of the apex is apparent, rendering it very similar to a single horn. Doubtless this peculiarity has caused the steeple to be classified under the common name of " Hennins," a word rather forcibly derived by some

French writers from the old verb *gehenner* (modern *gener*), to trouble or incommode. In Fig. 242, Pl., used above, four varieties of the steeple are given, from which it will be gathered that the correct angle at which it was *de rigueur* to wear it was at 45° from the perpendicular. This, of course, entailed a great strain upon the hair growing upon the forehead, and in order to ease this tension it was customary for ladies of high rank to wear the frontlet. This was composed of a piece of rigid wire netting covered with black material, which passed over the head and allowed a small loop to appear upon the forehead, as seen in Fig. 244, Pl. During the period we find a sump-tuary law was passed which permitted only the wives and daughters of persons having possessions of the yearly value of £10 to use and wear frontlets of black velvet, or of any other cloth of silk of a black colour. Frontlets of gold are mentioned in the wardrobe accounts of

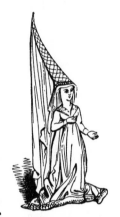

FIG. 243.—Steeple head-dress. From "The Comte d'Artois."

the princesses of the House of Tudor. It is quite remark-able to find how many different varieties of this particular style were evolved, differing in material, length, width, &c., but all based upon one general plan. In order to increase the weight, strain, and general inconvenience of this head-dress, a veil more or less voluminous was attached to it, pre-ferably near its upper extremity, where the maximum of leverage would be obtained; these are represented as of a very fine texture as a rule, but this was certainly not always the case. The tension caused by even a thin lace

veil, in conjunction with the general awkwardness of the
head-gear, can only be adequately appreciated by those
who have worn a modern reproduction.   The Lady of the
Tournament represented in Fig. 245, Pl., gives us an idea of
the great length of rich veiling which at times depended
from the head-gear; the pattern upon it may be readily
seen, while the richness of the clothes generally will com-
mend itself to the attention of the reader.   During the later

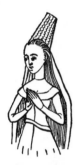

years of their use the veil appears to have
been distended by wires, as may be seen
in Fig. 246, Pl.   This interesting picture,
executed *c.* 1480, represents a masque of
Charles VI. of France, in which certain
knights disguised themselves in close-fitting
hairy garments and masks for the amuse-
ment of the Court.   Thinking to heighten
the effect, two courtiers set the pseudo-
skins on fire: the picture represents two of
the sufferers plunging into a bath and one
being saved by a lady, who enveloped him

FIG. 247.—Daughter
of Sir T. Urswick,
1479.   Dagenham
Church, Essex.

in her robe.   Four, however, died.   The broad bands encircling the faces of the ladies and falling upon their shoulders
is the inception of the subsequent *Pyramidal* head-dress.
The frontlets are well defined.   In Fig. 247 we have an
interesting representation from a brass of this period,
showing the long flowing hair under the steeple head-
dress.   This style with the butterflies' wings is still to be
seen in Normandy, and is known there by the name of
Cauchoise, from its being principally worn by the women
of Caux.

The Lamp-shade Head-dress.—This is a variety of the

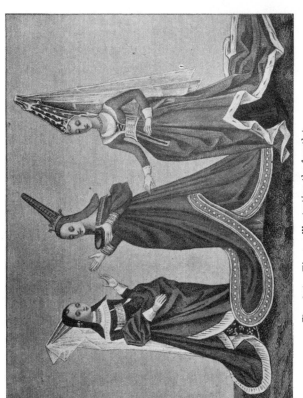

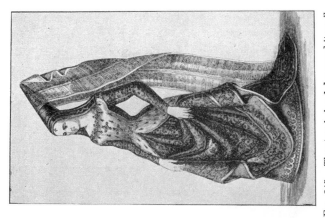

Fig. 245.—The steeple head-dress and its veil.

Fig. 244.—Figures illustrating the frontlet.
Roy. MSS. 14 E ii. and 14 E v.; Harl. MS. 4873.

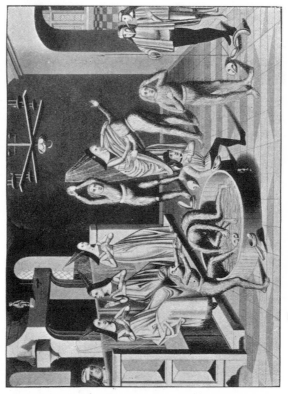

FIG. 246.—Masque of Charles VI. of France, c. 1480.

steeple, and contemporaneous. It is so named from its similarity to an inverted candle- or lamp-shade (Fig. 242, Pl.). A distinguishing feature is the remarkable arrangement of wire round the face, distending a gauze veil; the same peculiarity may be seen in the steeple head-dress borne by the lady behind the kneeling figure. In Fig. 248, Pl., three ladies are represented in head-dresses, of which only one can be accurately termed the steeple; the centre is a truncated parody, whilst the third is an extraordinary hybrid, embodying the funda-

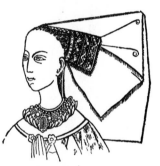

mental principles of the old-fashioned horned head-dress combined with an undeveloped steeple.

In Harl. MSS. 4379-80, which are illuminated copies of Froissart's "Chronicles," the artist has satirised the ladies by drawing a pig, rampant, on stilts in the margin

FIG. 250.—Lady Say, 1473. Broxbourne Church, Herts.

(Fig. 249, Pl.), and playing upon a harp; he, she, or it wears a steeple head-dress with a very pronounced veil.

The Butterfly Head-dress.—The first appearance of this style may be ascribed to about the year 1470; we find it represented upon the brass of Lady Say, 1473, wife of Sir John Say, Broxbourne Church, Herts (Fig. 250). As will be seen, it consisted of a truncated steeple, around which wires were arranged to carry gauze veiling of large dimensions. The "Scratch-back" style of hair then prevailing is well represented in this figure, and a prominent feature is the magnificent necklace of elaborate goldsmith's work. The

omission of a frontlet is probably due to an error on the part
of the engraver.

A lady of the Clopton family, represented upon a brass
in Melford Church, Suffolk, *c.* 1480, exhibits this style of

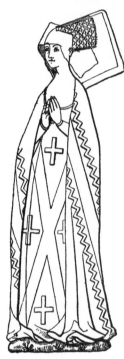

head-dress in great perfection; the
whole of the figure is given here
(Fig. 251), in order to represent the
fashion of wearing armorial bearings,
those upon the mantle being the
arms of Clopton, and those upon the
super côte-hardi of her own family,
Francis.

Two well-known examples of the
head-dress are those of Lady Elizabeth FitzGeoffrey, 1480, at Sandon,
and one in St. Stephen's Church, St.
Albans. An example of the butterfly will also be seen upon referring
to Fig. 241. Another, showing the
frontlet, is given in Fig. 252, Pl.,
where the extremely rich material of
the dresses of the time is well indicated. While speaking upon this

FIG. 251.—Lady of the Clopton family, *c.* 1480. Melford
Church, Suffolk.

subject it may be advisable to introduce one of the most elaborate dresses
with which we are acquainted relating
to this period, which shows to what extent bold and elaborate design were used, and also affords a good example of
the butterfly. It is shown upon the brass of Margaret,
Lady Peyton, *c.* 1484, at Iselham Church, Cambridgeshire
(Fig. 253, Pl.). The butterfly head-dresses are generally

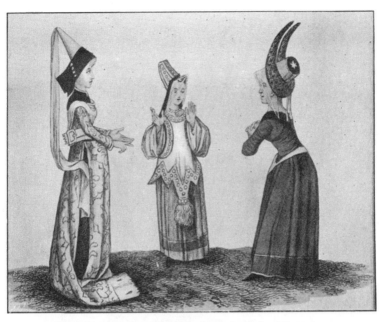

FIG. 248.—Varieties of the horned and steeple head-dresses.

Harl. MS. 4375.   Roy. MS. 15 D i.   Roy. MS. 15 E iv.

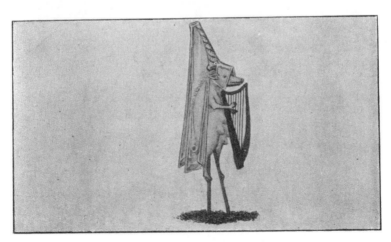

FIG. 249.—A caricature upon the steeple head-dress. (Harl. MSS. 4379–80.)

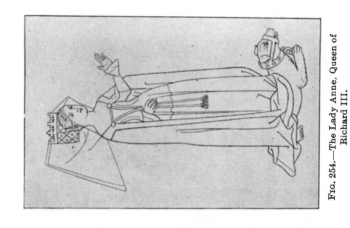

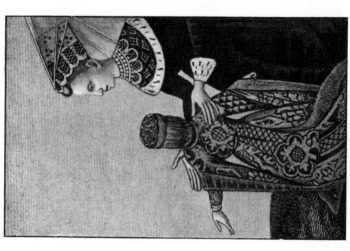

Fig. 254.—The Lady Anne, Queen of Richard III.

Fig. 252.—The butterfly head-dress, Edward IV.–Richard III. (Roy. MS. 16 F ii.)

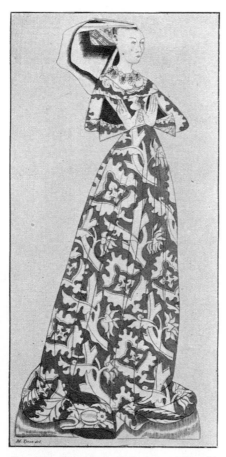

Fig. 253.—Margaret, Lady Peyton, *c.* 1484. At
Iselham Church, Cambridgeshire.

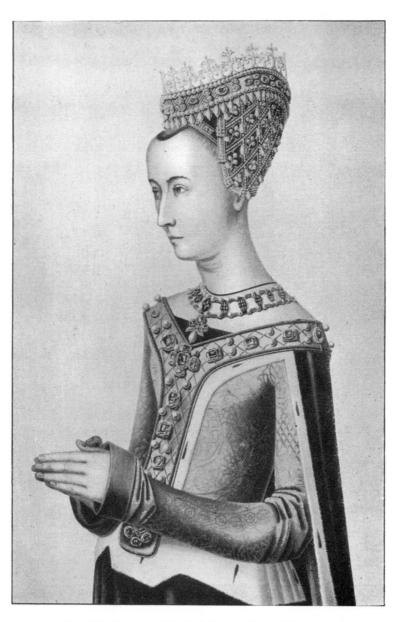

FIG. 255.—Margaret of Scotland, Queen of James III., *c.* 1483.

associated with the reign of Richard III., although, as we have seen, they were introduced much earlier. Probably this is because the Lady Anne, Queen of that monarch, is shown habited in this style in the Warwick Roll, a copy of which we append in Fig. 254, Pl. This illustration, together with that of Margaret of Scotland, referred to below, afford examples of the extraordinary persistence of the super côte-hardi, to which we are now to bid "adieu"; it has accompanied us for over one hundred years in the course of this work.

We have seen that fashions developed in England at a much later period than on the Continent, and that thirty or forty years may safely be allowed for a French fashion to become general here. With regard to Scotland, one hardly knows what interval to assign, inasmuch as the intimate connection then subsisting between that country and France must be kept in mind; for example, a head-dress prevalent in France, and occupying an intermediate position between the butterfly and the pyramidal, is seen in the accompanying illustration representing Margaret of Scotland, and approximately of the date 1483 (Fig. 255, Pl.). Its development from the horned, or rather the forked, head-dress is easily discernible, the cleft at the upper part being now closed up. Around the neck is a rich jewelled necklace, an example of which we have seen upon the brass of Isabella Cheyne (Fig. 241). The beautiful nature of the embellished cauls, in which pearls play a predominant part, is very striking.

A contemporary example of this head-dress is that of Joan, daughter of Richard Neville, Earl of Salisbury, afterwards Countess of William Fitz-Alan, Earl of Arundel, who died 1487, in Arundel Church, Sussex (Figs. 256, 257, Pl.). We give two representations of it, so that it may be compared with that of Queen Margaret. In the three-quarter face illustration the cushion must not be mistaken for the head-dress.

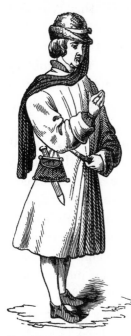

FIG. 258.—Gentleman, *temp.* Henry VII. From the "Romance of the Rose."

Respecting the dress of the middle classes, it is not to be supposed that the exceedingly awkward head-dresses and extremely long garments were closely imitated; we have reason to suppose that they adopted a modified style in order to allow of their avocations being pursued. Thus the ordinary civilian costumes may be judged from Fig. 258, which represents a personage in comfortable circumstances, judging from the gold band with buckle which encircles his bycocket, the pendent cloth streamer to which should be noticed. The dagger thrust through the gypcière is of old fashion, as we have seen. Although there are suggestions of pour-pointerie in his coat, we may classify him as one unspoilt by the prevailing fopperies. The beggar of the period also shows the leading characteristics of the costume in fashion, as may be seen by Fig. 259, taken from Roy. MS. 15 E ii. In precisely the same way as the middle-class man modified his dress to suit his circumstances, so the woman of the period proceeded on the same lines. In Fig. 260 we have a representation of Cicely

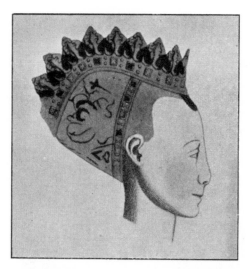

FIG. 256.—Joan, daughter of Richard Neville, Earl of Salisbury, Countess of William Fitz-Alan, Earl of Arundel, d. 1487.

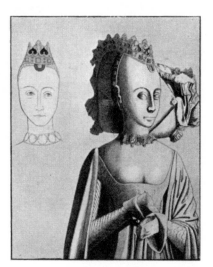

FIG. 257.—Joan, daughter of Richard Neville, Earl of Salisbury.

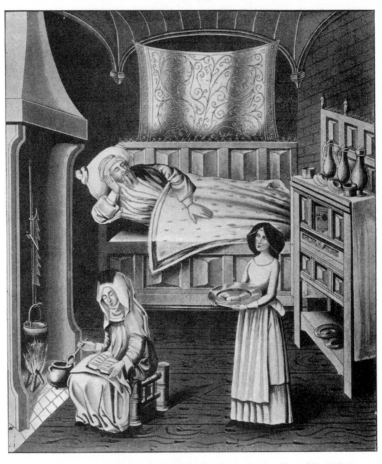

FIG. 262.—Matron and servant in the sick-chamber, *c.* 1470.   (Roy. MS. 15 D i.)

Roleston, in Swarkstone Church, Derbyshire, 1482, whose head-dress is extremely reasonable when compared with those we have previously cited. It is a simple dome-like cap exhibiting flutings after the manner of the pourpoint, to which is attached a plain hood of cloth.

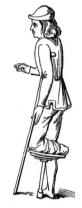

Another example is seen in Fig. 261, which comes from the same source, but is three years later. It suggests the lower portion of the steeple head-dress, fitted in a more comfortable manner upon the head. The matron and maid-servant of the period are represented in Fig. 262, Pl., taken from Roy. MS. 15 D i., dating from 1470; the picture also shows the interior arrangements of a sick-chamber. From Roy. MS. 15 E iv. we gather that a very common dress for the

Fig. 259.—Beggar, *temp.* Edward IV. (Roy. MS. 15 E ii.)

lower classes of the period consisted of a striped material, which is shown in Fig. 263; the girl's head is simply covered by the old-fashioned wimple, although she wears the cuffs

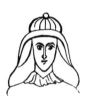

Fig. 260.—Cicely Roleston, 1482.

Fig. 261. — Mary Roleston, 1485.

of the period. The woodman's dress (Fig. 264) needs no description. As for the female beggar of the time, it is probable that no more pathetic figure can be adduced than that shown in the accompanying illustration, which is taken from the fifteenth century illuminated manuscript of the "Romance of the Rose," and is an allegorical representation of "Poverty." The ragged cloak and gown, the worn-out cloth hose, the coarse shaggy hat, the beggar's dish, and the spoon which we see stuck in the band of the hat, are all eloquent reminders of the subject (Fig. 265, Pl.).

During the short reign of Richard III. no essential variation was made in the national costume; a few fresh ideas were introduced which are distinctly features of the reign of Henry VII., and as such will be described in the following chapter. We may mention that the wardrobe

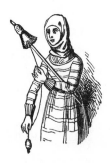

FIG. 263.—Country woman in rayed dress, *temp.* Edward IV.

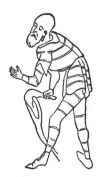

FIG. 264.—Husbandman in rayed dress, *temp.* Edward IV.

lists left by this King are of great value in enumerating the different articles of dress worn by the nobility, and frequent appeals to these have been made in the compilation of this book. Richard III. appears to have been almost as much a fop as was his namesake Richard II.; he and Buckingham apparently rivalled each other in the richness and ostentation of their civil dresses, the extreme elaboration of which are almost beyond description. As for the reign of the ill-fated boy Edward V., no historical records are preserved relating to dress except some unimportant details respecting coronation robes.

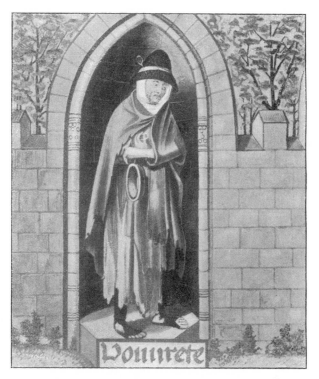

Fig. 265.—"Poverty."

CHAPTER XIV

HENRY VII., 1485-1509

THE reign of Henry VII. may be looked upon as a transition period for the evolution of the true Tudor dress which is so indelibly impressed upon our minds and memories by the numberless representations of costumes in the time of Henry VIII. and his children.

The King was of a miserly disposition, and his penurious habits were not conducive to the formation of a brilliant court and the evolution of magnificent dress. Consequently we find a certain amount of forced sobriety and rigid sombreness in costume during this reign, but, as fops always have been, and always will be, so a parsimonious King could not restrain numerous extravagances bursting forth into the light of day. With the advent of printing, the era of the priceless manuscripts which have descended to us necessarily comes to an end; one copy, however, the "Romance of the Rose," 1479, and almost the last of the series, is in the highest degree remarkable for the beauty of its execution and the fidelity to detail of its workmanship. From it our chief authorities are gleaned for the earlier portion of this reign.

THE MEN

The effigy of King Henry VII. upon his tomb in Westminster Abbey is simply habited in a fur gown and cap,

very similar and in no degree more kingly than that shown
in the portraits of many contemporary gentlemen.

A general idea of the usual dress of the monarch may be
deduced from the accompanying portrait (Fig. 266), where,

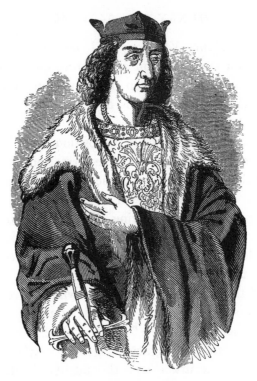

FIG. 266.—Henry VII.

however, the only garment seen is the very full fur-lined
cloak over the stomacher, which will subsequently be
alluded to.

It is perhaps possible to refer to the garments worn by
the gentlemen of the period in regular sequence, inasmuch

as to a great extent a certain degree of uniformity was
being evolved at this time out of the chaos of Plantagenet
costume.   We will deal with these garments in the order
in which they would be assumed by the wearer.

The Shirt.—This garment, viewed as a means of adornment, was not in use earlier than this reign, although as an
article of use it had been prevalent since the Saxon Period.
It was now, however, decorated with
elaborate embroidery, and portions of it
were exposed to view by the shape of
the superimposed garments.

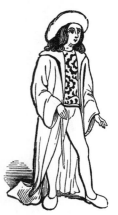

The Stomacher was an addition introduced during the reign of Richard
III., and probably the only important
innovation in that period.   It reached
from the throat to the waist, and was
invariably of the most elaborate workmanship, as seen upon the portrait of
the King.   It was probably padded, as
creases never appear in its representation.   The ornamental neckband per-

Fig. 267.—Figure from
Winchester Cathedral,
1489.

taining to his shirt appears above this stomacher, and
so unseemly low did the gallants wear the open neck
that the critical busybodies, prevalent in that age as in
every other, seized upon it as a subject for their sarcasms.
An example of these elaborate stomachers may be gleaned
from Fig. 267, taken from a painting on the walls of Winchester Cathedral, and executed in 1489.   The pattern
exhibited may be considered as rather loud, but it is in
the most approved taste of the age.   Another example
from Harl. MS. 4939 (Fig. 268) shows the stomacher of

less aggressive design, and finished with a band at the neck
and waist.

The Doublet.—This garment took the place of the
pourpoint of the preceding reigns and the côte-hardi of
the fourteenth century. It fitted tightly to the figure, but
was cut away in front over the chest in order to show the

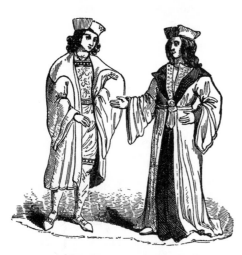

stomacher, lacing being
substituted for the
cloth removed. To this
doublet sleeves were
attached either in one
or two pieces, the first
covering the upper arm
and the second the
lower; they were se-
cured to each other and
to the doublet by the
universal lacing, which
we may mention is one
of the leading points,
both practically and
mnemonically, to be

FIG. 268.—Costume, *temp.* Henry VII.

Harl. MS. 4939.   Roy. MS. 19 C viii., A.D. 1496.

remembered for this period. The object of this lacing was
to show the fine shirt beneath, and undoubtedly suggested
the fashion of "slashing" which subsequently became
all the rage. It is shown in many paintings; one by
Memling at Leipzig clearly depicts the sleeve separated
from the shoulder. The doublet as a rule terminated just
below the waist with a small base, basque, or skirt, and to
it the breeches or chausses, as the case might be, were
attached by points.

The *Petti-cotte* (or petticoat) was worn over the doublet. It was a loose garment falling from the shoulders on either side, and apparently not fastened in any way. We rarely find it furnished with sleeves, those of the doublet taking their place; if, however, the outer coat was not worn, it was permissible to attach long sleeves to the petti-cotte by points.

The *Long-Cotte or Cloak*, as the outermost garment was termed, was of varying proportions, sometimes trailing on the ground, as seen in Fig. 268, where the second personage represented—taken from Roy. MS. 19 C viii., dated 1496—is habited in one. The chief features of this outer cotte were the cylindrical sleeve, with its slit for the emergence of the arm, and the broad lapelles, which as a rule fell from the shoulders and ornamented the neck and front. The shape is well defined in the last illustration. Another example of the cylindrical

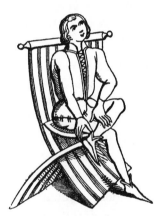

FIG. 269.—The lacing of points.

sleeve was combined with an elaborate pourpointed long-cotte, where also the wide lapelles were a special feature.

The Breeches.—The chausses, which up to this time had been in universal wear, now began to disappear and give place to breeches and hose. A late example of chausses attached to the doublet by points is seen in the accompanying sketch (Fig. 269). In order to correct a very common error which prevails respecting the mediæval chausses, it may be stated here that they were made of cloth and in many cases lined, and thus differed essentially from the stockingette trunk-hose by which they are represented upon the stage and elsewhere at the present day. In a picture by Memling preserved in the Museum at Brussels, and representing the martyrdom of St. Sebastian, the body part of the chausses is turned down a little, and exposes a white lining, and the button or lace holes for fixing the same. The chausses are made of a dark-coloured cloth. The breeches were extremely tight to the person, the upper part being laced to the doublet in a manner similar to the chausses; to the lower part, which reached to about mid-thigh, the nether-stocks or stockings were attached by points; they were parti-coloured, pied, or striped.

The Boots.—A peculiar fashion was the wearing of soft leather boots which came to about the knees or a little higher; or the feet thrust into a pair of the broad-toed "duck-bill" shoes, which superseded the poleyns. These broad-toed shoes, or *Sabbatons*, became subsequently of such preposterous width, that they almost rivalled in one measurement what the poleyns did in another.

The Head-gear.—A very characteristic hat of the reign, which underwent many subsequent alterations and additions, but may invariably be traced back to this period, is the square example shown upon the head of the King (Fig. 266), and also upon the two personages in Fig. 268. It is remarkably like the ecclesiastical biretta, but possesses a lower crown. This hat, however, was very modest when compared with that of the dandy of the period, as seen in Fig. 270, Pl., which represents the same person under three aspects. Upon the right he is finishing his toilet; taking a silver needle from the needle-case, he is about to make the points

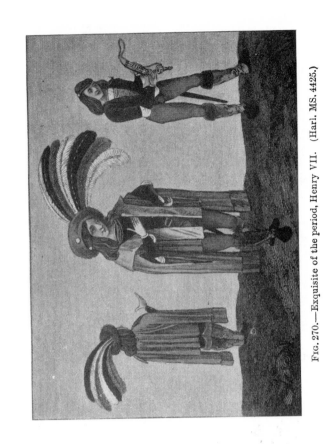

Fig. 270.—Exquisite of the period, Henry VII. (Harl. MS. 4425.)

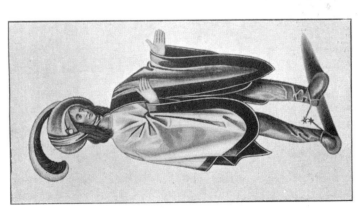

Fig. 271.—Head-gear, Henry VII
(Roy. MS. 19 E viii.)

which fix the different portions of his sleeves together. The small skull-cap that he wears appears to have been general, as we see it in many illustrations. In the centre he is delineated in full war-paint, the hat being seen worn over the skull-cap previously mentioned. It appears to be made of a stiff rough felt, and bears seven feathers of a preposterous   length, which are of varying colours and ornamented with pearls up the quills. The figure upon the left is a back view of this striking   personage, upon which it will be noticed that the lapelles do not meet behind.   That the beaux of the time experienced a certain amount of inconveni-

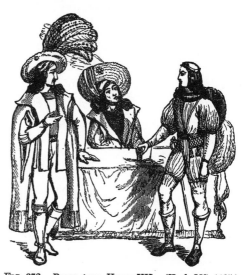

Fig. 272.—Dress, *temp.* Henry VII.   (Harl. MS. 4425.)

ence in keeping their huge hats upon their heads may readily be conceived, and in Fig. 271, Pl., we have an exquisite represented, who has tied a red silk scarf over the top of the hat and knotted it under the chin. He is booted and spurred and wears a horseman's cloak. It is taken from Roy. MS. 19 C viii. A peculiarity of this reign, which it shares with that of Edward II., is the habit of suspending the hat down the back and wearing the small cap only, as seen in Fig. 272, and Fig. 273, Pl., though occasionally it was simply held

under the arm, as in Fig. 274, Pl.   One of the most interesting pictures from that marvellous manuscript "The
Romance of the Rose" is that depicting three minstrels,
probably servants of persons of high degree.   It is given in
Fig. 275, Pl., and shows the first personage habited in a court-
pie with large dagged sleeves, the others being dressed in
the long cottes of the period.   The chief thing to be noticed
is the pied character of the garments ; for instance, the left
arm of the leading character is black, and the right
green.   The legs are alternately in black and violet, and the
adaptation of points as an ornamental device is very conspicuously shown.   In all three cases a ridiculously small
cap surmounts a mass of long hair.

THE WOMEN

THE PYRAMIDAL HEAD-DRESS, 1490–1550

So far as royalty is concerned, the effigy of Elizabeth of
York in Westminster Abbey does not possess any points
distinguishing it from that of a lady of rank of the period,
and therefore does not necessitate a separate description.

The Robe.—This still continued to be short-waisted, but
not to such a degree as formerly ; it was cut square at the
neck, high or low, or else open from the waist upwards,
displaying the stomacher, across which it was laced.   The
large full sleeves, which may be termed the bishop's sleeve,
were loose and easy, as seen in Fig. 273, Pl. ; they were confined at the wrist, and during the later part of this period
a fashion prevailed of tying them at intervals between the
wrist and elbow.   Another fashion in sleeves was imitated
from the men's costume, in being tight to the arm, but

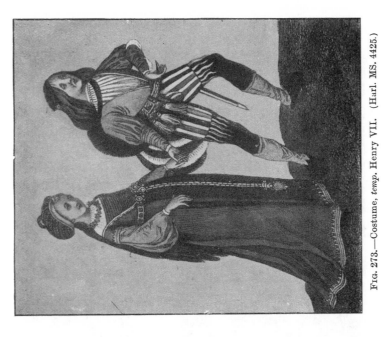

Fig. 273.—Costume, *temp.* Henry VII. (Harl. MS. 4425.)

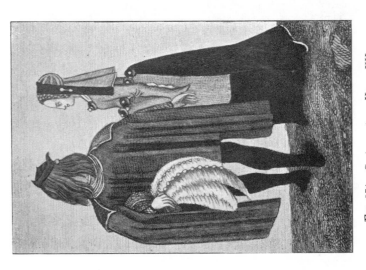

Fig. 274.—Costume, *temp.* Henry VII.
(Harl. MS. 4425.)

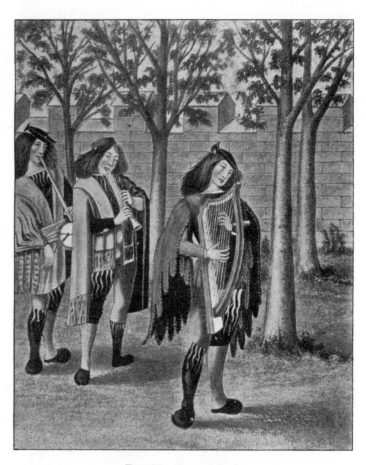

Fig. 275.—Three minstrels.

long to cover the hands. Similarly it was sometimes in
separate pieces at the elbow and shoulder, and laced with
points, the opening at the wrist being also laced, and
showing a white under sleeve (Fig. 276, Pl.). With regard
to the train, the fashion of having a double one no longer
prevailed; that in front was abolished, and a style was
introduced whereby the train pure and simple was looped
up through the girdle at the back. See Fig. 277, Pl.

The Shoes worn by the ladies are very seldom seen in
illustrations in consequence of the long dress; they were
wide at the toes, but do not seem to have attained very
broad proportions.

The Stockings worn at this time were not always cloth,
as we read of "calaber web hose" being in use for both
sexes. These in common language may be termed cotton
stockings.

Girdles of the most elaborate workmanship were in use
during this reign and prevailed for many years. The general
fashion of the waist-belt was remarkably similar to that of
the hip-belt of the time of Richard II.; a long pendant of
different design hung from the clasp in front. A good
example of this style is seen in Fig. 273, Pl. Coupled also
with this, we may cite the beautiful necklaces, one of which
may be seen upon the figure alluded to.

The Cloak.—An interesting little group from Roy. MS.
16 F ii., a work probably executed for King Henry VII.,
illustrates the capacious cloaks of the time; the very large
open sleeves are a distinctive feature.

The Pyramidal Head-dress.—Undoubtedly this form of
head-dress was derived directly from the broad band of the
steeple, which rested upon the forehead and fell on either side

of the face.　During the first part of its existence an ornamental crown was in use, as represented in Fig. 276, Pl., but
subsequently this developed into a simple hood, as is plainly
seen in the first figure of our illustration (Fig. 278), which
represents Margaret, Countess of Richmond, the mother of
Henry VII.　The second figure, Elizabeth of York, the Queen
of Henry VII., wears the same style, but much more ornamented.　It is lined with ermine, and decorated with jewels

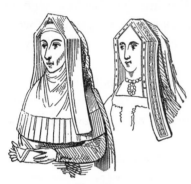

FIG. 278.

Margaret, Countess of
Richmond, mother of
King Henry VII.

Elizabeth of York,
by Holbein.

and embroidery.　Numberless
examples of this style occur
upon brasses, and also upon
effigies.　The bands were
frequently edged with pearls
and most elaborately decorated with precious stones,
so much so that we occasionally read of them being mentioned in wills as special
bequests.　Although appar-
ently so inconvenient in
shape, this style retained its
ascendency in the world of fashion for more than half a
century.　The simple character of its early form may be
gleaned from Fig. 279, Pl., where the lady wears a piece
of reticulated wire-work enclosing the hair, while over it
the head-dress is seen bearing a remarkable resemblance to
the earlier capuchon, with the front thrown back showing
the interior lining.　An excellent representation of this
head-dress, showing the hood portion at the back, is seen in
Fig. 274, Pl., where the remarkable belt and necklace are
also worthy of notice.　It should be mentioned that common

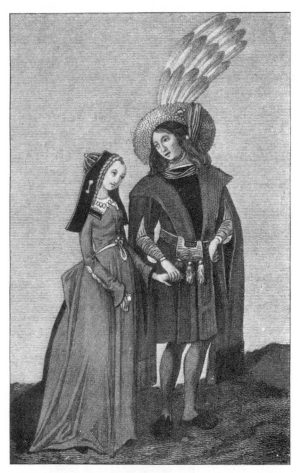

FIG. 276.—Costume, *temp*. Henry VII. (Harl. MS. 4425.)

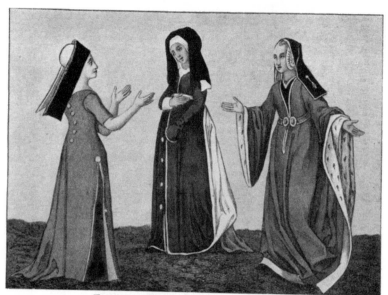

FIG. 277.—Ladies' costume, *temp.* Henry VII.
(Harl. MSS. 621 and 4425; Roy. MS. 19 C viii.)

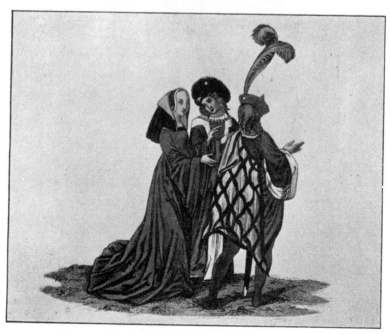

FIG. 279.—Early pyramidal head-dress. (Roy. MS. 20 D viii.)

names for the Pyramidal Head-dress are the Angular, the
Pedimental, and also the Kennel, the derivations being
obvious. The idea that the pyramidal only was in vogue
during this reign must not be entertained, as it took some
little time to ensure universal adoption; a contemporary

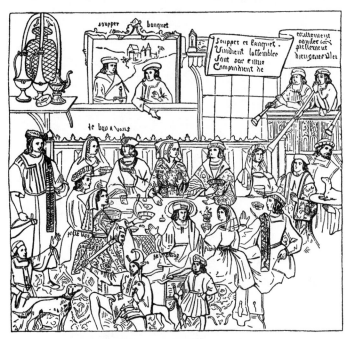

FIG. 280.—A dinner party, late fifteenth century.

style may be seen in Fig. 273, Pl., and probably one or
two other nondescript varieties may be gathered from the
numerous illustrations given in this chapter.

The general tone and feeling of a high class assembly
during this reign may be gleaned from the accompanying
illustrations, where nearly all the characteristics which we
have been careful to explain are exemplified. They are

of extreme interest to the student, inasmuch as the re-

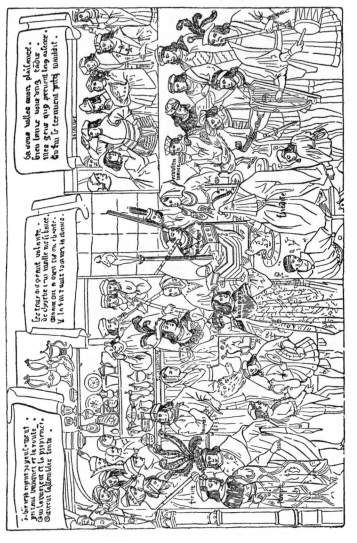

FIG. 281.—A banquet, late fifteenth century.

markable variety of the hats of the men, the pourpoints

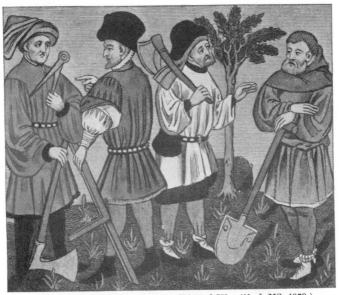

Fig. 282.—Artificers, &c., *temp.* Edward IV. (Harl. MS. 4379.)

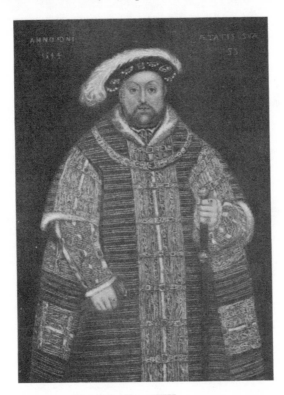

Fig. 286.—Henry VIII.

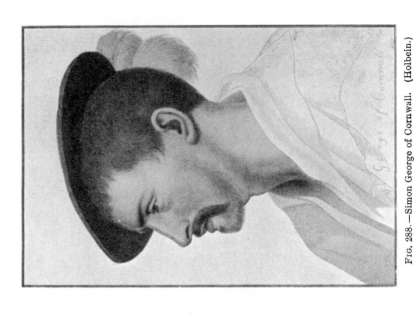

FIG. 288.—Simon George of Cornwall. (Holbein.)

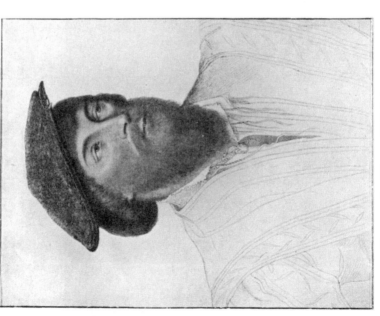

FIG. 287.—Lord Vaux. (Holbein.)

and sleeves, the women's dress, and especially the head-gear, are all well defined, and a careful examination should prove of fascinating interest to the earnest student (Figs. 280, 281).

In Fig. 282, Pl., a group of workmen is represented, the vocation of each being readily perceived from the implements carried, although it is very much open to question whether artificers at that time were habited in clothes so eminently respectable as those here shown.   The value of

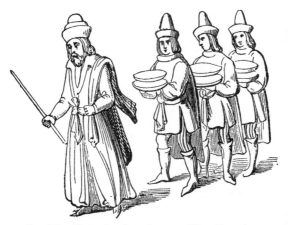

FIG. 283.—Steward and serving men, fifteenth century.

the figure lies, however, in furnishing us with particulars respecting the cut of garments for the working classes. The preceding (Fig. 283) represents the servants of the hall, headed by the steward with his rod of office, bringing the dishes to the table in formal procession. The pied hose and sugar-loaf caps are prominent features.

The mourning habits of the sixteenth century were regulated by the law, the most stringent orders being enforced respecting the cut and amount of material employed according to the rank of the wearer. The chief

point of interest in the mourning habits of the women
lies in the wearing of the *barbe*, the long pleated arrangement seen in the accompanying figure (Fig. 284), from
Harl. MS. 6464, and often represented upon monumental
brasses.   From a Baroness upwards the barbe was worn
above the chin, other estates under the chin; while inferior

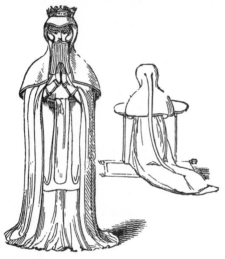 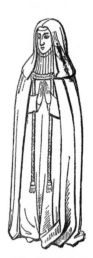

FIG. 284.—Sixteenth century mourning habit.   FIG. 285.—Elizabeth Porte,
(Harl. MS. 6464.)   1516.   Etwall Church,
Derbyshire.

gentry wore it below the "throat goyll," or gullet, the
lowest part of the throat.

   These subtle distinctions are well shown, so far as
two are concerned, in the illustration previously given and
that of Elizabeth Porte, 1516, Etwall Church, Derbyshire (Fig. 285), for if they are compared it will be seen
that the lady wearing the coronet has the barbe above the
chin, in contradistinction to her more humble sister.

CHAPTER XV

HENRY VIII., 1509–1547

In books dealing with costume the authors frequently make the assertion that it is quite unnecessary to introduce a portrait of King Henry VIII., giving as a reason that the proverbial schoolboy is fully acquainted with his dress. It is readily granted that the said schoolboy recognises "Bluff King Hal" at the first glance, but if desired to write an essay upon his apparel we fear it would be more interesting than accurate. Beyond the broad characteristics of the period few could give a detailed description, inasmuch as the many portraits extant invariably depict him in a different costume. The configuration of a male dress distinguishing the reign of Henry VIII. was directly derived from the broad-shouldered doublet of Henry VII., which again was undoubtedly of German origin; the burly frame of the English monarch set off this Teutonic costume to the fullest advantage, and it naturally followed that court and country alike quickly adopted it. There is to a certain extent no great change perceivable in men's dress during this reign, and the coronation of Henry VIII., as shown on the Islip Roll, fully exemplifies this; a stereotyped fashion appears to have been adopted in the first part of it, and almost rigidly adhered to during the succeeding years. It may be briefly summed up as an aggregation of extreme breadth combined with narrowness; great width of body made the lower limbs appear attenuated, extreme width of the toes made the ankles appear ludicrously small. Such width of body has never been surpassed in English costume, and we can fully appreciate the dismay of those who had been blessed by nature with a spare habit of body. The portrait of the King reproduced here (Fig. 286, Pl.), and attributed by different authorities to Holbein, Da Treviso, Janet, and other artists, exemplifies this great width of shoulder, and it may be readily seen in other portraits reproduced in this chapter. Dealing seriatim with the separate articles of attire we have the following :—

The Shirt (or French " Chemay ").—The fashion introduced during the previous reigns of rendering this article of attire ornamental as well as useful was developed to the fullest extent. These garments were ornamented with gold, with silver, and, what was very fashionable, with designs of needlework in black silk. It was made of fine linen or silk, and the collar exhibited a great variety of forms. In the picture before us it is finished with a frill, which is caused by the shirt being gathered in at the neck. This fashion was the pioneer of the subsequent ruff, the development of which may be traced from this early conception. Frills similarly produced may also be seen upon the wrists. In the portrait of the Lord Vaux (Fig. 287, Pl.), the shirt collar is seen to be worked with an ornamental design ; the fastening cords are also shown, while the edge of the collar is indented. The shirt was often worn open at the neck, as will be seen in Holbein's portrait of Simon George of Cornwall (Fig. 288, Pl.), and at times was furnished with a turn-down collar. It must not be supposed that ornamentation was entirely confined to the collar.

The Stomacher or Waistcoat.—Over the shirt and under

the doublet was occasionally worn the decorated stomacher or waistcoat, as seen in the portrait of the King, where it is slashed in order to exhibit the shirt. It had sleeves, and was made of rich materials, such as cloth of silver, quilted with black silk, and these must have been occasionally visible in consequence of the excess of slashing.

As this is distinctly the age of puffing and slashing, it may not be out of place to give the origin of this fashion as detailed by Henry Peacham in "The Truth of our Times," 1638:—"At that time the Duke of Burgundy received his overthrow (*i.e.* at Nancy in 1477), and the Swiss recovered their liberty; he entered the field in all the state and pomp he could possibly devise. He brought with him all his plate and jewels; all his tents were of silk, of several colours, which, the battle being ended, being all torn to pieces by the Swiss soldiers, of a part of one colour they made their doublets, of the rest of the colours breeches, stockings, and caps, returning home in that habit; so ever in remembrance of that famous victory by them achieved, and their liberty recovered, even to this day they go still in their party-colours," and which he further says, "consists of doublets and breeches, drawn out with huge puffs of taffatee or linen, and their stockings (like the knaves of our cards), party-coloured of red and yellow, and other colours." This rage for slashing was carried to such an extent that it was imitated in armour, and a splendid suit in the Wallace Collection is one of the finest examples ("Arms and Armour," page 289 *et seq.*). It is worthy of notice that slashes were never made in a straight line; they all possessed more or less the wavy nature which distinguishes a capital S.

The Doublet.—The name appears to have been derived from the garment being made of double material, often padded between. At the time of Henry VIII. it was made so as to open down the front, thereby disclosing the ornamented shirt. It was as a rule girded round the waist, and the skirts reached nearly to the knees, but subsequently became much shorter. The sleeves were generally separate articles, and could be attached by points. Holbein's portrait of the Earl of Surrey (which by some has been attributed to Strete) shows the doublet open in front, dis-

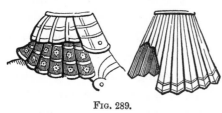

FIG. 289.

Lamboys or bases.   Imitation in steel.

closing a white shirt ornamented with black silk. The skirts of the garment reach nearly to the knees, and distinctly show the fluting, called bases, so characteristic of this time, and which could only have been produced in padded garments.

In one description of the King's dress it is stated that " his garment was of cloth of silver, of damask, ribbed with cloth of gold, so thick as might be ; the garment was large and pleated very thick, and cantled of very good intail [designs], of such shape and making that it was marvellous to behold."

The preceding illustration gives perhaps the perfection of this mode of ornamentation, which was also copied in the armour of the period (see " bases," p. 289, " Arms and Armour "). The Emperor Maximilian of Germany introduced this fashion (Fig. 289).

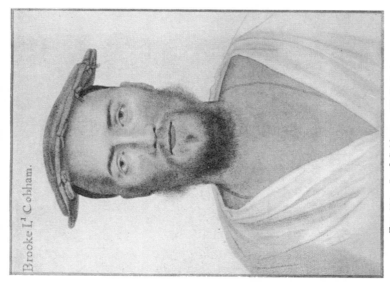

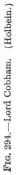

Brooke L[d] Cobham.

Fig. 294.—Lord Cobham.   (Holbein.)

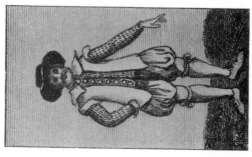

Fig. 290.—Citizen.   From Harl.
MS. 2014.

The Jerkin, Coat, Gown, &c.—This garment was the outermost then worn, and may be seen upon the representation of Henry Howard, Earl of Surrey the poet, as being abnormally broad in the shoulders. The sleeves still further accentuate the width of the figure, as they are slashed, gathered, and puffed in the height of fashion then prevailing. The cape (or lapelles) is a striking characteristic of this jerkin, being very wide and broad upon the shoulders. It was often made of costly fur, as may be seen upon the portraits of the King and other personages. In Harl. MS. 2284, we find half a yard of purple cloth of gold baudekyn is allowed to make a cape to a gown of baudekyn for the King; and a Spanish cape of crimson satin, embroidered all over with Venice gold tissue, and lined with crimson velvet, having five pairs of large aglets of gold, is named as the Queen's gift. There is a bewildering variety of jerkins or coats mentioned at this period, such as short-coats, demi-coats, riding coats, coats with bases, tunic coats, leather coats, coats like a frock, &c. ; while gowns are distinguished as half, strait, loose, Turkey, Spanish, &c.—all referring to the outer garment. The sleeve prevailing during the early portion of the reign consisted of a large puff covering the humeral portion of the arm, and another shaped puff covering the forearm, at times almost fitting the limb. It terminated in a cuff, beneath which lace ruffles were fixed, falling over the hands. In the latter half of the reign the sleeve assumed an ungainly bolster-shape, as seen on the portrait of the King (Fig. 286, Pl.). Here one half of the sleeve of the doublet is shown, the upper part in this case being covered by the jerkin sleeve. This sleeve is best seen upon the ladies of the period.

A cloak much in use towards the end of the reign was called a *Mandevile*. It fitted loosely to the body, and at times was furnished with a collar, but the great distinction seems to have been the lack of sleeves. This statement, however, must be qualified, for about 1540 sleeves were partly attached to it by the usual points and hung down the back, being known as the "manches perdues." A citizen of the better class wearing a mandevile is shown in Fig. 290, Pl.

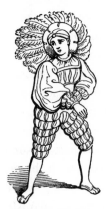

The shapes of the mandevile were many, and varied similarly to the majority of outer garments at this period.

Breeches.—For probably the first time in the history of English dress the breeches became quite distinct from the hose, and as such have remained to the present period. They were short, bolstered, and slashed, projecting at times to a considerable distance from the body; they were often termed "Slopes" during this and subsequent periods. The bolstered breeches may well be seen on Fig. 291, where they reach to the knee.

Fig. 291.—Puffed and slashed costume. Hôtel du Bourgtheroulde, Rouen.

" It is generally understood that stockings of silk were an article of dress unknown in this country before the middle of the sixteenth century; and a pair of long Spanish silk hose, at that period, was considered as a donation worthy of the acceptance of a monarch, and accordingly was presented to King Edward VI. by Sir Thomas Gresham. This record, though it be indisputable in itself, does not prove by any means that silk stockings were not worn in England prior to the reign of that prince, notwithstanding that it seems to have been considered so by Howe, the continuator of Stow's 'Chronicle,' who, at the same time, assures us that Henry VIII. never wore any hose but such as were made of cloth. Had he spoken in general terms, or confined his observations to the early part of Henry's reign, we should readily have agreed with him ; but in the present case he is certainly mistaken; stockings of silk were not only known by that monarch, but worn by him, and several pairs were found in his wardrobe after his decease. We shall notice only the following articles of this kind, taken from an inventory, in manuscript preserved at the British Museum, Harl. MSS. 1419, 1420 :—' One pair of short hose of black silk and gold woven together; one pair of hose of purple silk and Venice gold, woven like unto a caul, and lined with blue silver sarsenet, edged with a passemain of purple silk and of gold, wrought at Milan ; one pair of hose of white silk and gold knit, bought of Christopher Millener ; six pairs of black silk hose knit. The 'short hose' were, we presume, for the use of the Queen ; for the article occurs among others appropriated to the women. We have also before us another inventory of the wardrobe belonging to the same monarch, taken in the eighth year of his reign, Harl. MS. 2284. The hose for his *own use* are frequently mentioned, and the materials specified to be cloth of various kinds and colours; from which it appears that stockings of silk formed no part of his dress at that period."

The Trunk-Hose or Stocks.—A fashion prevailed of making the upper part of the long hose of much thicker material than the lower portion. For example, crimson velvet elaborately slashed and puffed and provided with ornamental bands would serve for the upper stocks, while

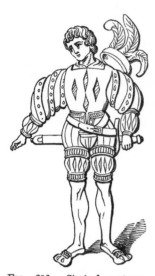

FIG. 292. — Slashed costume, from the Ware Chantry, 1532. Boxgrove Church, Sussex.

crimson cloth of a finer texture occurred for the nether. This is very clearly shown in Fig. 292. It is copied from a figure on one of the columns of the Ware Chantry (dated 1532) in Boxgrove Church, Sussex. This fashion, however, did not prevail for long, for we soon find that plain stockings were attached by points directly to the lower part of the breeches, or to the doublet. These points were really laces furnished with tags at the extremities called aiglets (*aiguillettes*); in one inventory we read of "a white doublet cut upon cloth of gold, embraudered, with hose to the same, and clasps and auglettes of golde, delivered to the Duke of Buckingham."

The Sabbatons or shoes during the reign of Henry VIII. preserved the same characteristics which developed during the time of his predecessors. They became excessively wide at the toes, and were remarkable for the very small amount of protection given to the feet, the

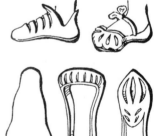

FIG. 293.—Shoes, Henry VIII.

toes having only the slight covering which was afforded by the puffed silk inserted in the slashings of the leather, though frequently the latter were left open to show part of the coloured nether stock inside.

Different shapes prevailed, as will be seen in the accompanying figures. They were made of black velvet cloth or leather (Fig. 293).

Hats.—The flat cap was the universal head-gear for men, which was undoubtedly derived from the style prevailing in the preceding reign. The cap may be seen upon the portraits of the Lord Vaux and Simon George in Figs. 287, 288, Pls.; but probably the most ludicrous example of this covering is that shown upon Holbein's portrait of Brook, Lord Cobham (Fig. 294, Pl.), which is not even relieved by the small feathers shown in the portrait previously mentioned. But although little change was made in the shape of the hat, there was great variety both in colour and material. For example, we read of "a hatte of greene velvette embrowdered with grene silke lace, and lyned with grene sarcenette," as occurring in an inventory of Henry VIII.'s wardrobe. And again, "Item for making of three cappes of velvette, the one yalowe, the other orange coloure, and the thirde greene," from the same source. Upon these caps clasps were often worn and, as illustrated upon the three accompanying examples, brooches of great variety and value. Hall mentions Henry VIII. as wearing a "chapeau Montaubyn with a rich coronal, the folde of the chapeau lined with crimson satin, and on that a brooche with the image of St. George." Some contemporary hats, including that worn by Sir Thomas More, are inserted here (Fig. 295). In a number of cases we find the coif worn under the flat cap (Fig. 296).

One great feature by which the student of dress is enabled

to fix approximately the period of an illustration is by the mode of wearing the hair, and the reigns of Edward IV., Richard III., and Henry VII. are all distinguished by the hair flowing straight to the shoulders and then terminating in an upward curl. This characteristic lasted approximately

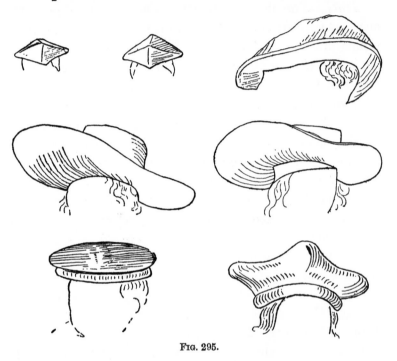

FIG. 295.

until the time of the Reformation, although upon the Continent short hair had been in fashion since *circa* 1520, and its influence was felt in England shortly after that time, though it did not become general. It will be noticed that all portraits by Holbein represent the men with short hair. The fashion of wearing a beard appears to have been introduced by the King, and was naturally adopted by the court ; among continental nations the old fashion of being clean shaven was retained, thus affording us another example of the strong individuality of the King.

Gloves.—These were chiefly made in France and Spain, and were not in general use by the men.

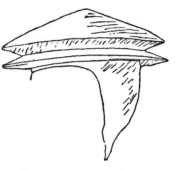

FIG. 296.—Coif under flat cap.

It will readily be seen by the foregoing description of the garments worn by the nobles that they were many and varied, and the accessories to these garments were multitudinous. It was fashionable to wear everything open in front in order to show the superposition of the various articles and the richness of the material of which they were made, also for greater ease in wearing them. One writer, FitzHerbert, states that "men had so many pleats upon their breasts and such puffed sleeves, that they could not draw a bow when habited in their coats."

> " My doublet is unlaced before
>   A stomacher of satin and no more ;
>   Rain it, snow it, never so sore
>   Me thinketh I am too hot.
>   Then have I such a short gown
>   With wide sleeves that hang adown
>   They would make some lad in this town
>   A doublet and a coat."

The passion for dress so prevalent among the upper classes soon spread to the lower orders, and by the middle of the century we find that the serving man who had formerly been contented with a frieze coat in winter and a Kendal coat during the rest of the year became arrayed in a doublet of the best cloth to be had in the market, with hose of new and startling dyes imported from abroad. They even went so far as to use embroidery and fancy stitching.

The accompanying figure (Fig. 297) exhibits the costume of the ordinary citizen, where the plain doublet is furnished with attenuated hanging sleeves; the breeches are puffed to the knees, and the universal flat cap is worn upon the side of the head. Another citizen, taken from the frontispiece to the Great Bible of Henry VIII., is armed with sword and buckler; his flat cap hangs upon his shoulder by a cord. The body of his doublet exhibits numerous slashes, and the skirt shows an attempt at pleating, while the hanging sleeve is more fully developed than in the last figure (Fig. 298, Pl.).

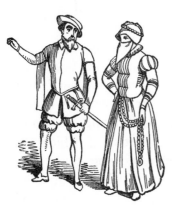

Fig. 297.—Costume, *temp.* Henry VIII.

The ordinary dress of a plain countryman is well described as having been worn by the uncle of Will Somers, the King's jester, who visited his nephew at the court. He was "a plain old man of three-score years, with a buttoned cap" (*i.e.* the flaps, that fell over the ears, could be turned up and fastened with a button). "A lockram falling band" (which was a narrow collar of coarse linen, turned down round the neck), "coarse but clean; a russet coat; a white belt of a horse-hide, right horse-collar white leather; a close round breech of russet sheep's wool, with a long stock of white kersey, and a high shoe with yellow buckles."

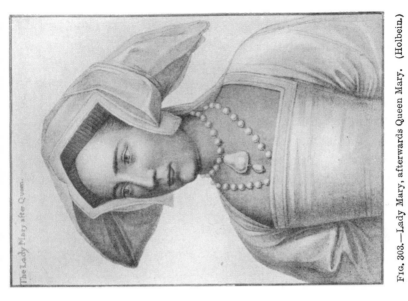

The Lady Mary after Queen.

FIG. 303.—Lady Mary, afterwards Queen Mary. (Holbein.)

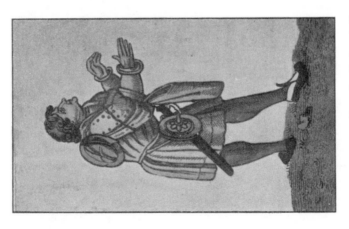

FIG. 298.—Citizen. From frontispiece to the
Great Bible of Henry VIII.

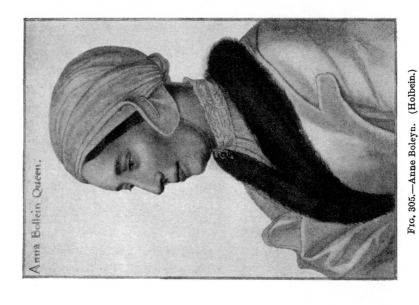

FIG. 305.—Anne Boleyn. (Holbein.)

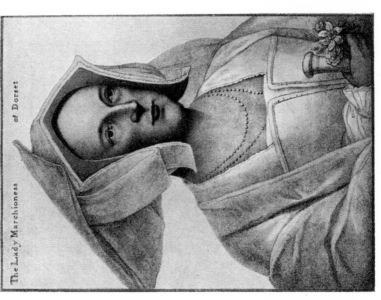

FIG. 304.— Marchioness of Dorset. (Holbein.)

THE WOMEN

The extraordinary penchant exhibited by Henry VIII.
for matrimonial entanglements has resulted in a rich harvest
of pictorial representations of women's attire, and it would
be exceedingly strange if we were unable to make a definite
conception of the style of feminine costume during this era.

If we take the lady's dress in its entirety, we find that
no radical changes occurred during the whole reign upon

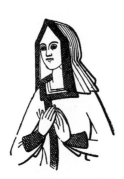

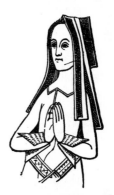

FIG. 299.—Margaret Pettwode, 1514.   FIG. 300.—Jane Sylan, 1516.
St. Clement's Church, Norwich.   Luton Church, Beds.

that which had descended from Henry VII.'s time; in fact,
if we had nothing but historical brasses by which to judge,
we might probably say there was no change worth speaking
of with the exception of the head-dress.

The Head-dress.—The pyramidal form of head-gear
was almost universal until the divorce of Catherine of
Arragon; with the accession of Anne Boleyn modifications
began to appear; but if we take the entire range of head-
dresses, and compare the last style evolved with the first, we
readily perceive the direct derivation of the whole of them

from the kennel.   An early example during this reign is
seen upon the brass of Margaret Pettwode, 1514 (Fig. 299),
St. Clement's Church, Norwich, and also upon that of
Jane Sylan, 1516, Luton, Beds (Fig. 300).   A later example
is that of Mistress Goodwyn, 1532 (Fig. 301), Necton Church,
Norfolk.   Fig. 302 is copied from Holbein's portrait of
Catherine of Arragon, and shows the acme of simplicity;
vis-à-vis with her is a representation of Anne Boleyn,
where the kennel head-dress is seen to be much less cum-

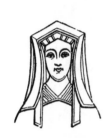

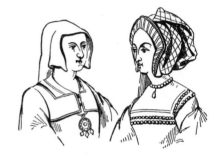

Fig. 301.—Wife of Robert
Goodwyn, 1532. Necton
Church, Norfolk.

Fig. 302.

Catherine of Arragon.   Anne Boleyn.

brous than formerly.   Of the portraits by Holbein, who
was portrait painter to the King from 1537 until his
death in 1543, we have a range of fashions which may be
divided as follows :—

1. *Pyramidal Style.*—The Lady Mary, afterwards Queen
Mary (Fig. 303, Pl.), is shown with ribbed bands of brown
silk upon the forehead forming the foundation, a small
portion of the hair appearing from underneath it.   Round
the face is a wired framework of the kennel form, over
which is the usual broad band which formerly fell down
to the shoulders, but is now looped up on either side and

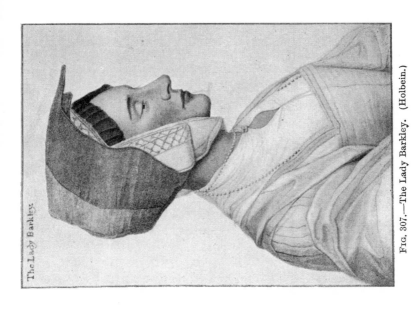

The Lady Audley.

Fig. 306.—Lady Audley.   (Holbein.)

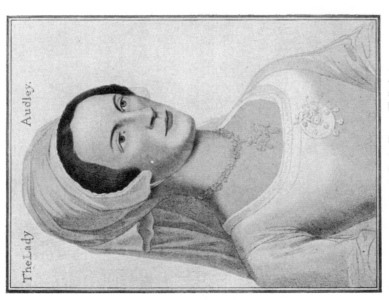

The Lady Barkley.

Fig. 307.—The Lady Barkley.   (Holbein.)

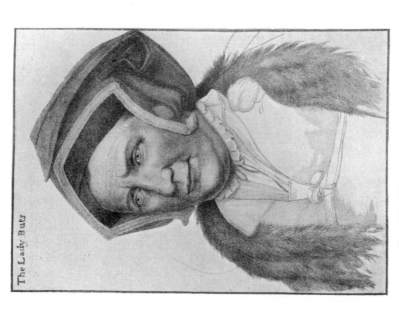

The Lady Buts

Fig. 308.—The Lady Buts.   (Holbein.)

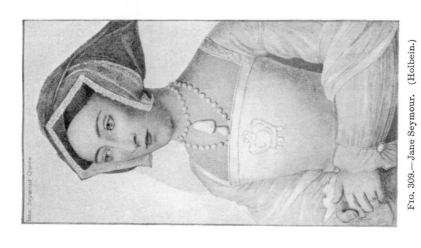

Jane Seymour Queen

Fig. 309.—Jane Seymour.   (Holbein.)

pinned upon the top of the head. The bag which previously hung at the back of the head is also brought up to the top and pinned there, and, being stiffened, presents a rather ungainly appearance as it projects on either side. At times only one part of the bag was looped up, as in the case of the Lady Marchioness of Dorset (Fig. 304, Pl.).

2. *The Coif.*—Anne Boleyn is represented in this engraving as very plainly attired in a tightly-fitting coif tied under the chin; this was undoubtedly the progenitor of the French hood. It was probably adapted for indoor wear (Fig. 305, Pl.).

3. *Coif and Flat Cap.*—In this illustration we see a copy of the universal flat cap worn by the men appearing over the coif (Fig. 296).

4. *The Transition Style.*—In this we may discern the last lingering traces of the kennel head-dress. Lady Audley (Fig. 306, Pl.) exhibits a combination of the coif and the kennel, but the latter can be more distinctly traced in the two following illustrations, Lady Barkley and Lady Buts (Figs. 307, 308, Pls.).

The Partlet.—This was an innovation peculiar to the reign. It took the place of the modern habit shirt, and is plainly seen upon the portrait of the Lady Buts. At times it was provided with sleeves, and was generally made of very rich material. In an inventory we find "two partlets of Venice gold, caul fashion; two partlets of white thread; and two partlets of white lawn, wrought with gold about the collars." These sleeves form the puffs which appear through the slashings of the sleeve proper. Round the necks of some of the ladies in Holbein's pictures a band of frilling appears as a separate article of attire, and it is

fair to surmise that in this we have the parent of the subsequent *bands* so prevalent in the seventeenth century.

The Waistcoat or Surcoat.—This was a garment similar
to that worn by the men, and succeeded the stomacher.
"Two wastcotes for women, being of clothe of silver,
embroidered, both of them having sleeves." "Then proceeded forth the queene, in a circote and robe of purple
velvet, furred with ermine, in her hayre coife and circlet.
After her followed ladies, being lords' wives, which had
circotes of scarlet, with narrow sleeves, the breast all lettice
(a kind of fur resembling ermine) with barres of pouders,
according to their degrees; and over that they had mantles
of scarlet, furred, and every mantle had lettice about the
necke, like a neckerchiefe, likewise poudered, so that by their
pouderings their degrees might be knowne. Then followed
ladies, being knights' wives, in gowns of scarlet, with narrow
sleeves, without traines, only edged with lettice."

The Kirtle.—The kirtle reached from the waist to the
ground, and took the place of the modern petticoat, and
was often of the richest material, being exposed in front by
reason of the opening in the robe.

The Robe or Gown was the outermost garment, and is
invariably shown opening down the front, thus exposing the
kirtle and the waistcoat over which it was laced. The
length of the garment was long or short according to the
rank of the wearer; thus a Countess was compelled to wear
it of sufficient length that she could carry the train over her
arm; the Baroness and all under that degree were prohibited this badge of distinction. Undoubtedly one of the
most remarkable features of female attire in this reign
was the extraordinary sleeve. The under sleeve has been

already mentioned as being fastened to the partlet; over it was a puffed, padded, and slashed example attached to the kirtle or waistcoat, and at times of the same material. Above all was a bell-shaped sleeve of large dimensions, the cuff of which was turned back upon the arm showing the lining, which at times was of rich fur.   The portrait of Jane

Seymour by Holbein shows a variation of the sleeve (Fig. 309, Pl.). In the early part of the reign we are told that " gowns of blue velvet, cut and lined with cloth of gold, made after the fashion of Savoy," were worn by ladies at a regal masque. In later years Anne of Cleves, upon her first arrival in England, is said to have worn " a rich gown of cloth of gold raised, made round, without any train, after the Dutch fashion " (Fig. 310, Pl.). Among the inventories and wardrobe accounts we find "three pairs of purple satin sleeves for

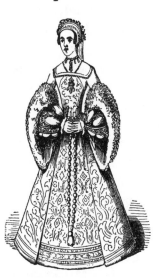

FIG. 311.—Catherine Parr.

women; one pair of sleeves of purple gold tissue damask wire tied with aiglets of gold; one pair of crimson satin sleeves, four buttons of gold being set on each sleeve, and in every button nine pearls." A kirtle for Queen Catherine of Arragon took seven yards of purple cloth of damask gold. Catherine Parr's dress (Fig. 311) is described as of cloth of gold, with sleeves lined with crimson satin and trimmed with three-pile crimson velvet; while the Princess Mary was dressed in a kirtle of cloth of gold, with a gown of violet-coloured three-piled velvet, with a head-dress of many precious stones.   Holbein's portrait of the King, Princess Mary, and Will Somers the jester (Fig. 312, Pl.), will afford the reader some idea of the display of jewellery we have mentioned.   It will be noticed that the sombre-minded Mary was not averse at that period to rings, pendants, and jewelled head-dresses.   The extravagant richness of the court dresses at this time are unparalleled; we read of garments embroidered and fretted with gold worked upon satin, damask, velvet of all colours, together with the universal cloth of gold and silver.   As for the head-dresses, they are stated in one description to have been all of gold; we know they were enriched with every variety of precious stone and every art of the goldsmith's work.   The passion for jewels was carried to a strange excess by both men and women.   The King and his nobles wore chains, brooches, pendants, jewelled girdles, &c.   The King, even upon ordinary occasions, wore a collar of rubies; diamonds ornamented his flat cap, and many rings clustered upon his fingers.   The clergy followed the example of the court, and Roy says that the shoes of Cardinal Wolsey were

> " Of gold and stones precious,
> Costing many a thousand pounds."

Those were the times when it might be said that a nobleman would

> " Wear a farm in shoe-strings edged with gold,
> And spangled garters worth a copyhold ;
> A hose and doublet which a lordship cost,
> A gaudy cloak three mansions' price almost,
> A beaver hat and feather for the head,
> Prized at the church's tithe."

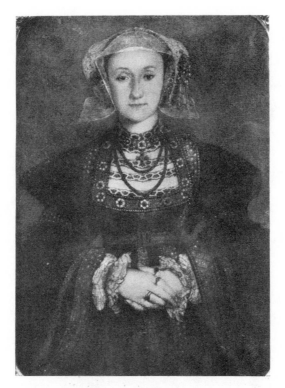

Fig. 310.—Anne of Cleves. (Holbein.)

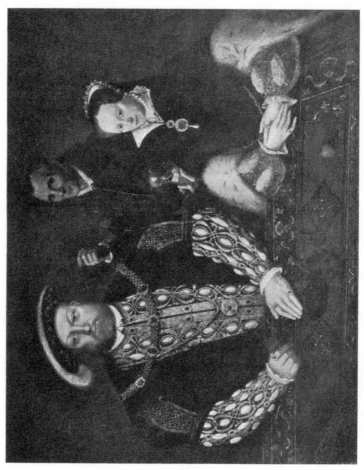

FIG. 312.—Henry VIII, Will Somers the jester, and Princess Mary. (Holbein.)

A woman of the period is seen in Fig. 313, upon the brass of Dorothea Peckham, 1512, Wrotham, Kent, where the dress is represented as being very simple; the cuffs worn are very characteristic, as is the ornamental waist-belt with the long hanging tab. In Fig. 297 a woman of the middle class is represented; she wears a close hood, and affords us an example of the muffler. This article of attire became fashionable during the reign, and continued so among elderly ladies until the reign of Charles I. It formed part of the disguise of Falstaff when impersonating the fat woman of Brentford. The pendent waist-belt consists of two strings of beads terminating in a large jewel. The front of the dress and also the sleeves are slashed and puffed. Towards the end of the reign persons in the middle rank of life began to dress with greater simplicity, thus following the fashion of the court, for we find no such extraordinary extravagances in dress marking Henry's declining years as that which distinguished the Field of the Cloth-of-Gold.

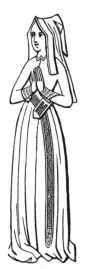

FIG. 313.—Dorothea Peckham, 1512. Wrotham Church, Kent.

The widow of John Winchcomb, the famous clothier, is described, after having laid aside her beads, as coming out of the kitchen in a fair train gown stuck full of silver pins, having a white cap upon her head, with cuts of curious needlework under the same, and an apron before her as white as driven snow. Her wedding dress is also specified in the following manner: "The bride, being habited in a gown of sheep's russet and a kirtle of fine worsted, her

head attired with a *billiment* (habiliment) of gold, and her
hair as yellow as gold hanging down behind her, which was
curiously combed and plaited according to the manner of
those days."

A rural dance taken from the " Chapter-House Treatise,"
Public Record Offices, is appended, which also shows the
simple dress of the peasantry (Fig. 314, Pl.).

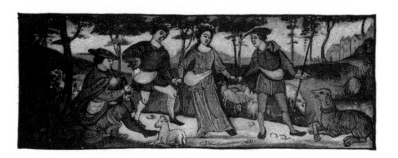

FIG. 314.—A rural dance, *temp.* Henry VIII.

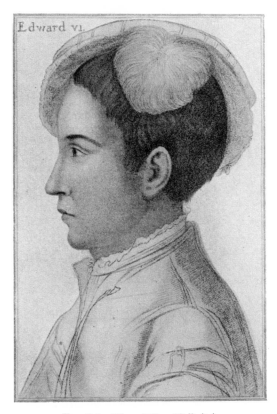

FIG. 315.—Edward VI.   (Holbein.)

CHAPTER XVI

EDWARD VI., 1547–1553. MARY, 1553–1558

THE brief reigns of these two monarchs do not furnish us with any marked originality in the costume of either sex, but only modifications of that which preceded them; the simplification of dress towards the end of the reign of Henry VIII. was carried still further in these eleven years. Men were too anxious and occupied during the time of Edward in endeavouring to settle the many religious questions which the Reformation had raised to devote much time or attention to frivolities of dress; and although the marriage of Queen Mary to the Spanish monarch naturally introduced some innovation, yet the general feeling was one of sombreness, owing to the terrible persecution for conscience' sake which prevailed in her reign. The portrait of Edward VI. by Holbein (Fig. 315, Pl.) represents him in the same kind of hat which his father affected, with a feather lying round the brim and a few ornamental brooches. The hair is cut close, and round the neck the partlet shows plainly. The jerkin is now no longer open to display the under garments, and the sleeves of the doublet do not present the exaggerated fulness of the preceding style, but fall closer to the arms. In Queen Mary's portrait, by Sir Antonio More, we have presented a dress which is eminently typical of the last days of Henry VIII., and is almost identical with that by Holbein (see

Fig. 312, Pl.).   A difference is perceivable in the sleeve,
which, like that of the young King, is no longer distended to
such an extent as formerly.   The kirtle is of elaborate workmanship, and the pendent chain from the waist, with its huge

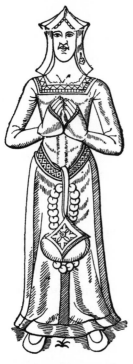

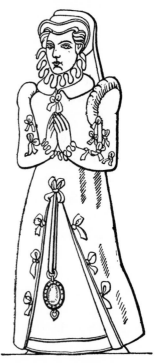

FIG. 316.—Anne Duke, in Frense
Church, Norfolk.   The brass
dates from *c.* 1551.

FIG. 317.—Anne Rede, formerly
Anne Duke, 1577.

termination, is very striking.   We give here a figure from the
brass of Anne, daughter of Sir Thomas Blenerhaysett (Fig.
316), who first married George Duke, on whose decease,
1551, her effigy, with that of her husband, was laid down
in Frense Church, Norfolk; she subsequently married Peter

Rede, and died 1577, and her second effigy is also given
here (Fig. 317).   The first of these interesting figures, which belongs to the period with
which we are now concerned, shows extraordinary cuffs falling over the hands.   Round
the waist is the usual ornamental girdle, from
which depends a huge rosary and a still larger
aulmonière.   The late survival of the pedimental or pyramidal head-dress with long
tabs still pendent is remarkable.   The figure
of Anne Rede will be alluded to in its proper
place.   The following figure is from an incised stone slab to the memory of Laurence
Colston, 1550, in Colston Church, Stafford-
shire (Fig. 318), and shows the dress of a
gentleman of that time with a long gown

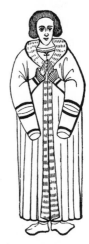

FIG. 318.—Laurence
Colston, 1550.

and hanging sleeves entirely covering the under dress.   In
Fig. 319 we have some costumes of the ordinary people

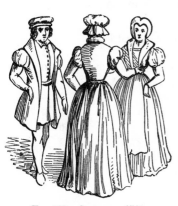

FIG. 319.—Costumes, 1549.

taken from the coronation procession of King Edward VI.
The dresses of the women are
extremely plain, the sleeves
being tight-fitting and furnished
only with a slight puff at the
shoulder.   The cap worn by
one is still reminiscent of the
pyramidal, but strongly suggestive of the subsequent hat
known as the Mary Stuart,
while the open gown discloses
the partlet.   The male figure is clad in doublet, jerkin,

and hose, and wears the flat cap which was universally termed the "Statute-cap" in the time of Elizabeth. This figure very strongly reminds us of the Blue-coat Boy, whose quaint dress is always sufficiently startling to attract attention wherever it is seen. His costume has descended from the time of Edward VI. to the present with but very little alteration, and although he no longer wears anything upon his head, the flat cap formed a part of his attire until the early years of Queen Victoria. The many portraits and effigies of citizens existing in our metropolitan churches and elsewhere afford us examples of this particular style of dress.

The prices of wearing apparel in England at this period may be gathered from the bill of expenses of the famous Peter Martyr and Bernardus Ochin, in 1547, who were invited to this country from Basle by Archbishop Cranmer. The original bill is in the Ashmolean Museum; it has been printed in the "Archæologia," volume xxi., whence the following few extracts have been obtained:—

	s.	d.
Payd for two payer of hose for Bernardus and Petrus Martyr	11	4
Pd. for a payer of nether stocks for his servant .	2	0
Pd. for three payer of shooe for them and their servant	2	4
Pd. for two nyght cappes of vellvet for them . .	8	0
Pd. for two round cappes for them . . .	6	0
Pd. for two payer of tunbrydg' knyves for them .	2	8
Pd. for two payer garters of sylke ryband .	2	6
For ryband for a gyrdyll for Petrus Martyr . .	1	2
For two payer of glovys for them	1	0

CHAPTER XVII

ELIZABETH, 1558–1603

THE accession to the throne of England of a monarch possessing a strong individuality has always resulted in that particular peculiarity being stamped upon the nation, and Elizabeth stands pre-eminently in the van. Her force of will, her strong business qualities, her intense love of pleasure, her passion for display, her love and encouragement of everything that added to the greatness of England, are all marked upon the progress of the nation during her reign, and upon none more so than upon costume. It was not to be expected that a woman of her force of character would be content with the same garments her grandmother affected, and consequently at an early period in her reign we find those changes inaugurated which resulted finally in a complete upheaval and entire revolution of the dress of the English nation. Hitherto innovations had invariably come from abroad, but now all that was altered as by the stroke of a pen, and sartorial and other extravagances occurred in constant and rapid succession, which led the continental nations to think that England had become demented upon the subject of dress. The term "Elizabethan" aptly describes it; it possesses a distinctive individuality shared by no other period; it was not beautiful, it was a frank distortion of the human frame; it was fantastical and extreme in its daring conceptions; but it stands out boldly and distinctly from all kinds of costume which preceded or succeeded it. It was a bold age, and an age of daring adventure in the regions of discovery, literature, art, drama, and other branches which tend to build up national life, and this daring spirit when let loose in the realm of dress resulted in the wild extravagance which is now so familiar to us.

Elizabethan dress may for purposes of description be divided into two chronological periods preceding and succeeding the year 1580. This date must not be taken as *rigidly* dividing two distinct styles, but the careful observer will perceive that in many parts of the costume of both sexes there are styles which mark these two divisions. So far as the men are concerned, it approximately forms the boundary between the ordinary doublet and the peascod variety; with women, before and after the farthingale.

MEN

First Period to 1580

The Doublet was now made tight to the figure, and the sleeves also tight to the arm; the huge puffing which had previously distorted the latter crept up the arm until it assumed the form of a crescent-shaped roll which was fairly persistent throughout the whole reign. The narrow band round the waist, which had previously been worn horizontally, now began to work downwards in front to a point— one of the marked characteristics of Elizabethan dress. In the " Art of Faulconrie," 1575, by Turberville (Fig. 320), the doublets are shown with innumerable slashings, the white shirt protruding through the panes, and a small ruffle at the wrists. Stubbs tells us that the doublets were so hard-quilted, stuffed, bombasted, and sewed that men could neither work nor yet play in them. The collar is now high

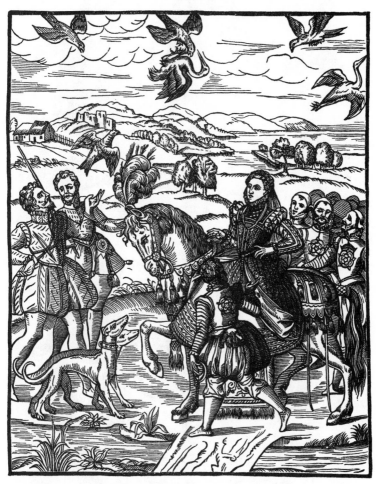

Fig. 320.—Queen Elizabeth hawking, 1575.

and close to the neck, being surmounted by an incipient ruff, the descendant of the band or frill of the previous reigns.

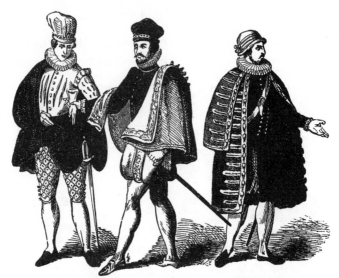

Venetian, 1590.   Spanish, 1577.   French, 1581.

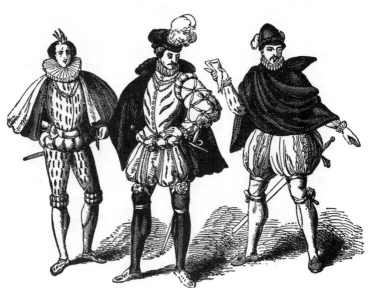

French, 1574.   German, 1577.   Burgundian, 1577.

FIG. 321.—Continental costumes, *temp*. Elizabeth.

The Breeches.—By this time these articles of dress had become enormously distended or bombasted; they reached to the knees, where *canions* were attached round the legs above the calf, or to mid-thigh.   These styles were in accordance with continental fashions; the first, reaching to the knees, being French.   They were ornamented by being paned (similar to lattice windows), or slashed, and finished with two rolls beneath the knee, the canions.   The English fashion was the second enumerated above, reaching half-

way down the thigh, and was apparently copied from the German, Burgundian, or Spanish.   The preceding figures will sufficiently explain these foreign fashions, with which the English costume should be compared (Fig. 321). From the previous illustration, and also

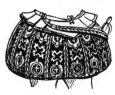

FIG. 322.—Breeches as worn by Lord Darnley.

from others given, these distinct styles may be easily perceived.   A good representation of the highly ornamental breeches is appended (Fig. 322).   In 1562 a proclamation was issued against the wearing of great breeches, and no one was permitted to have more than a yard and a half of kersey in them.   The stockings may, perhaps, be best seen in a portrait of Sir Philip Sidney and his brother, where the fashion of gartering them with a band round the knees is clearly shown.   Small rosettes upon the flat-soled shoes are also a feature of the picture, as is also a falling band or collar edged with lace.   It should be distinctly noted that rosettes upon the shoes were not a feature of the earlier period, and probably those of Sidney and his brother, Lord Lysle, are among the earliest shown.

Hats.—The men's hats at this period were distinguished by high crowns and broad brims, the latter being either flat or waved. They are shown in Fig. 323 furnished with a feather, but this fashion does not appear to have been universal; for instance, the hat of Douglas, Earl of Morton, Sir Philip Sidney (from Oliver), and one from the Court of

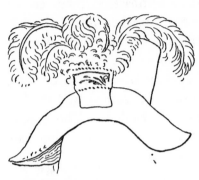

FIG. 323.—Copotain hat with feathers.

Wards (*Vetust. Monum.*), are shown without feathers (Fig.

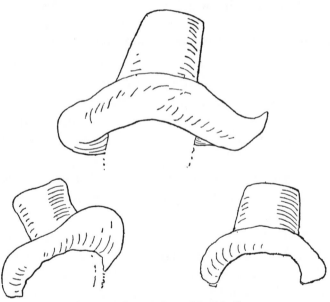

FIG. 324.—Copotain hats without feathers.

324), but that of a Yeoman of the Guard (Fig. 325) has no

less than three. In a woodcut (Fig. 326), from Weigel's
Habitus præcipuorum Populorum, 1577, an English nobleman and an English gentleman are delineated; they both

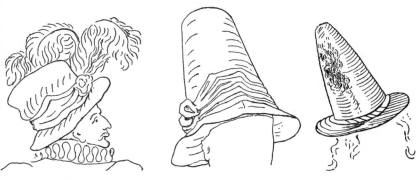

Fig. 325.—Hat : Yeoman of   Fig. 326.—Examples of the copotain hat.
      the Guard.

wear the *copotain* hat, as it was termed, one with a
feather in it. These hats were at times ornamented with
patterns (Fig. 327); they were generally made of velvet or

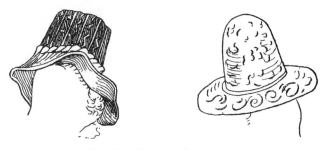

Fig. 327.—Ornamented copotains.

felt, the latter being often *thrummed, i.e.* having a long nap
upon it. This is the earliest form of the beaver hat. Stubbs,
writing at this period, states that men " are content with
no kind of hat withoute a great bunche of feathers of divers

and sundrie colours. Many get good living dying and sellying of them, and not a few prove themselves fooles by wearing them."

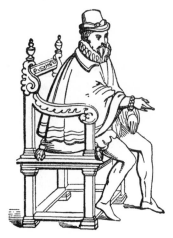

Fig. 328.—Louis de Gonzagues, Duke de Nivernois, 1587.

Cloak.—The cloaks worn at this time were made of cloth, silk, velvet, or taffeta, and of every colour then known. There were Spanish, French, and Dutch fashions for cutting the cloak, all having their own peculiarities, some reaching to the waist, some to the knee, and others trailing upon the ground. They were guarded with velvet or else faced with costly lace of gold, silver, or silk. Sometimes beads, bugles, and spangles were used to heighten the effect, and we are told that the linings at times cost as much as the cloak itself. In some cases sleeves were fixed to them and hoods also. The Spanish shape is shown in Fig. 328, representing Louis de Gonzagues.

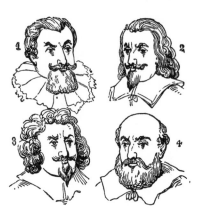

Fig. 329.—Military beards.

1. Spade beard. 2 and 3. Stiletto beards. 4. Falstaff beard.

Beards became fashionable during the reign of Henry VIII., and were continued during that of Elizabeth.

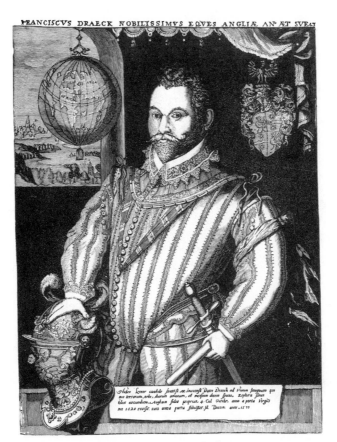

Fig. 331.—Sir Francis Drake.

The Cathedral beard was affected by Churchmen, and consisted of beard and moustaches long and flowing upon the chest. The military beards were the spade beard and the stiletto beard, being Nos. 1 and 2 (Fig. 329). No. 3 may be considered as a variety of the stiletto beard. No. 4 was a sufficiently common fashion among the soldiers of the period, and might do for Falstaff, inasmuch as we see the "great round beard like a glover's paring-knife."

Second Period, 1580 to 1603

The latter half of the reign of Queen Elizabeth is noticeable for the exaggerations of the style prevailing in the former. The doublets, which had always fitted the body very closely, and had been invariably stuffed and padded, gradually acquired a ridge down the front with a point in it; this point crept lower and lower, until it finally assumed that shape which is known as the peascod doublet. The exact shape which it eventually assumed may perhaps be better gleaned from the breast-plates of that time, which have

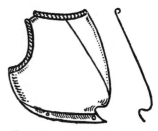

Fig. 330.—Peascod breastplate. (Tower of London.)

preserved to us in rigid metal the forms which the civil garments displayed. The accompanying sketch (Fig. 330) of a peascod breastplate in the Tower of London (from "Arms and Armour, British and Foreign") clearly demonstrates the shape. Sir Francis Drake, as represented in the accompanying sketch (Fig. 331, Pl.), wears a doublet of this character. This part of the dress now, in addition to

being padded, became bombasted, and, allowing a little for
caricature, assumed the familiar shape with which we
associate Punch, that costume being a direct descendant of
the Italian variety of this period (Fig. 332).   A fine full-
length portrait of a noble-
man is that of Sir William
Russell (Fig. 333).   He

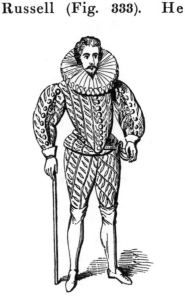

FIG. 332.—Dwarf, in peascod doublet   FIG. 333.—Sir William Russell,
        and copotain hat.   c. 1580.

shows a peascod doublet, slashed and bombasted, and
apparently of the richest material, the point of the waist
hanging over the sword-belt.   The sleeves now are
much fuller than in the earlier years, and the crescent-
shape rolls at the shoulders have almost, if not entirely,
disappeared.   The sleeves have large slashes down the
front, exposing a rich lining underneath, while rows of

large buttons upon one side, and loops on the other, suggest that the slashings could be brought together if required.   His breeches are of the Venetian type and slashed like the doublet, and his stockings made of the

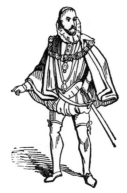

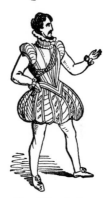

Fig. 334.—Costume, Lord Howard of Effingham, 1600.

Fig. 335.—Costume, 1575.

finest black yarn.   These long stockings without garters were introduced by the Earl of Leicester.   Peacham speaks of the wide saucy sleeves that would be in every dish before their master, with buttons as big as table men, *i.e.* the men used upon draught-boards.

> " His doublet was of sattin very fine,
> And it was cut and stitched very thick ;
> Of silke it had a costly enterlyne :
> His shirt had bands and ruffe of pure cambrick."

The costume at the end of the reign is well illustrated in Fig. 334, representing Lord Howard of Effingham in 1600.

Hats.—With respect to the hats, a number are given here which are chiefly taken from a representation showing the funeral of Queen Elizabeth, which will sufficiently illustrate the rich choice of head-gear prevailing at that time (Fig. 336).

Breeches.—The very wide breeches will be seen upon Fig. 335, taken from the "Book of Hawking," and were

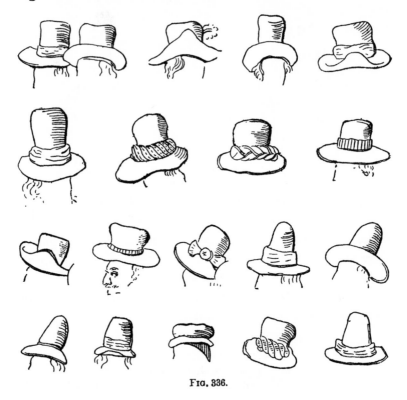

FIG. 336.

very much objected to by the satirists of the day. Douce quotes a ballad which speaks of them in strong terms, and all those folk who

> " Furnyshe forthe their pryde
> With woole, with flaxe, with hair also,
> To make their bryches wyde."

It is in the Harleian MSS., and entitled "A lamentable complaint of the countrymen for the loss of their cattelle's tails," which were used for stuffing such breeches.

A good description of a gallant of the period is found in the following:—

"Behold a most accomplished cavaleere
  That the world's Ape of fashions doth appeare,
  Walking the streetes his humours to disclose,
  In the French doublet and the German hose :
  The muffes, cloake, Spanish hat, Toledo blade,
  Italian ruffe, a shooe right Flemish made ;
  Like Lord of Misrule, where he comes hee'le revell,
  And lie for wagers, with the lying'st devill."

Two walking-canes of the latter part of the century, generally affected by gentlemen, are illustrated here (Fig. 337).

At the end of the reign the dress of the well-to-do citizen is shown on the brass of John Barley, burgess of Hastings, 1601, in St. Clement's Church, Hastings (Fig. 338). The dress of the agricultural labourer may be seen in Fig. 339, taken from "The Shepherd's Calendar," 1579. If we except the hat, it differs in no essential from preceding periods. The two illustrations appended are those of Tarlton, the famous actor, and Banks, the proprietor of a learned horse, which was subsequently burnt alive together with his master by the Italian peasantry, who deemed both possessed of evil spirits. Tarlton appears in trousers and a close-fitting doublet, while the other figure is simply a

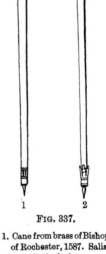

1   2

FIG. 337.

1. Cane from brass of Bishop of Rochester, 1587. Salisbury Cathedral.
2. From portrait of Sir F. Hart, 1587. Lullingstone, Kent.

modification of the prevailing costume (Fig. 340). In
1592, Greene's "Quip for an Upstart Courtier" appeared,
the frontispiece of which, "Velvet Breeches and Cloth

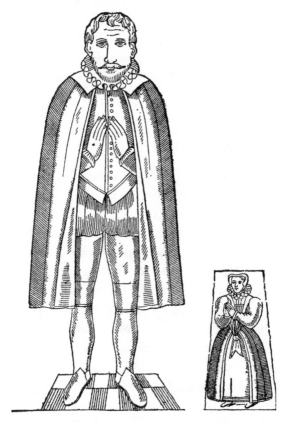

FIG. 338.—John Barley, 1601, and his daughter Alice, 1592. St. Clement's
Church, Hastings.

Breeches," is here given (Fig. 341). The feathered hat of
the courtier may be compared with that of the labourer,
the peascod doublet with its imitation, but there the re-

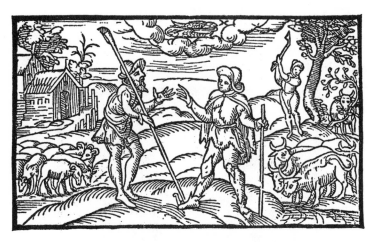

FIG. 339.—From "The Shepherd's Calendar," 1579.

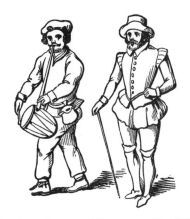

FIG. 340.—Costume of the commonalty, 1595.

semblance ends. The trousers of the labourer and the
rough boots will be noticed.

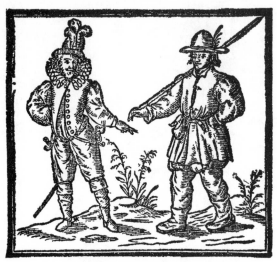

FIG. 341.—"Velvet breeches and cloth breeches," 1592.

THE WOMEN

FIRST PERIOD TO 1580

The first few years of the reign of Queen Elizabeth form
a transition period, but by about 1570 the leading features of
the first half had asserted themselves.

A very interesting panel picture, in the possession of
Earl Brownlow at Ashridge, Herts, represents Elizabeth just
before her accession to the throne. Her hat is of the
plainest description.

An out-door hat affected by the Queen, and somewhat
similar in shape to the one previously mentioned, is well
shown in the "Noble Arte of Venerie," by Turberville,
1575, where she is represented with her huntsmen. It

merely consists of a tall cylindrical crown inserted in a flat
brim, ornamented with plumes and jewels.   In another book

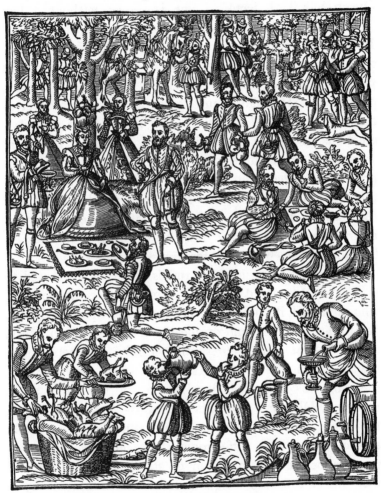

FIG. 342.—A royal picnic, 1575.

by the same author a royal picnic is delineated which is full
of interest to the student of costume (Fig. 342).   The Queen's

hat is of the same design as the preceding, but the brim is bent downwards in front.   In Fig. 320, representing Queen Elizabeth hawking, she is shown without a hat. The indoor coiffure of the Queen is well illustrated in the Penshurst portrait, presented by her to Sir Henry Sidney and reproduced here (Fig. 343, Pl.).   The emblematical portrait of Queen Elizabeth, painted by Zucchero, *c.* 1580, preserved at Hatfield House, gives us the fullest development of the head-dress, which, like most of her Majesty's erections, is almost indescribable by reason of the great wealth of ornamentation upon it.   Elizabeth was very proud of her hair, and it was no doubt owing to this fact that the hat is perched so high upon the head.   It was the fashion during the early part of the reign for un-married women to wear low-necked dresses, as seen in this picture, even out of doors.

Ruffs.—The origin of the ruff is generally attributed to a Spanish lady about the middle of the fifteenth century, who invented it to hide a disfigurement upon her neck. It appeared in England during the reign of Queen Mary, as the Great Seal representing Philip and herself dis-tinctly shows small ruffs.   It may be taken, however, that the ruff was a gradual development of the band, as in many of Holbein's portraits the shirt-band appearing at the neck frequently has the edges ruffled and delicately embroidered.   The ruff proper, however, was quite im-possible before the invention of starch, and in 1564 this was introduced into England from the Continent by a Madame Dingham Van der Plasse.   Stubbs waxes wroth over this starch, which he terms " devil's liquor."   He tells us it was made of wheat flour, bran, or other grains,

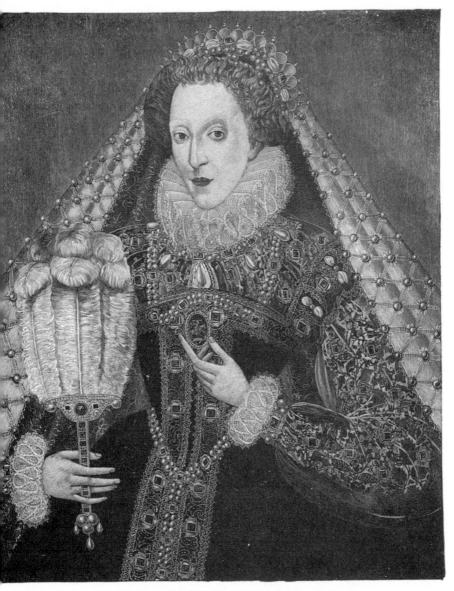

FIG. 343.—Queen Elizabeth, from the Penshurst portrait.

and was all colours and hues, such as white, red, blue, purple, &c.

Queen Elizabeth, whose ruffs were always of larger dimensions than those of her ladies, was troubled to find a laundress who could undertake the difficult task of starching her cambric and lawn ruffs; for her Majesty disdained to encircle her royal throat with those made of holland, usually worn by her subjects; she therefore sent abroad for a Dutchwoman, whose knowledge of this art was celebrated. "There is a certain liquid matter which they call starch, wherein the devil," says Stubbs, "hath learned them to wash and dive their ruffs, which, being dry, will then stand stiff and inflexible about their necks." He also alludes to a device made of wire, "crested for the purpose, and whipped all over either with gold, thread, silver or silk, called a supper-tasse, or under-propper" (Fig. 344).

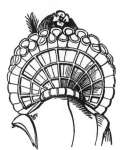

FIG. 344.—Under-proper.

These great ruffs or neckerchiefs were made of lawn, holland, and cambric, "so fine that the thickest thread shall not be so big as the least hair that is," three or four sometimes being placed under the "master devil ruff," "which was often loaded and adorned with gold, silver, and needlework." They must have been most wonderful structures, particularly when they expanded like wings as high as the head, or fell over the shoulders like flags. The ruff to a certain extent gives us a chronological clue to this reign, as they gradually grew in size and attained their maximum dimensions about 1580, retaining them to about the end of the century, when they began to decrease in size. In the Ashridge portrait, it is small and close to the neck; the Penshurst painting (Fig. 343, Pl.) exhibits it not very much larger; while in the Hatfield House portrait the ruff is dwarfed by the lace collar. From the back of her gown two wings, probably of fine lawn, edged with a border of jewels, and stiffened with wire, rise in semi-

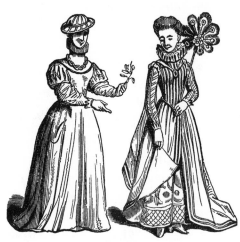

FIG. 345.

Lady, 1577.   Lady, 1588.

circular sweeps as high as the top of the head-dress, and, turning down to the ears, form the general shape of a heart, with the face, encircled with the ruff, set in the midst. The brass of Anna Rede (see page 230), dated 1577, shows us a ruff of ordinary dimensions, as also does the figure of an English lady of quality, 1577, in Fig. 345. The pleats in the ruffs were made by goffering tongs or "poking sticks," as they were termed; the earliest were of wood and bone, and were inserted into the ruff after its emergence from the starch which then dried in the required form. Subsequently steel sticks came into use which were heated, and thus expedited the process.

The Partlet.—At the commencement of this reign unmarried women wore the neck bare, even when in the open, but finally adopted the partlet like their married sisters, until the growing size of the ruff abolished it.

Stomacher.—As Queen Elizabeth was long-waisted and narrow-chested, it became somewhat difficult to imitate the regal figure; the stomacher, however, approximated all figures to the ideal. To imitate the royal complexion, which was pale and fair, the ladies were in the habit of swallowing ashes, gravel, and tallow to produce the " pale bleake colour" they so much desired. This anæmic appearance was powerfully aided by the stomacher, which "cribb'd, cabin'd and confin'd" the body within its steel embrace. It was brought down to a peak in front which gradually lengthened, as we have noticed in the case of the men.

Petticoat.—This began to occupy the same position in women's dress as it does at the present time. Although under ordinary circumstances it was hidden by the kirtle, yet we are told that it was, as a rule, made of the best cloth, silk, grograin, &c., and fringed about the skirts with shot silk.

The Kirtle.—This very important article was, as a rule, exposed to view by the opening in the front of the robe. They were made of silk, velvet, taffeta, grograin, satin or scarlet, bordered with guards, lace, fringe, &c.; by its general appearance, we may infer that it was padded.

The Robe.—The great feature of the first division of the reign is the spread of the skirts, which are not padded to a great extent, if at all, upon the hips, and generally present a bell-shaped figure. This is well noted in the hunting scene previously referred to. In Fig. 346 a group of burgher women and one country woman is given, which clearly shows no distention whatever of the skirts, in marked contrast to that exhibited at the end of the reign by the same class of persons.

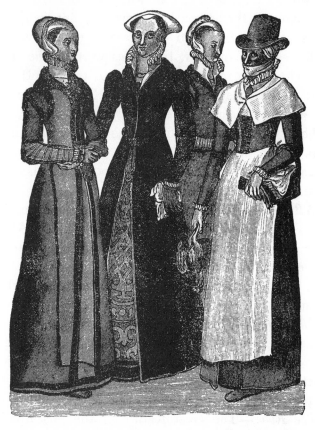

FIG. 346.—Costumes of town women and a country woman, in the time of "The Merry Wives of Windsor." (Add. MS. 28,330.)

Corsets.—During the reign of Elizabeth these were worn by both men and women. The following lines are descriptive and satirical:—

" These privie coates by art made strong
  With bones, with paste, with such like ware,
Whereby their backe and sides grew long,
  And now they harnest gallants are ;
Were they for use against the foe,
Our dames for Amazones might goe.

But seeing they doe only stay
  The course that nature doth intend,
And mothers often by them slay
  Their daughters yoong, and worke their end ;
What are they els but armours stout,
Wherein like gyants Jove they flout ? "

Hair.—About the middle of the reign the Queen began
to wear false hair, and Stow informs us that women's
periwigs were first brought into England at the time of
the massacre of Paris; Stubbs says that about the year
1595, when the fashion became general in England of
wearing a greater quantity of hair than was ever the produce of a single head, it was dangerous for any child to
wander, as nothing was more common than for women to
entice such as had fine locks into out-of-the-way places,
and there cut them off. The same author adds, "And if
any have haire of her owne naturall growing, which is not
faire ynough, then will they *die* it in divers colours." The
dyeing of hair was frequently severely censured from the
pulpit during this reign, and two books were published
against perukes and peruke-makers. It was fashionable
to dye it yellow out of compliment to the Queen; both
Elizabeth and Mary Queen of Scots patronised wigs,
Elizabeth having eighty attires of false hair at one time.
It was customary to dress the hair over wire frames or
padding, precisely similar to those worn at the present day.

Curling tongs were used among the upper classes. Stubbs describes women's hair as "frizzled and crisped, laid out on wreaths and borders from ear to ear propped with forks and wire," and says that "on this bolstered hair, which standeth crested round about their frontiers, they apply gold wreaths, bugles, and gewgaws."

Gloves are frequently mentioned during this period, and were commonly worn. We read of "five or six pair of the white innocent wedding-gloves" in Dekker's "Untrussing of the Humourous Poet," 1599; and gloves of leather, silk, and worsted are described at the same period. They were decorated with fringe and embroidery, and often perfumed. In one portrait of Queen Elizabeth she wears on her left hand a dark-coloured leather glove, the back of the hand and fingers of which appear to be stamped with patterns, and ornamented with small stones and pearls. Walton in his "Compleat Angler" speaks of otter skins as being excellent for gloves. Perfumed gloves were brought as presents from Italy at this time, a custom which continued till the middle of the eighteenth century. Perfumes are said to have been introduced into England by Edward Vere, Earl of Oxford. He also brought Elizabeth a pair of embroidered gloves scented with sweet perfume from Italy. They were trimmed with four tufts, or roses, of coloured silk, and her Majesty was so much delighted with this new fashion, that in one of her pictures she is painted with them upon her hands.

Wharton says that gloves were often presented to persons of distinction during this reign.

Fans were generally made of ostrich feathers, or the bright-coloured feathers from the peacock's tail. They

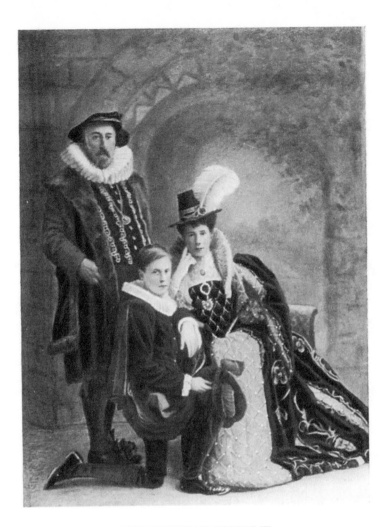

ELIZABETHAN COSTUME

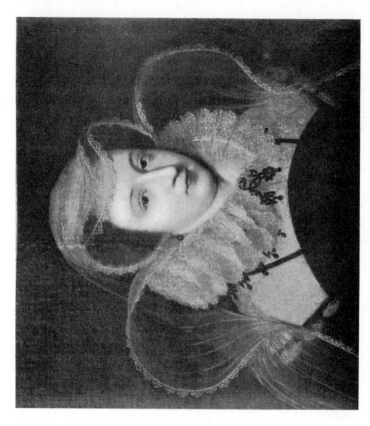

FIG. 349.—Mary, Queen of Scots, by Mytens, 1580.

were suspended together with a looking-glass from the girdle by a gold or silver chain. Wharton mentions a fan presented to Elizabeth, the handle of which was studded with diamonds. The most costly were made of ostrich feathers, fastened into handles composed of gold, silver, or ivory curiously worked. In a portrait at Ditchley, Oxon, of Queen Elizabeth, painted about 1592, she has a fan of the modern shape, suspended from her waist by pink ribands; we know also that she possessed "two fannes of strawe, wrought with silke of sondry collours." Goscon says they used them

> "In house, in field, in church, in street;
> In summer, winter, water, land;
> In colde, in heate, in drie, in weet,—
> I judge they are for wives such tooles
> As bables are in plays for fooles."

A reproduction of a group is introduced here, for the purpose of illustrating the general features of costume prevailing during the early part of the reign of Elizabeth, and approximately of the date 1572. It embodies many of the principal features characteristic of the costume of that period, and it is hoped that the accentuations of these points by means of colour may prove of material assistance to the student.

THE WOMEN

Second Period, 1580–1603

It was during this second period that the true Elizabethan costume was evolved, and gave it that emphatic and remarkable character which distinctly stamps it. The

essential evolutions distinguishing it occurred chiefly in connection with the stomacher and the robe.   In order to
produce the desired length of body, a corset was worn con-

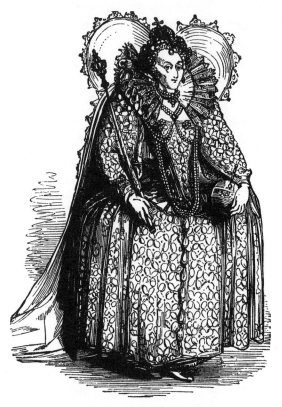

FIG. 347.—Elizabeth, 1588.

sisting of whalebone and leather, rigid and inflexible; to
the lower part of this a horizontal shelf of the same unbend-
ing material was firmly affixed, projecting more at the sides
than in front or at the back.

The shelf thus presented an irregular oval to a bird's-eye

view. Having tightly encased the human form within this rigid prison-house, the stomacher was laid upon and tightly laced to the support thus afforded, while the kirtle and robe were draped over the projection. Thus was the *Vardingale* or *Farthingale* evolved, one of the most hideous distortions that has ever obsessed the imagination, and distorted the lines of human beauty. Upon the stage and elsewhere the farthingale is often seen as a simple hoop distending the dress and swaying freely with the movements of the wearer. Needless to say this is quite incorrect. Fig. 347, representing the Queen as she appeared when returning thanks for the defeat of the Spanish Armada, in 1588, fully exhibits this distortion; at the same time it should be noticed that the

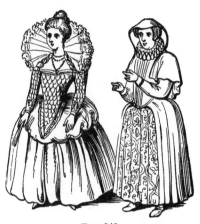

FIG. 348.

c. 1600.   1596.

sleeves have become much fuller and somewhat like those worn by her parents. The ludicrous effect produced by the farthingale in the apparent shortening of the lower limbs is painfully apparent. The partlet was now discarded, and an enormous ruff, rising gradually from the front of the shoulders to about the height of the head behind, further accentuated by the two wings, rising higher still and forming a heart-shaped background for the head, helped to complete the presentment of the Queen in all her glory. One can hardly help thinking of

Walpole's caustic remark of "a sharp-eyed lady with a hooked nose, red hair, loaded with jewels, an enormous ruff, a vaster farthingale, and a bushel of pearls bestrewed over the entire figure." The figure (Fig. 348), supposed to be that of Lady Herbert, afterwards Marchioness of Worcester, dates from the year 1600, while the figure seen beside her is four years earlier.

To Mary, Queen of Scots, who played such a prominent

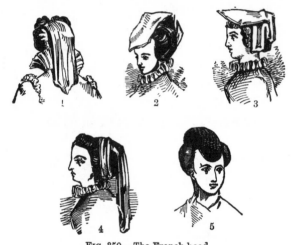

FIG. 350.—The French hood.

Nos. 1 and 2, 1582.   Nos. 3 and 4, 1596.   No. 5, 1653.

part in the second part of the reign, has been ascribed the pretty head-dress which goes by her name. A portrait painted by Mytens in 1580 is reproduced here (Fig. 349, Pl.). One of the head-dresses of this style is represented, but the special objects of interest are the two wings at the sides, which are formed by stiffening the upper portions of the cloak. If the portrait of Elizabeth by Zucchero is examined, it will be seen that the two wings in that case

are also attached to a gauze cloak.   French hoods were
now the mode, and continued fashionable till the reign of
Charles I.   Stubbs says: "Then on toppes of their stately
turrets (I mean heades, wherein is
more vanitie than true philosophie now
and then) stand their capitall ornaments, as French
hood, hatte, cappe,
kercher, and such
like; whereof some
be of velvet, some
of taffatie, some
(but few) of wooll;
someofthisfashion,

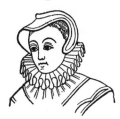

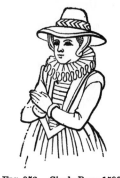

FIG. 351.—Julian Clippesby, 1594. Clippesby Church.

FIG. 352.—Cicely Page, 1598. Bray Church, Bucks.

some of that, some of this colour, some of that, according
to the variable phantasies of their serpentine minds.   And
to such excess is it growne, as every artificer's wife (almost)

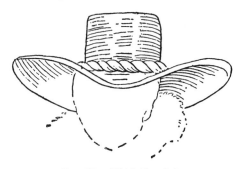

FIG. 353.—Elizabethan hat.

will not stick to goe in her hatte of velvet every day; every
merchant's wife and meane gentlewoman in her French hood
—and every poore cottager's wife in her taffatie hatte, or else
of wool at least" (Fig. 350).   We also read of their being

worn among the lower classes: "Frances, I'll have thee go like a citizen, in a guarded gown, and a French hood." The French hood so often alluded to, and sometimes termed the Paris-hede, is seen upon the brass of Julian Clippesby, 1594, in Clippesby Church, Norfolk (Fig. 351); while the broad-brimmed hat worn over the hood is well exemplified upon the brass of Cicely Page, 1598, in the church at Bray, Bucks (Fig. 352). Another example of an Elizabethan hat is given in Fig. 353.

CHAPTER XVIII

JAMES I., 1603–1625

THE MEN

Costume under James I. was in a state of transition. At the commencement we have all the absurdities of the Elizabethan period in their highest accentuation carefully adopted by the King, and for a time further developed. James I., amongst other qualities, possessed cowardice in a very marked form, and the thickly-padded doublet and bombasted breeches strongly appealed to him as being effective against the point of a dagger or a rapier. A representation of his Majesty, executed in 1614, may give some idea of the length to which this padding could go (Fig. 354). Corsets were in use by gentlemen at this period to give the necessary shape to chest and waist, while the nether garments, "the great round abominable breech," as the cynics termed it, tapered towards the knee, and presented hundreds of slashes, being otherwise decorated with lace and embroidery.

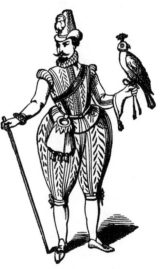

FIG. 354.—King James I., 1614.

To show to what an extent this fashion was followed, we may cite the following. There was a law in force against wearing "*bags stuffed in their sacks*," and a person is described as being brought before a court of justice: he is charged by the judges with being habited contrary to the statute, but he convinced them that the stuffing was not composed of any prohibited article, inasmuch as it consisted merely of a pair of sheets, two tablecloths, ten napkins, four shirts, a brush, a glass, a comb and a nightcap!

The *Hat* has a brim turned up only on one side; it is the latest fashion in the crown, *i.e.* a truncated cone, and is decorated with a feather. The sleeves are tight to the arms, and have the crescent puff at the shoulders. It was chiefly in the accessories of costume that the Jacobean exquisite sought relief for his yearnings towards style; he was careful in the choice of colours and their contrasts, also in the selection of materials. Pearl and peach colour, white satin hand-worked in silver and gold, flame colour and orange tawny were among the favourites. Many anxious problems had to be solved respecting the jewel, band, and feathers for the hat; while boot fringes, shoe roses, and the exact length, width, and pattern of garter were objects of intense and earnest thought. When we add to these the cut of the doublet and the cloak, the points of the shoes, the curl of the love-lock, the ribbons with which it should be tied, the particular style of earrings, and the hundred and one things that rule that "bush of vanity whereby the devil leads and holds men captive," it will be readily seen that the *rôle* of a Jacobean dandy was no sinecure.

The *Hair* also was a matter for consideration, inasmuch

as there were many methods for treating it. Greene, in his "Quip for an Upstart Courtier," makes a barber ask: "Sir, will you have your worship's hair cut after the Italian manner, short and round, and then frounst with the curling-iron to make it look like a half-moon in a mist? Or like a Spaniard, long at the ears, and curled like the two ends of an old cast periwig? Or will you be Frenchified, with a love-lock down to your shoulders, wherein you may weave your mistress's favour?" These locks were of French origin. When Christian IV. of Denmark visited England in 1606, he wore a love-lock upon the left side adorned with a bow of ribbons. In Lyly's "Midas" a barber says: "Will you have a low curl upon your head like a bull, or a dangling locke like a spaniell? Your love-lockes wreathed with a silken twist, or

Fig. 355.—Love-lock of Sir T. Meautys, *temp.* James I.

shaggie to fall on your shoulders?" In the "Return from Parnassus," 1606, "An upstart must take tobacco and must wear a lock"; and in Rich's "Opinion Deified," 1613, "Some by wearing a long lock that hangs dangling by his ear, do think by that commodity to be esteemed by the opinion of foolery." In the time of James I. this fashion appears in the height of its extravagance.

Sir Thomas Meautys, secretary to Sir Francis Bacon, wore a waved love-lock reaching to his elbow (Fig. 355). In "Follie's Anatomie," 1619, we read—

> "Correct your frizled locks, and in your glasse
> Behold the picture of a foolish asse."

This refers to the fashion, prevalent among the men, as the women, of wearing a pocket mirror.

The extraordinary variety of beards which mark the latter part of the reign of Elizabeth was continued in that of James. One, however, in which the moustache was brushed upwards from the lips (Fig. 356), appears to have become nearly obsolete, although in "Cynthia's Revels," 1601, Mercury says to the barber, "Come, invert my mustachio."

Fig. 356.—Inverted moustache, 1587.

Greene, in his "Quip for an Upstart Courtier," more clearly denotes the form of these fashions. Speaking of the barber, after dressing the head, he says: "He descends as low as his beard, and asketh whether he please to be shaven or no? whether he will have his peak cut short and sharp, amiable like an *inamorato;* or broade pendant, like a spade, to be terrible like a warrior and soldado? Whether he will have his *crates* cut low, like a juniper bush; or his *suberche* taken away with a razor? If it be his pleasure to have his *appendices* primed; or his *mouchaches* fostered, or turned about his ears like the branches of a vine, or cut down to the lip with the Italian lash, to make him look like a half-faced baby in brass?" The following woodcuts illustrate some of the varieties of beards in use :—

Fig. 357, No. 1, is the *pique devant*, or *pick-a-devant*, noticed by Hutton in his "Follie's Anatomie," 1619 :—

> "With what grace bold, actor like he speaks,
> Having his beard precisely cut i' th' peake.
> How neat's mouchatoes do at a distance stand,
> Lest they disturbe his lips or saffron band.'"

No. 2, the screw beard, was worn by Taylor, the Water
Poet.

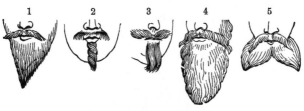

FIG. 357.—Beards.

| Pique devant, c. 1620. | Screw, c. 1600. | T-shape, or Hammercut, Charles I. | Sugar-loaf, Elizabethan and James I. | Swallow-tail, late Elizabethan. |

No. 3 is the T-shaped beard, or hammercut, which is
just appearing at the end of the reign.

No. 4 is the sugar-loaf beard, as worn by many distinguished men of the end of the reign of
Elizabeth and during that of James I.

No. 5 is the swallow-tail cut, as mentioned by Tom Nash. In "Cynthia's
Revels," 1601, Anaides says: "Sir, you
with the *pencil* on your chin," probably
a delicate and playful allusion to a beard
cut like a pencel or pennonçel (the small
flag at the end of the lance). We also
read of tile beards, something like cathedral
beards before mentioned, and a perfumed
beard is alluded to. Brushes were especially kept for the use of the beard; in
Dekker's play, "Match Me in London,"
one of the characters exclaims, "I like this beard-brush,
but that the haire's too stiff."

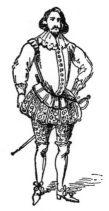

FIG. 358.—Sir G. Hart, 1600.

In Fig. 358, being a representation of Sir G. Hart,

the peascod doublet is of plain white silk with white lace
falling band and cuffs, the bombasted breeches and hose
are of white silk with needlework crescents, the stockings
of white silk rolled over the knees, and the shoes are also
white.   There is only one bit of colour in the whole

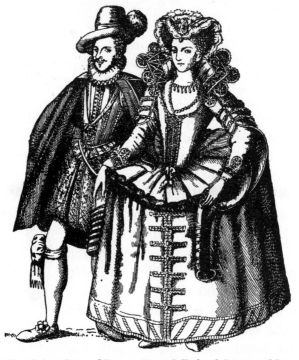

FIG. 359.—Robert Carr and Frances Howard, Earl and Countess of Somerset.

dress—the red heels to the shoes.   The taste for pure
white prevailed for a time, and in 1607 we have a gentleman's wardrobe described as a cloak lined with rich taffeta,
a white satin suit, the jerkin covered with gold lace, a
chain of pearl, a gilt rapier in an embroidered hanger, pearl-
coloured silk stockings, and a pair of silver spurs.

The costume of a nobleman about the middle of the reign may be judged from the preceding figure of the Earl and Countess of Somerset (Fig. 359), from a print in the British Museum. The chief points to notice are the ruff, which is still very large, and the garter, which at

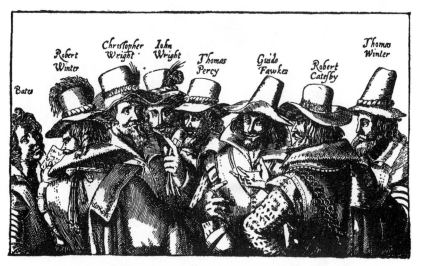

FIG. 361.—The Gunpowder Plotters. From a picture painted in 1606.

this time consisted of a large sash with lace ends. The cloak is also fairly voluminous.

Towards the end of the reign the extravagantly rich clothes of the Duke of Buckingham (Fig. 360, Pl.) called forth special comment. "It was common with him at any ordinary dancing to have his clothes trimmed with great diamond buttons, and to have diamond hat-bands, cockades, and earrings; to be yoked with great and manifold knots of pearl. . . . At his going over to Paris in 1625 he had twenty-seven suits of clothes made, the richest that embroidery, lace, silk, velvet, gold, and gems could contribute; one of which was a white, uncut velvet, set all over, both

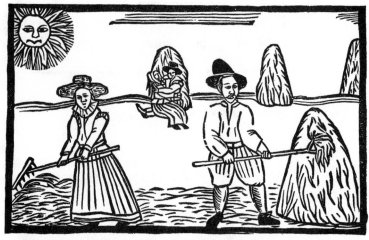

FIG. 362.—Haymaking. Early seventeenth century.

suit and cloak, with diamonds, valued at £14,000, besides a great feather, stuck all over with diamonds, as were also his sword, girdle, hat-band and spurs."

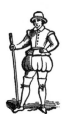

Respecting the dress of ordinary persons, we may include that of the Gunpowder Plotters (Fig. 361), where the hats, the falling bands, and the tightly-fitting doublets are distinctive features, if we omit the unkempt hair.

Among the labouring classes, "Haymaking" (Fig. 362) affords us a glimpse of agricultural attire. A small figure of a yeoman is given here

FIG. 363.—Yeo-man, 1682.

(Fig. 363), and we read that they affected "narrow-brimmed hats with flat crowns, doublets with large wings and short skirts, and girdles about their waists, trunk breeches, with hosen drawn up to the thighs and gartered under the knees."

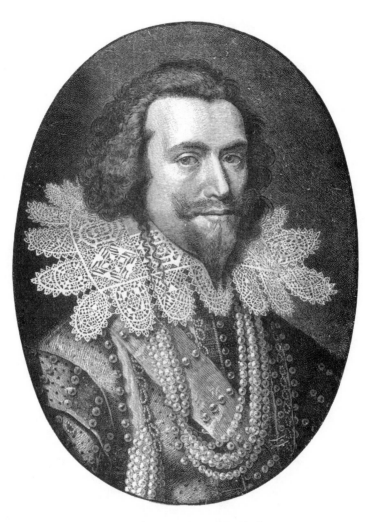

Fig. 360.—The Duke of Buckingham.

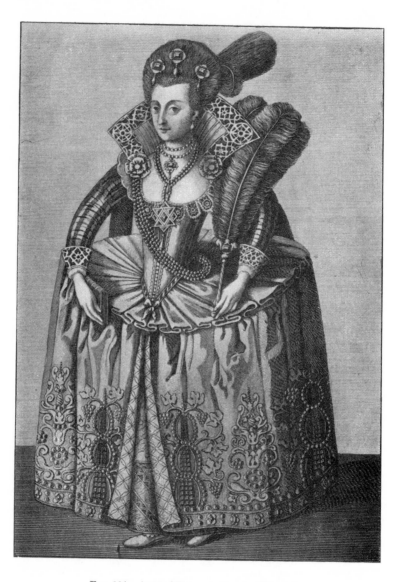

FIG. 364.—Anne of Denmark, Queen of James I.

THE WOMEN

The portrait of Anne of Denmark, Queen of James I. (Fig. 364, Pl.), gives us a clear insight into the style of female costume prevailing amongst court ladies during this period, and, as will be seen, it differs in no way from that of the latter part of the time of Queen Elizabeth. One point, however, ought perhaps to be emphasized, namely, the absolutely flat projection of the farthingale with its table-like edge, and the series of radiating plaits upon the surface of it. The exquisite design in needlework upon the robe is well shown in the illustration. The fact, which has been insisted upon before in this work, that the farthingale projected considerably more at the sides, and to a lesser extent at the back, than towards the front is well defined in this case. The Queen carries

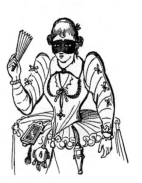

FIG. 365.—Fan, &c., *temp.* James I.

a long feathered fan and also a book, and is thus somewhat in contrast with the many articles borne by ladies at that time. For example, in Fig. 365 a lady is represented with a folding bone fan, a looking-glass attached to her girdle, a pomander in the form of a ball with tassels hanging from it, containing perfume (much in use at that time as a preventative against the plague and other infection); and also a case, probably of silver, containing articles of toilet, but possibly a " casting-bottle " of liquid perfume.

In a dissolute court like that of James I. the mask was an essential, and was worn upon all public occasions, even in the chase. The few ladies who dared to appear in public without this disfigurement were termed "bare-faced." One lady in particular, the Countess of Bedford, braved the court remarks, and, in 1613, Chamberlain wrote that she forbears painting, which makes her look somewhat strange among so many vizards, which with their frizzled powdered hair makes the ladies look all alike. Masks were small, and did not cover much of the face. Sir John Harington, in 1606, says: "The great ladies do go well masked, and indeed it be the only show of their modesty, to conceal their countenance." Ben Jonson alludes to

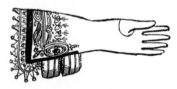

them, and Middleton, in 1611, makes various references to women's masks in "The Roaring Girl." Painting and patching, as well as masking, were fashionable.

FIG. 366.—Tudor glove in Saffron Walden Museum.

Gloves were extremely fashionable, and we hear of a lady taking off no less than three pairs of gloves which were worn one over the other. In Saffron Walden Museum is a specimen of a richly decorated glove of the period, beautifully ornamented with needlework in gold and silver thread, and the silk opening at the wrist (Fig. 366). In the Ashmolean Museum at Oxford is a pair reputed to have belonged to Queen Anne of Denmark possessing a very handsome lace edging.

A lady's costume of the middle of the reign is well shown in Fig. 367, Pl., representing Hester, daughter of the first Sir T. Myddelton, and first wife of Sir Henry Salusbury, who died in 1614, and was buried in Stanstead-Mountfitchet Church. The very high hat with its cable

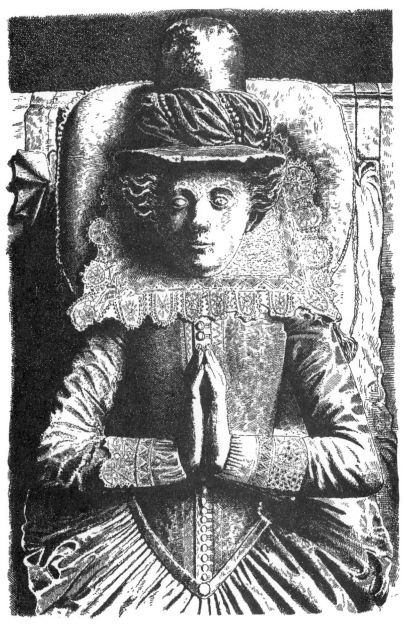

FIG. 367.—Hester, daughter of Sir T. Myddelton, 1614. Stanstead-Mountfitchet Church.

trimming, the tight sleeves with their lace cuffs, the peaked stomacher and its many buttons, and the size of the farthingale at that time are worthy of notice; also the lace collar or falling band, which is remarkable for the beauty of its design.

At the close of the reign of James the farthingale had become modified as shown in Fig. 868, which represents the daughter of John Harpur in Swarkestone Church, Derbyshire, dated 1622. The robe has commenced to assume the form of a loose gown, like that of succeeding reigns; the stomacher is still tight with a long waist, and the sleeves are wider. The small hood worn over the brushed-back hair has a frontlet which at times was pendent down the back, but could be brought forward when required to shade the face, as in this case. The frontlets were

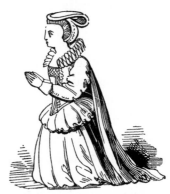

Fig. 368.—Daughter of John Harpur, 1622. Swarkestone Church, Derbyshire.

sometimes embroidered and ornamented with precious stones. It is probable that this example is the last we shall find of a fashion which had survived from the days of Henry VIII., and possibly this is also the end of the farthingale. Planché tells us an amusing story with regard to this "unnatural disguisement." When Sir Peter Wych was sent ambassador to the Grand Seignior from James I., his lady accompanied him to Constantinople, and the Sultana, having heard much of her, desired to see her; whereupon Lady Wych, attended by her waiting-women, all of them dressed in their great varthingales, which was the court dress of the English ladies at that time, waited upon her Highness. The Sultana received her visitor with great respect, but, struck with the extraordinary extension of the hips of the whole party, seriously inquired if that shape was peculiar to the natural formation of English women. Lady Wych was obliged to explain the whole mystery of the dress in order to convince her that she and her companions were not really so deformed as they appeared to be. In "Lingua, or the Combat of the Tongue and the Five Senses for Superiority," 1607, an account is given by one of the characters of the articles comprising a fashionable lady's dress, and the length of time required for arranging the same. He says: "Five hours ago I set a dozen maids to attire a boy like a nice gentlewoman; but there is such doing with their looking-glasses, pinning, unpinning, setting, unsetting, formings, and unformings, painting blew vains and cheeks; such stir with sticks and combs, cascanets, dressings, purles, falles, squares, buskes, bodies, scarfs, necklaces, carcanets, rebatoes, borders, tires, fans, palisa-does, puffs, ruffs, cuffs, muffs, pusles, fusles, partlets, frislets, bandlets, fillets, croslets, pendulets, amulets, annulets, bracelets, and so many lets, that yet she is scarce drest to the girdle; and now there's such calling for farthingales, kirtlets, busk-points, shoe-ties, &c., that seven pedlars' shops—nay, all Sturbridge fair—will scarce furnish her: a ship is sooner rigged by far than a gentlewoman made ready." [1]

---

[1] An interesting list of the clothing for gentlemen, and also for ladies, is afforded by the Chirk Castle accounts, 1605–1666, compiled by

William M. Myddelton and privately printed. The following extracts deal with the accounts during the reign of James I. :—

9 yds. of tawney satton in grayn @ 15s. yd.

4 els taffete sasnet @ 8s. yd.

7 yds. fustian lining, 7s.

Pointes to your collar, 1s. 5d.

Waste band for your hose, 3d.

Rybbon to tye your girdle, 6d.

1 pr. carnacŏ silck stockings, £2, 6s.

1 pr. garters and roses, 8s.

1 falling bande with lace and cuffes, £1.

1 pr. gloves with fringe, £1, 3s.

1 black bever hat, £2, 4s.

1 doz. Holland handkerchiefs, 14s.

1 pr. pearle coloured stockings, 11s.

1 pr. embroidered gloves (ladies'), £2, 10s.

1¼ yds. watchet velvet, £1, 7s. 6d.

9 yds. watchet and gold lace, £2, 16s. 10d.

1 pr. sarsenet garters and roses, £1, 13s.

1 white beavor hatte and gold band, for a lady, £3, 2s.

3 yds. silver grograin for a doublet @ 22s. yd.

8 yds. crimson satton to make your hose @ 16s. yd.

3 ells white taffete sasnet to draw out your hose, 8s. yd.

3 ells rich black taffete to make your cloak, 15s. 6d.

1000 white pins, 1s.

1000 red pins, 6d.

1 pr. Spanish leather shoes, 3s. 6d.

For wedding gloves for the Lady Savell, £22, 8s.

2 yds. of gallowne lace [galloon], 7d.

1 pr. of Spanishe showes, 3s. 6d.

Gould lace for a quoiffe, 5s. 3d.

12 ells (15 yds.) of rich taffaty, £9.

CHAPTER XIX

CHARLES I. AND THE COMMONWEALTH, 1625–1660

THE simple and elegant costumes with which we associate this reign were undoubtedly the most picturesque of English dresses since the reign of Edward III., inasmuch as they followed more closely the natural lines of beauty than any that had preceded them in the interval. The uncouth monstrosities which had prevailed served to accentuate the graceful lines of the dress when finally evolved. This evolution, as may be expected, did not take place at once, and for five or ten years after Charles came to the throne the old vanities still persisted and clung obstinately to life. Thus in "The Young Gallant's Whirligig," 1629, we find an exquisite is described with

> "The Estridge [ostrich feather] on his head with Beaver rare,
> Upon his hands a Spanish Sent to weare,
> Haire's curl'd, ears pearl'd, with Bristows brave and bright
> Bought for true Diamonds in his false sight;
> All are perfumed, and as for him 'tis meete
> His body's clad i' th' Silkworms winding sheete."

And Sir Samuel Rowland, speaking of the "Roaring Boys" of his time, says:

> "And what our neat fantasticks newest hatch,
> That at the second hand hee's sure to catch,
> If it be feather time, he weares a feather,
> A golden hat-band or a silver either

A beastly bushie head of tousled haire,
A horse-taile locke most dreadful he doth weare.

.   .   .   .   .   .

An elbow cloake, because wide hose and garters
May be apparent in the lower quarters.

.   .   .   .   .

His cabage ruffe, of the outrageouse size,
Starched in colour to beholders' eyes."

We may ascribe the change from the bombasted breeches and cart-wheel farthingale, to the elegant Carolean costume, to two chief causes. One was the cultivated and refined taste of the King, which was in marked contrast with the boorish mind of his father, and the conception of artistic feeling which Henrietta Maria undoubtedly possessed compared with the utter lack of the appreciation of the beautiful shown by Anne of Denmark. The other was the strong influence which the Puritan movement was manifesting in the feelings of the nation in all matters, including that of dress. Perhaps the inconveniences attendant upon distended garments had no small part in their abolition, for during the reign of James it had been found necessary to forbid ladies and gentlemen from attending masques in their expanded costume, because of the impossibility of finding seating accommodation when each spectator occupied the place of three.

THE MEN

A broadside dating 1630 shows the flight of the towns-people into the country to escape from the plague, and upon careful examination will show many points of interest in this transition stage of costume (Fig. 369).

The Doublet as a rule reached to nearly mid-thigh, the

lower part from the hips sometimes forming a kind of skirt. At the waist it displayed the undershirt, but from thence buttoned up the front until it disappeared under the white falling band or lace collar. The sleeves were full, and made tight to the wrists, where a plain white cuff of the gauntlet shape, or else one of lace, formed the finish. If desired, the hands could be withdrawn through the cuffs and thrust through the openings which can be plainly seen, thus forming hanging sleeves. This is well shown in Fig. 370, dating from 1645.

Breeches.—These had now lost all their padding; they were of uniform width, and hung loosely to the knees, where they were fastened with sash-like garters, either loose, or running in a case round the leg. Tight stockings, and square-toed shoes, with large roses or bows upon them, were worn.

The *Hat* was of felt, and generally large and wide in

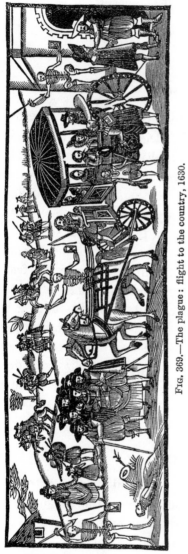

Fig. 369.—The plague: flight to the country, 1630.

the brim. The hair was long, and hung in apparently natural curls upon the shoulders. With regard to this costume, we can only say that it was dignified and graceful by reason of its simplicity; but, as there are always certain minds to whom mediocrity is an abomination, we discover that even this simple attire could be made fantastic and absurd by the exquisite of the time. A first-class example of a gentleman possessing this type of mind is shown in Fig.

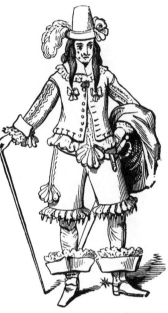

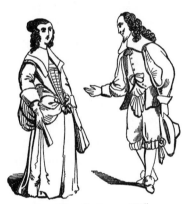

FIG. 370.—Costumes, 1645.

FIG. 371.—An exquisite of 1646.

371, where nearly every point previously described has become distorted. Thus the hat now suffers from a feather and a bunch of ribbons; the love-locks on either side of the face, tied up with fancy bows, distort the beauty of the hair; the doublet, despoiled of its skirt, discloses an appalling array of shirt, while the stiff pair of cylinders which serve for breeches are finished with frills exhibiting a superfluity of points. The boots are suggestive of the modern bouquet, and necessitated an ambling straddle as he perambulated the streets singing. The toes of these boots were as a rule about two inches longer than necessary. In addition to the above vagaries, these "extremists" also adopted bunches of riband, lace, feathers, embroidery, and gold lace, fans, mirrors, patches, masks, and a short cloak hung over the left arm, while their rapiers were of an excessive length, and their walking-sticks peculiarly aggressive. With reference to the patches, Glapthorne, in his "Lady's Privilege," 1640, says: "Look you, signor, if 't be a lover's part you are to act, take a black spot or two. I can furnish you; 'twill make your face more amórous, and appear more gracious in your mistress' eyes."

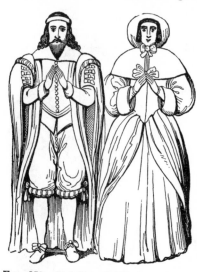

Fig. 372.—Jacinth and Elizabeth Sacheverell, 1657. Morley Church, Derbyshire.

In Morley Church, Derbyshire, are the monumental effigies of Jacinth and Elizabeth Sacheverell, 1657 (Fig. 372), which afford us examples of the dresses of an elderly gentleman and his wife at the end of this period. The long open gown with hanging sleeves, with bows from the shoulder, the close skull-cap, falling band, tight vest, and loose breeches have a quiet simplicity which bespeaks the age.

THE WOMEN

A most remarkable series of drawings of women of all classes was made by the engraver Hollar at this period, and from them we may glean practically every detail.

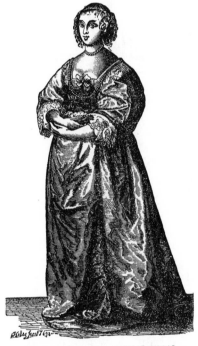

FIG. 373.—English court lady, 1643.

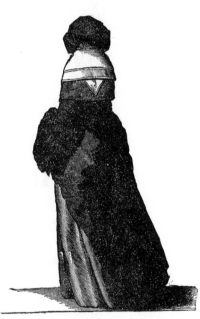

FIG. 374.—English lady: winter costume, 1644.

For instance, we learn that all traces of the Mary Stuart cap, the ruff, and the farthingale had disappeared by about 1640. The dresses were made with very full sleeves, either reaching to the elbow or to the wrists, but generally drawn in at the centre so as to form two puffs. At the termination a wide cuff of the gauntlet shape appears as a rule

edged with lace.   The bodice was tight-fitting, and a
marked characteristic was the tabs of various shapes and
sizes depending from the lower portions.   The bodice was
brought to a point in front, or else terminated at the natural
waist.   The long petticoat was generally made of rich

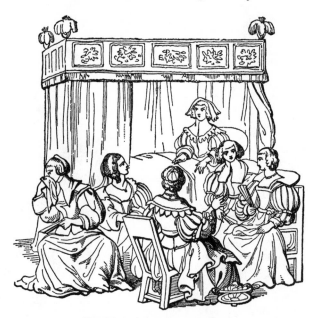

FIG. 375.—A bedroom party, 1631.

material, and was partly or largely displayed by the robe,
which at times was gathered up to the waist, as may be
seen in Fig. 370.   A lady of the court is shown in Fig. 373,
where the lace collar surrounding the low-cut neck
is seen, and where also the robe is not draped.   The
distinguishing mode of doing the hair may be noted;
at the sides it is allowed to flow freely, while from the
forehead it is tightly combed back and gathered in close

rolls behind. A fringe of small curls upon the forehead was a later development. An English lady in winter dress (Fig. 374) is seen to be provided with a close hood and cape, with the indispensable muff, and having the robe turned back and pinned. The broad-brimmed hat was almost universal with or without the coif underneath.

A very interesting print of the date 1631 affords us a glimpse of domestic manners of the first half of this century. It represents one of the fashionable bedroom parties, which formed the subject of many popular sarcastic remarks (Fig. 375).

The fashion of patching introduced in the last reign was developed to a ludicrous extent in this reign. Bulwer in his " Artificial Changeling," 1650, has favoured us with a representation of a lady's face, which is reproduced here (Fig. 376). He says : " Our ladies

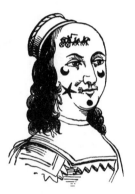

FIG. 376.—Patching, 1650.

have lately entertained a vague custom of spotting their faces out of an affectation of a mole, to set off their beauty, such as Venus had ; and it is well if one black patch will serve to make their faces remarkable, for some fill their visages full of them, varied into all manner of shapes and figures." In " Wit Restored," 1658, we read :

> " Their faces are besmear'd and pierc'd
>   With severall sorts of patches,
> As if some cats their skins had flead
>   With scarres, half moons, and notches."

We also find in Beaumont and Fletcher's "Elder Brother," 1637 : "Your black patches you wear variously, some cut like stars, some in half moons, some in lozenges."

The apparel and ornaments of a lady of fashion may be

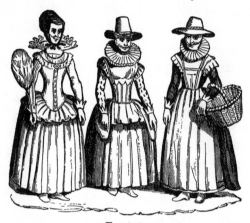

FIG. 377.

Gentlewoman.   Burgher's wife.   Countrywoman.
(From Speed's *Map of England*.)

gathered from a pastoral play first acted in 1631, where they are enumerated as follows :—

" Chains, coronets, pendants, bracelets, and ear-rings;
  Pins, girdles, spangles, embroyderies, and rings;
  Shadowes, rebatoes, ribbands, ruffs, cuffs, falls,
  Scarfes, feathers, fans, maskes, muffs, laces, cauls,
  Thin taffanies, cobweb lawn, and fardingales,
  Sweet fals, vayles, wimples, glasses, crisping-pins,
  Pots of ointment, combes, with poking sticks, and bodkines,
  Coyfes, gorgets, fringes, rowles, fillets, and hair laces,
  Silks, damasks, velvets, tinsels, cloth of gold,
  Of tissues with colours of a hundred fold."

The costume of the generality of people may be learnt from various figures taken from Speed's *Map of England*, published early in the reign, and given in Fig. 377. One

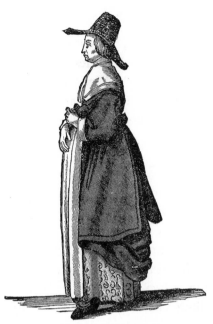

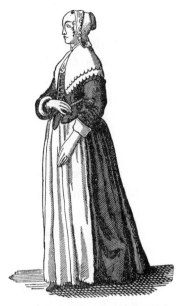

FIG. 378.—English tradesman's wife, 1649.   FIG. 379.—Citizen's daughter, 1649.

Citizen.   *Country Man.*

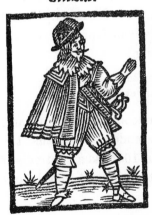

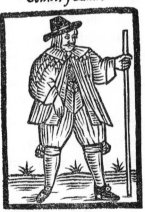

Printed at London for T. B. 1641.

FIG. 380.—From a tract, 1641.

of these, the centre, is the citizen's wife; for comparison of
the alteration in costume, we give Hollar's tradesman's wife
and citizen's daughter of the year 1649 (Figs. 378, 379).
With regard to the men, a citizen and countryman of 1641
are shown in the preceding rough woodcut (Fig. 380).

THE PURITANS

The general idea concerning the Puritan dress is that
which was evolved under the Commonwealth, but we may
discover distinctly Puritanical forms of costume long before
that period. These outward manifestations of different
religious belief generally took the form of opposites or nega-
tives to prevailing styles; thus, when ruffs were in fashion
the Puritan wore a large falling band; when wide falling
bands of delicate lace came in, he wore a very small band.
The fashionable hose were always coloured—he wore black;
when shoes were wide at the toes, his were pointed. Even
as early as the end of the sixteenth century, short hair
was a distinguishing characteristic of Nonconformity. John
Jonson speaks of their possessing

> " Religion in their garments, and their hair
>   Cut shorter than their eyebrows."

There was nothing more hideous in the Puritan's eyes
than the Stuart love-lock. Clarendon tells us that the term
" Roundhead " came into use in 1641, as a contradistinction
to " Cavalier." A complimentary couplet may be quoted:

> "What creature's this, with his short hairs,
>   His little band and huge long ears?"

Dramatic writers were never tired of poking fun at the

Puritans of their time, and it is peculiarly ironical that a very large proportion of the latter gained their livelihood by making the very articles which they so mercilessly condemned. Thus feather-making, bugle-making, confect-makers, and French fashioners were chiefly of the Puritan persuasion, as were also many tirewomen and starchers. The Puritans were loud in their denunciations of starch on delicate linen, but they allowed their shirts to be embroidered

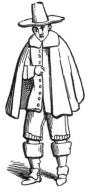

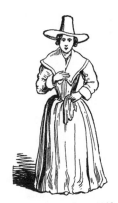

FIG. 381.—Roundhead, 1649.   FIG. 382.—Puritan, 1646.

with texts from Scripture. The precision of dress affected by the male members may be judged from a print of the date, 1649 (Fig. 381); that of the ladies from the second figure, dating from 1646 (Fig. 382). It must not, however, be supposed that this extreme simplicity of dress produced an equal humility in the mind ; for we are told by contemporary writers that the Puritans were as inordinately vain of any little departure in their clothes, either in texture or in style, as the opposite section whom they affected to despise. Although this gloomy Puritanism, which strangled all natural cheerfulness, depressed a large proportion of the

population, it must not be supposed that a general humilia-
tion in dress followed.   There was a very large part of the

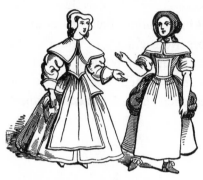

community who, in spite
of the danger of the pro-
ceeding, maintained the
Cavalier's style of dress and
living, and who practically
said, with Sir Toby Belch,
"Dost thou think, because
thou art virtuous, there
shall be no more cakes and
ale?"   Two members of the
humbler classes are repre-

FIG. 383.—The "milkmaid" costume, 1744.

sented here (Fig. 383) of the non-Puritanical order; the
costumes shown date from 1744, when a revival of the
dress occurred, and was termed the "milkmaid" style.
It will be seen that some of the children's dresses of the
lower orders at the present day have the Cromwellian style
for their prototype.

CHAPTER XX

CHARLES II., 1660-1685

THE delirious burst of joy with which the English nation welcomed the advent of Charles II. to the throne was the natural reaction after twenty years of uncertainty, gloom, and fanatical oppression. Probably this rebound to life and gaiety, inherent and natural qualities of the human mind, was in no way more plainly manifested that in articles of dress, for the love of beautiful colours and brightness generally is as natural to the ordinary human being as is the joy of living. Unfortunately, however, the new monarch had been reared in the French court, and possessed neither the will nor the inclination to restrain the excesses which went to such extremes during his time; the consequence was that extravagant fashions, chiefly from continental sources, poured over the land like a flood, and completely revolutionised the styles of dress which had obtained hitherto.

THE MEN

The doublet and the long coat passed out of fashion, and were succeeded by the

Tunic or Surcoat.—At the accession the fashion for men may be judged from the following (Fig. 384), which are taken from the figures shown in the procession of the coronation. The tunic is represented as a loose garment reaching below the hips and crossed by an ornamental baldrick; the sleeves are long and large, with a wide lace cuff.   In a print dating from 1662, the tunic is seen furnished with a petticoat pleated and ornamented.

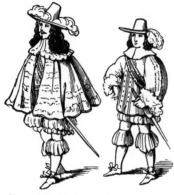

FIG. 384.—Early Charles I. costume.

The Petticoat Breeches, now introduced for the first time into England, were ornamented with rows of ribands above the knees, and deep lace ruffles beneath them.   These petticoat breeches, together with the petticoat skirt of the tunic, are admirably shown in a sketch by Randall Holme, the Chester Herald, in his note-book in the British Museum, and date from about 1658 and 1659 (Fig. 385).   The first he calls a short-waisted doublet and petticoat breeches, the lining lower than the breeches being tied above the knee, ribbon up to

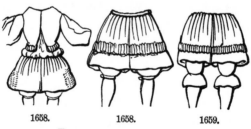

1658.   1658.   1659.

FIG. 385.—Petticoat breeches.

the pocket holes half the breadth of the breeches, then ribbons all about waist-band, and the shirt hanging out.   In the next year he notes a variety of this dress, and illustrates it in the second figure, describing it as "long stirrup hose, two

yards wide at the top, with points through several eyelet
holes, made fast to the petticoat breeches; a single row
of pointed ribbon hangs at the bottom of the breeches."
In the third figure, August 1659, he says: "The said large
stirrup hose were tied to the breeches, and another pair of
hose drawn over them to the calf of the leg and so turned
down." Sometimes the upper part of the hose was worn
bagging over the garter of the ribbons so extensively used,
he says they were, "first at the knees, then at the waist,
then at the hands, next about the neck."

Such is his description of a fashion which
became universal in England at the
Restoration.

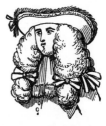

The Hat.—This was worn with a
broad brim, upon which reposed a heap
of feathers; the crown was of the cone
variety.

FIG. 386.—Periwig, *temp.*
King Charles II.

Periwig.—It must not be imagined
that the periwig was a new introduction into England at
this time; it had been known for many years before, but did
not become fashionable until the time of Charles II. They
are mentioned in the reign of Henry VIII., where there
occurs an entry of 20s. for a periwig for the King's fool, and
they were common at the time of Elizabeth. Hall in his
Satires, 1598, mentions a courtier as losing his periwinke in
a gust of wind; and in 1607, in "Cupid's Whirligig," a gentleman is mentioned as having his wig in pawn. A specimen
of one worn by an officer is given here (Fig. 386), where the
ends are seen to be tied up with ribbons. When introduced at the Reformation they were, however, of such a size
as to throw the wig of any modern judge completely into

the shade, and it was correct form for a man to be seen combing his wig in public while walking in the Mall or at the theatre. This act of gallantry was performed with combs of a very large size, which were carried in the pockets as constantly as the snuff-box. Pictures exist representing gentlemen conversing in public and combing their periwigs. In 1666, a type of dress was introduced

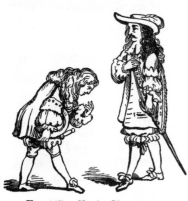

FIG. 387.—Charles II. costume.

by the King which he considered to be less costly and extravagant than the first. It consisted of a vest which, in different shapes and sizes, has lasted from that period down to the present time. The garment was tight to the body and without sleeves; it was of black cloth, and showed white silk under the pinking.

The tunic or coat worn over it was of the shape seen in the illustration (Fig. 387). The remainder of the costume was practically the same as before, except that the petticoat breeches were modified. Pepys says: "The court is full of vests; only my Lord St. Albans not pinked, but plain black; and they say the King says, the pinking upon white makes them look too much like magpies, and hath bespoken one of plain velvet."

The expenses of a gentleman's suit dated 1672 are here given:—

For making a dove-color'd and silk brocade coat, Rhingrave breeches and cannons, the coat lined with white lutestring, and interlined

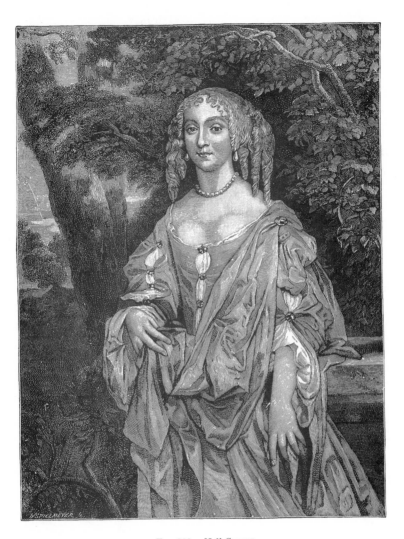

Fig. 388.—Nell Gwynn.

with camblett; the breeches lined with lutestring, and lutestring drawers, seamed all over with a scarlet and silver lace; sleeves and cannons whipt and laced with a scarlet and silver lace and a point lace; trimmed with a scarlet figured and plain satin ribbon, and scarlet and silver twist, £2.

Canvas, buckram, silk, thread, galloon and shamey pockets, 11s. 6d.

For fine camblet to interline the coat, 6s.

For silver thread for button holes, 3s.

For 6 dozen of scarlet and silver vellam buttons, £1, 1s.

For ½ doz. breast buttons, 6d.

10 yds. rich brocade at 28s. per yd.

8 yds. lutestring to line the coat, breeches, and drawers at 8s. per yd.

1 pair silk stockings at 12s.

An embroidered belt and garters, £3, 15s.

22 yds. scarlet and silver vellam lace for coat and cannons, 18s. per yd.

A black beaver hat, £2, 10s.

For a scarlet and silver edging to the hat, £1, 10s.

36 yds. of scarlet taffaty ribbon at 6d. per yd.[1]

---

[1] Following are further extracts from the Chirk Castle accounts to 1666:—

Paid for a paior of Spaynishe leather shoes for you, 4s. 6d., for ribon to the shoes, 8d., ribon for garters and cuffestrings, 2s. 6d.

Paid Mistress Mary Wilson for several things she bought for my lady at Chester, viz., a peice of Dimmity, 19s. 6d., 8 yards of Dowlas at 1s. 10d. per yard.

A lace for a primer, 7s.

Paid for weaveing 60 yds. of fine flaxen at 4d. per yd.

   ,,   ,,   ,,   60 yds. of another sorte of linen at 3d. per yd.

   ,,   ,,   ,,   60 yds. of Diaper at 8d. per yd.

26 yds. of coarse linen at 3d. per yd.

Paid for a pair of pumpes (slippers), 2s.

16 yds. of black Shaloone at 2s. 2d. per yd.

70 yds. of serge at 4s. 8d. per yd.

16 yds. of 3 piled velvet at 29s. per yd.

3 ells and a halfe of white Sarsnett at 11s. 8d. per ell.

Paid for a pair of worsted hose, 4s. 8d.

5 yds. of fine black Flaunders serge at 6s. 6d. per yd.

12 yds. black galloon, 3s. 4d. per yd.

One black lace peake, 8d.

1 black necklace, 4d.

In 1675, we are told that a London fop is composed of compliments, cringes, knots, fancies, perfumes, and a thousand French apish tricks. The universal costume at the end of the reign was generally plainer, and the vest and tunic were worn considerably longer. In 1670, the funeral procession of General Monk was illustrated, in which a great number of male figures are represented, and a careful examination of the costume will afford more instruction than pages of description.

40 yards of fine black cloth for women at 26s. 6d. per yd.
130 yds. black cloth at 21s. 6d. per yd.
65 yds. black cloth at 13s. per yd.
48 yds. black cloth at 11s. per yd.
1 lutestring handkercheefe, 6s.
1 pair shammy gloves, 6s.
1 pair of love shoe knotts, and pins, 8s.
1 pair of shoes, 3s.
2 prs. woollen and 1 of wolstead hose, 9s.
2 prs. silk stockings, 28s.
2 doz. prs. shammy gloves, 42s.
2 prs. gloves at 3s. 6d. per pair.
For making two coats, 22s.
1 long crape veil, £4, 10s.
1 band, 3s. 6d.
1 pinner (apron), 2s. 6d.
1 pr. stirrop stockings, 2s. 2d.
1 ell of ribbon for cuffstrings, 5d.
1 beaver hat, £3, 9s.
4 yds. yellow damask at 6s. per yd.
1 mourning hat band, 2s. 8d.
3 yds. silver lace for a petticoat, 16s.
1 crape hood, 3s. 6d.
1 pr. shamy gloves lined, 5s.
1 peake caul and border, 2s. 6d.
3 lutestring hoods, 21s.
1 short veil, 8s.
1 pr. boots, 12s.
  yds. gold and silver lace, £3, 18s.
6 doz. gold and silver buttons, 3s. per doz.
4 yds. galloon lace at 1s. per yd.
1 pr. shoes with galoshoes, 3s. 4d.

THE WOMEN

By this period starched ruffs, steeple-crowned hats, the rigid stomacher, and the stately farthingale were all banished to the region of forgetfulness, and a studied *négligé* style took the place of prim formality. It is true that when Catherine of Braganza arrived in England she wore her Portuguese farthingale, but it was soon discarded in favour of the English dress; she fought, however, gallantly to keep the dresses short, as she was particularly fond of showing her feet. The paintings of Sir Peter Lely acquaint us with every detail of the female dress, and we give in Fig. 388, Pl., a copy of a picture by that artist representing Nell Gwynn. The prevailing character of the costume is one of unconfined ease; her ringlets hang loosely upon her exposed neck, which is quite innocent of the transparent lawn of the band or the partlet. The gown is striking by its very simplicity, the sleeves being merely looped material covering the under sleeves of lawn. Trains became fashionable in 1663, and hats adorned with feathers were usual. In 1665 Mrs. Pepys paraded the streets in her fashionable "yellow bird's-eye hood."

In 1664 a bull-head fringe or "taure" was the mode, but in the majority of Lely's portraits, curls at irregular intervals upon the head form the fringe. Jewellery was not much in demand, with the exception of pearls. The buying of dozens of pairs of gloves was a fashionable form of extravagance (*vide* Chirk Castle accounts, pp. 295, &c.). About 1670, false locks came into fashion, which are termed puffs by Mrs. Pepys, who much admired them. Randall Holme gives the accompanying figure of a lady with a pair of locks

and curls (Fig. 389). He says they were set on wires to
make them stand out at a distance from the head. We can
hardly imagine that we have a representation here of the
much-talked-of Creve-cœurs (Heart-breakers) or Meurtriers

(Murderers), to which the gallants of the
court were always making sonnets. A specimen of a lady's dress about the middle of
the reign is here given (Fig. 390), which does
not call for special comment. The dresses
of the lower classes seem to point to the fact

FIG. 389.—Project-
ing locks. (Ran-
dall Holme.)

that they were of a thrifty nature, since the Grand Duke
Cosmo states that English women of the lowest rank wore
good clothes. Ladies frequently made their own costumes.
On Christmas Day in 1668 Mrs. Pepys sat up undressed
until ten o'clock at night, altering and
lacing a black petticoat; while one
gentleman, we are told, devised an in-
toxicating method of diversion by sitting
up unpicking dresses with his wife. The
female citizen wore a grograin gown, a
straight hood, little ringlets upon her
forehead, and a small pinner of lace—
"to make her look saint-like."

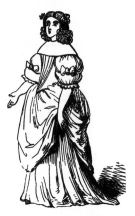

In the Duke of Newcastle's comedy,
"The Triumphant Widow," 1677, a
countryman's sweetheart is promised " a
white fustian waistcoat and a brave

FIG. 390.—Costume, c. 1675.

stammel petticoat, regarded with black velvet." In the
same comedy mention is made of " a Gingerline cloth cloke
with an olive plush cape bound about with a little silver
galloon lace."

A kind of large cloak or overall used by the ladies in 1676 was called the " semeare " or " mantua "; it had short sleeves, which were sometimes gathered up to the top of the shoulders, and there fastened with a jewel or button and loop.

CHAPTER XXI

JAMES II., 1685-1688. WILLIAM and MARY, 1688-1702

THE two reigns of James II. and William can hardly be separated so far as costume is concerned, for no appreciable novelty of a distinguishing character was introduced to differentiate it from the reign of Charles II. The only

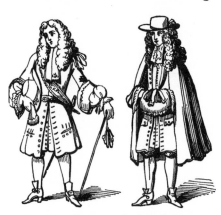

FIG. 391.—Summer and winter fashions, *temp.* William III.

remark that can be made is perhaps the following, —that so far as men's clothing is concerned, the reign of the precisian absolute had commenced. During the Mediæval Period it was quite possible for the tailoress to make the garments then worn; from Henry VII. to Charles II. the tailor and the tailoress could be employed; from James II. to the present day the tailor alone has been concerned. The exact cut of the cloth, and the indispensable pressing of seams and folds necessitated the art and strength of the precisian, and he has reigned indisputably since that period, even encroaching at times upon the domain of the tailoress.

The summer and winter costumes of a gentleman are well shown in Fig. 391. The petticoat breeches died a natural death, and were replaced by a more tightly fitting garment which reached below the knee. The stockings were made to draw over them, and sometimes reached to the middle of the thigh. The periwig became, if possible, more monstrous than ever, probably to compensate to some extent for the loss of the moustache, which now followed the way of the beard, which had disappeared some years previously. In Vanbrugh's " Relapse," 1697, Lord Foppington tells his wigmaker, who assures him that

he has put twenty ounces of hair into his wig: "A periwig to a man should be like a mask to a woman, nothing should be seen but his eyes." In 1698, Misson says of the gentlemen, " Their *perruques* and their habits were charged with powder, like millers, and their faces daubed with snuff."

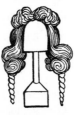

FIG. 392.—Campaign wig with dildoes on either side, 1684.

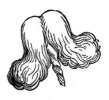

FIG. 393.—Wig showing the origin of the pig-tail.

In " Letters from the Dead to the Living," by Thomas Brown, we find the following choice morsel: " We met three flaming beaux of the first magnitude; he in the middle made a most magnificent figure,—his perriwig was large enough to have loaded a camel, and he had bestowed upon it at least a bushel of powder." A curious variety of robbery came into force; precautions were issued to those walking the streets of London to be careful of their wigs, as they were liable to be stolen from the head. Holme, in his " Academy of Armoury," has engraved a *campaign* wig, and says, "it hath knots or bobs, a *dildo* on each side, with a curl'd fore-

head," and is illustrated in Fig. 392.　These dildoes or pole-
locks, when hung from the centre of the long periwig,

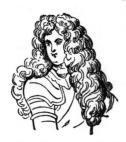

form without doubt the origin of the
pig-tail (Fig. 393).　For tightening the
curls of wigs, small rollers of pipeclay
called bilboquets or roulettes were used.
The curls were wound tightly round these
whilst very hot.　A fine specimen of the
voluminous periwig is shown in Fig.

FIG. 394.—George, Earl　394, whilst the utility of the article was
of Albemarle.　ably demonstrated by the wigmaker of
those days, who hired a sign-painter to depict Absalom
hanging on a tree, and relieved his soul in the following
choice lines :

> " O Absalom ! O Absalom !
> O Absalom, my son !
> If thou hadst worn a periwig,
> Thou hadst not been undone ! "

Hats.—The broad brims of the hats were now frequently turned up on two sides, and were ornamented by
several colours placed round them or by bows of ribbon.
There were different modes of cocking the hat, as it was
termed, one being called the Monmouth cock, after the
unfortunate Duke.　Hats were often carried under the left
arm, as the periwig sometimes rendered it awkward to
place it in its usual position.

Cravats of Brussels or Flanders lace were worn by the
nobility and men of fashion : they were of great length, and
the ends were generally passed through the button-holes
of the waistcoat.　Small bands were also introduced called
Geneva bands, and took the place of the previous wide

falling variety. Shoe buckles were substituted for roses
or rosettes. The accompanying print of William III.,
dating from 1694 (Fig. 395), will give an idea of the dress
of the King and of the nobility; while the costume of the
commonalty at the commencement of this period may be
gathered from Fig. 396. A beau of the later period is
described by Misson in his "Travels in England," 1697,

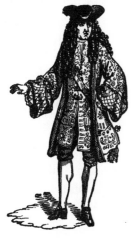

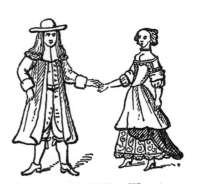

FIG. 396.—Early William III. costume.

FIG. 395.—King William
III., 1694.

as "a creature compounded of a perriwig and a coat laden
with powder as white as a miller's; a face besmeared with
snuff, and a few affected airs." The fashion of taking snuff
was universal. Tom Brown mentions one "whose long
lace cravat was most agreeably discoloured with snuff from
top to bottom." To take snuff and to offer a box gracefully was part of a beau's education. One, who is described
as being more periwig than man, has his occupation very
fairly defined; he has to chat an hour with a mask in a

side-box, then whip behind the scenes, bow to a fool in the pit, take snuff, and talk to the actresses. This intellectual ideal is represented in Fig. 397.

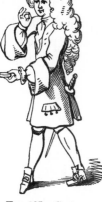

FIG. 397.—Costume, c. 1700.

THE WOMEN

During the reign of James II. the dress of the women underwent no alteration, but a few Dutch fashions were introduced, as was but natural, upon the accession of William III. The Queen is represented in Fig. 398, where her costume, from two prints of the period, is well seen. The bodice of the robe is worn higher in the neck, and the full sleeve of the robe was superseded by a tight one with the cuff above the elbow, in imitation of the coats of the gentlemen. From beneath the cuffs fell a

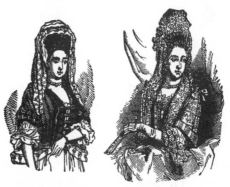

FIG. 398.—From two portraits of Queen Mary.

profusion of lace and lawn in the shape of ruffles and lappets, which partly covered a long glove.

Commode.—At this time the commode, which had been fashionable in France for about twenty years, appeared in England, and is shown in Fig. 399. It consisted of rows of lace stuck bolt upright over the forehead, and shooting upwards one over the other in a succession of plaits, diminishing in width as they rose. From these erections long streaming lappets hung down over the shoulders, while

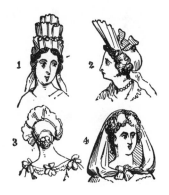

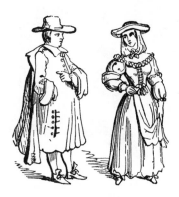

FIG. 399.—Head-dresses, *c.* 1685.

FIG. 400.—Costume of the commonalty, *c.* 1685.

the hair was combed upwards as if to give some support to the head-dress. Varieties are given in the illustration, the last one showing a hood which the ladies wore when the commode was absent. The other portions of the dress may be gleaned from the illustrations to this chapter. A milkmaid of the period is shown in Fig. 400 talking to a farmer, and the influence of the Dutch fashion in dress is well shown in the formality of the costumes of both. We append a selection from "Cryes of London," by Tempest, which appeared at this period; the illustrations depict the itinerant sellers and other characters to be seen in the

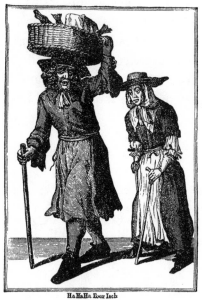

Ha Ha Ha Poor Iack

FIG. 401.—Tempest's "Cryes of London,"
1688–1711.

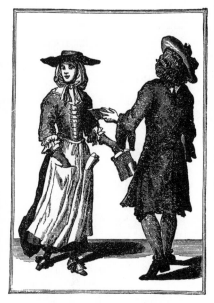

FIG. 402.—Tempest's "Cryes of London,"
1688–1711.

streets of London. They are extremely valuable by reason
of their evident fidelity (Figs. 401, 402).

CHAPTER XXII

ANNE, 1702–1714

THE MEN

THE square-cut coat was rather shorter than in the previous period, and the long flapped waistcoat to the knees remained in fashion during the reign of this Queen, the only innovation being the pockets inserted in them; both coats and waistcoats were embroidered, while the button-holes, as a rule, were beautifully frogged. A material composed of wool or linen twill, and faced with satin, which came into vogue during the time of Elizabeth, and termed Calimanco, now came into fashion for waistcoats, a rich design being worked on one side only. The stockings were still drawn up over the knee, and covered a considerable portion of the breeches—they were, however, gartered below the knee. Large turned-back cuffs, square and wide, and hanging lace ruffles distinguish the sleeves; while the skirts of the coat were stiffened out with wire, buckram, and whalebone, thus showing the hilt of the sword, which no longer depended from a baldrick. The stockings were generally

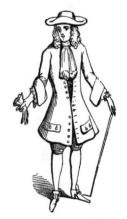

FIG. 403.—Reigns of Queen Anne and George I.

coloured, the prevailing tints being blues and reds; these were inserted in square-toed shoes with red heels and small buckles. Different kinds of wigs were in use, such as very long accurately curled perukes, bagwigs, nightcaps, wigs, and black riding wigs. The hats were small and three-cornered, and laced with gold or silver galloon, sometimes being decorated with feathers (Fig. 403). In 1703 a boy of the middle rank of life was missing, and the description of his dress was as follows: " He is of a fair complexion, light-brown lank hair, having on a dark brown frieze coat, double-breasted on each side, with black buttons and button-holes; a light drugget waistcoat, red shag breeches striped with black stripes, and black stockings."

THE WOMEN

During the first part of the reign the general aspect of the dress was identical with that of William and Mary. The towering erections upon their heads (the commode) were still in fashion, but the dress generally became flounced and furbelowed, so that every part appeared as if it had been subjected to a process of curling. Malcolm says in his anecdotes of " The Manners and Customs of London in the Eighteenth Century ": " The ladies must have exhibited a wonderful appearance in 1709 ; behold one equipped in a black silk petticoat, with a red and white calico border, cherry coloured stays trimmed with blue and silver, a red and dove coloured damask gown flowered with large trees, a yellow satin apron trimmed with white Persian (silk), and muslin head cloths with crow-foot edging, double ruffles with fine edging, a black silk furbelowed scarf, and a spotted hood!" About 1709 the ladies' dresses began to heave and swell, and attain to large proportions, and in 1710 hoops assisted in the distention. Addison says: "The whole sex is now dwarfed and shrunk into a race of beauties that seems almost another species. I remember several ladies who were once very near seven foot high, that at present want some inches to five. How they came to be thus curtailed I cannot learn; whether the whole sex be at present under any penance which we know nothing of, or whether they have cast their head-dresses in order to surprise us with something in that kind which shall be entirely new, though I find most are of opinion they are at present like trees lopped and pruned that

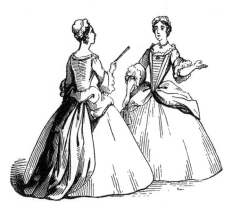

FIG. 404.—Costumes, 1718.

will certainly sprout up and flourish with greater heads than before." In 1711 Sir Roger de Coverley, referring to his family pictures, says: "You see, Sir, my great-great-grandmother has on the new fashioned petticoat, except that the modern is gathered at the waist; my grandmother appears as if she stood in a large drum, whereas the ladies now walk as if they were in a go-cart." The new-fashioned petticoat is engraved here (Fig. 404); it widens out gradually from the waist to the ground, while the dress is looped up round the body in front, and falls down in loose folds behind. A writer says: "Nothing can be imagined more unnatural, and consequently less agreeable.   When a slender woman stands upon a basis so exorbitantly wide, she resembles a funnel, a figure of no great elegancy." The general appearance of the ladies with commodes and hooped petticoats may be gathered from Sutton Nichol's view of Hampton Court Palace.

A lady's riding-dress was advertised in 1711, "of blue camlet, well laced with silver." With a petticoat of the same stuff, she wore a smartly-cocked beaver hat edged with silver, and rendered more sprightly by a feather; her hair was curled and powdered, and tied like that of a rakish young gentleman with a long streaming scarlet ribbon.   On these occasions they assumed the male periwig, in addition to the coat, hat, and feather, which fully excuses Sir Roger de Coverley when, upon looking at the hat, coat, and waistcoat of the young sporting lady, he was about to call her Sir, but luckily casting his eye lower, he saw the petticoat beneath, and addressed her as Madam.   A lady in 1712 advertised the following losses: " A green silk knit waistcoat, with gold and silver flowers all over it, and about fourteen yards of gold and silver thick lace on it, and a petticoat of rich strong flowered satin red and white, all in great flowers or leaves, and scarlet flowers with black specks brocaded in, raised high, like velvet or shag." How cheaply the poor could dress at this period can be seen from an entry in the parish accounts of Sprowston, Norfolk, 1719 : "Paid for clading of the Widow Bernard with a gown, petticoat, bodice, hose, shoes, apron, and stomacher, £0, 18s. 6d."

CHAPTER XXIII

GEORGE I., 1714–1727. GEORGE II., 1727–1760

THE reign of George I. did not see many marked peculiarities introduced. The King, naturally heavy and stolid, was not inclined to follow the freaks of fashion himself, or to encourage others to do so, while the absence of a Queen from the court hindered that habitual centre of fashion from producing anything noteworthy. The King was old, and the act preventing the granting of honours to foreigners did not encourage German nobility to visit England. It is true that the peace permitted intercourse with France, but it was seldom taken advantage of. An ex-

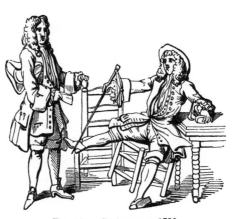

FIG. 405.—Costumes, c. 1720.

quisite of 1737 is stated to have been dressed in a "fine linen shirt, the ruffles and bosom of Mechlin lace; a small wig, with an enormous queue or tail; his coat well garnished with lace; black velvet breeches; red heels to his shoes, and gold clocks to his stockings; his hat beneath his arm, a sword by his side, and himself well scented!" In the foregoing figure (Fig. 405) we have an exquisite represented lolling upon two chairs with a tasselled cane in one hand and a snuff-box in the other. The heaviness of the whole costume is well shown upon the other figure, with its ample folds, large pockets, and wide cuffs. The seated figure has his coat buttoned at the waist in accordance with the fashion of the day, thereby showing a wide opening reaching to the neck, disclosing the lace cravat. A general idea of the ordinary costume, together with the well-dressed, may be formed from the following account of a company of all conditions assembled in "The Folly," a floating music-room and house of entertainment on the Thames, opposite Somerset House: "At the north end were a parcel of brawny fellows with mantles about their shoulders and blue caps upon their heads. Next to them sat a company of clownish-looking fellows, with leather breeches and hob-nailed shoes. Just about the organ, which stood in the south-east part of the room, stood a vast many dapper sparks, with huge powdered perrukes, red-heeled shoes, laced cravats, and brocade waistcoats, intermingled, like a chess board, with men in dark long habits, whose red faces were covered with large broad-brim'd hats."

The reign of George II. also was not distinguished by any innovations which may be termed national; variations only occurred in the prevailing mode of dress, which left them at the end of the reign not much altered in appearance from the commencement. The great rage during the reign for pastoral plays and court masques, wherein the simplicity of milkmaids was imitated by great ladies disporting diamonds, and simple shepherds acted by noblemen with golden crooks, caused for a time a modelling of the civil

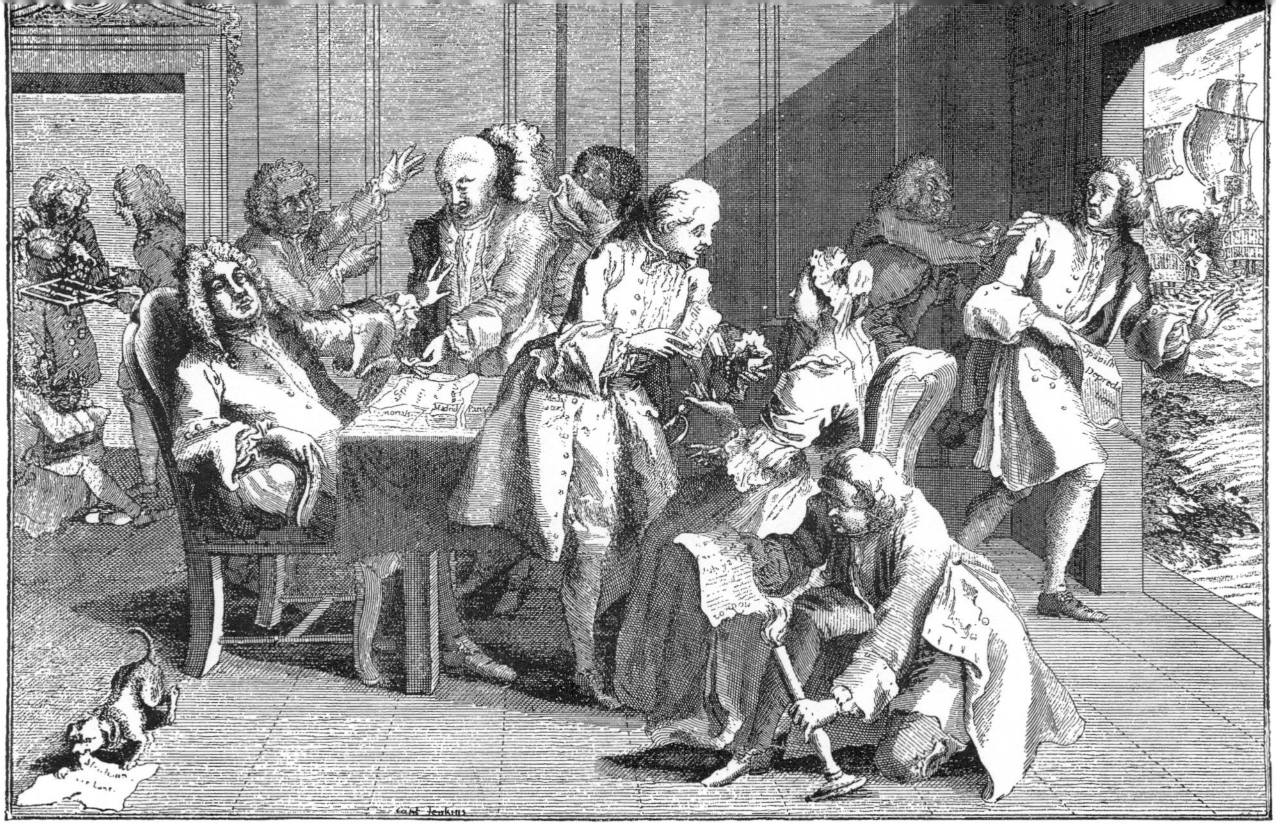

Fig. 408.—Satire on Walpole, 1738.

dress upon simpler lines, but this did not prevail throughout the reign however. In Fig. 406 we have a group dating from the year 1739, which affords us an excellent contrast

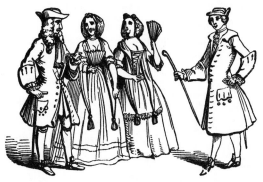

FIG. 406.—Costumes, 1739.

between an old gentleman who wears a full-bottomed tie-wig, a large cocked hat, and a laced cravat with ends which would do well for the year 1720. Opposite we have the fashion of the day as shown upon a young spark whose wig is exceedingly small, as likewise his hat; the coat collar turns over in a broad fold upon the shoulders, and the cuffs of his coat reach to above the elbow. But the great distinction between the two figures is the disproportionate length of the skirts, which are long and

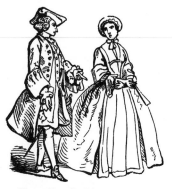

FIG. 407.—Costumes, c. 1744.

ample, and reach to the calf of the leg. A print dated 1744 is given (Fig. 407), which illustrates the progress made in costume during five years. The skirts of the coat are still very wide, and expanded by means of buckram or wire, but the cuffs and the hat have returned to the older fashion, the wig, however, still remaining small. A satire upon Walpole, dated 1738, may not be out of place here, as it affords valuable examples of costume (Fig. 408, Pl.).

The wigs and hats of the period form a study in themselves. No. 1 in Fig. 409 is the extreme of fashion about

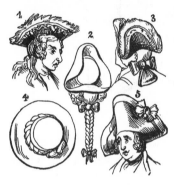

FIG. 409.

1. Fashionable hat, *c.* 1740. 2. Usual cocking, *c.* 1740. 3. Cocking and bagwig, 1745. 4. Clergyman's hat, 1745. Kevenhuller hat, 1745.

1740, and is worn by the dissipated husband in Hogarth's "Marriage à la Mode." A deep edging of gold lace ornaments the brim, which is further decorated by a row of feathers. No. 2 exhibits the form of cocking then adopted; the particular turn given to the brim is known as the Ramilie cock, and the wig, which is plaited in a queue with a black tie at the top and also at the bottom, is called the Ramilie wig. That this style was in fashion for many years may be gleaned from the fact that the battle of Ramilies was fought in 1706. No. 3 shows us a plainer and more decisively cocked hat in fashion in 1745, together with a bagwig below it. No. 4 is not cocked in any way; a broad band of twisted black cloth surrounds it, fastened by a bow at the side. It is represented by Hogarth upon the head of a clergyman. No. 5 is the large Kevenhuller hat; it was generally of extravagant proportions, and patronised by military men and bullies about town—the gentlemanly blackguards known as the

Mohocks, Bloods, &c., indigenous to that period. The particular cock to this hat generally indicated the disposition of the man who wore it. In 1753, the transformation of a country bumpkin into a full-blown blood is thus described :

"I cut off my hair and produced a brown bob periwig of Wilding, of the same colour, with a single row of curls just below the bottom, which I wore very nicely combed and without powder. My hat, which had been cocked with great exactness in an equilateral triangle, I discarded, and purchased one of a more fashionable size, the fore corner of which projected near two inches further than those on each side, and was moulded into the shape of a spout." However, we find he altered his hat, for we are told " it no longer resembled a spout, but the corner of a minced pye."

THE WOMEN

The fashions in women's dress are so multitudinous at this time, and change with such chameleon-like quickness, that we are only able to point out a few chief points among a host of others. The hoop petticoat, although it frequently changed its fashion, was persistent throughout, and the following three figures illustrate it at intervals of ten years, from 1735 (Fig. 410). Thus, in 1735,

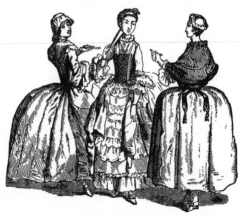

FIG. 410.—Costumes.

1. (Left), 1735.   2. (Centre), 1745.   3. (Right), 1755.

the petticoat was short, the gown was without a train, and the general appearance was that of a bell; it probably was the most hideous form of a hideous dress. By 1745 the hoop had considerably increased at the sides, and diminished in front; and a pamphlet of the time refers to it as "an enormous abomination." It is also seen in Fig. 411, and still further illustrated in Fig. 412, from which we can fully justify the caricaturists of the day in their assertions that ladies

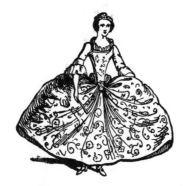

FIG. 411.—Costume, 1746.

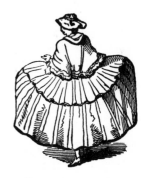

FIG. 412.—Costume, 1746.

looked like donkeys carrying panniers. But perhaps the greatest extent to which this fashion was carried is dealt with and illustrated in "The Review," from which we select a figure as a good sample (Fig. 412). The print exhibits the inconvenience of the hooped petticoat, and suggests methods to remedy it, such as a coach with a movable roof, and a derrick with ropes and pulleys to drop the lady into it, &c. The hoops were of whalebone, and had to be doubled up in front or lifted at the sides when the wearer entered a door; and when seated they occupied the space usually allotted for half-a-dozen of the male sex. Such a torrent of invective was levelled at the hooped petticoat, that ten years after it had almost disappeared (*vide* No. 3, Fig. 410); but before its departure it added one more atrocity to the long list of which it was guilty, in the *sacque*, a wide loose gown open in front, which hung free of the body from the shoulders to the ground, and was gathered up in great folds over the hooped petticoat. An idea of this caricature of dress may be gleaned from Fig.

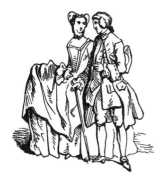 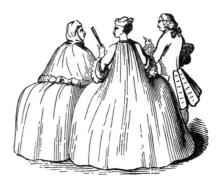

FIG. 413.—Costumes, 1750.

FIG. 414.—Costumes, end of reign of George II. (1753).

413. If we refer to Fig. 406, we note that the gowns in 1739 are extremely plain, and that scarves were worn with tasselled ends; the high commode has disappeared, and aprons or pinners are worn. This simplicity respecting the gown is due to the milkmaid fashion, and is still further shown in Fig. 383, dating from 1744. Before finally bidding adieu to the hooped petticoat, we append an illustration (Fig. 414) showing how this distortion appeared when viewed from the rear and covered with a sacque; it dates from 1753. Its popularity prob-

ably declined owing to a pamphlet which was published against it, entitled "The Enormous Abomination of the Hoop Petticoat as the Fashion now is."

Caps and straw hats flourished, and capuchons replaced the hoods of former reigns.

CHAPTER XXIV

GEORGE III., 1760-1820

THE MEN

THE style of dress for gentlemen in 1760 may be described as comparatively simple, differing in no essential particular from that preceding it, except as regards the large quantity of lace with which it was adorned, and by a small black cravat. A writer in the *St. James'* *Chronicle* of 1763 describes the costume of a man who was aping his betters and appeared in "a coat loaded with innumerable gilt buttons; the cuffs cut in the shape of a sea-officer's uniform, and, together with the pockets, mounting no less than twenty-four. The skirts were remarkably long, and the cape so contrived as to make him appear very round about the shoulders. To this he had a scarlet waistcoat, with a narrow gold lace, double lapelled; a pair of doe-skin breeches that came half-way down his leg, and were almost met by a pair of shoes that reached about three inches and a quarter above his ankles. His hat was of the true Kevenhuller size, and of course decorated with a gold button and loop. His hair was cropped very short behind, and thinned about the middle in such a manner as to make room for a stone stock-buckle of no ordinary dimensions. To complete the picture, he carried a little rattan cane in his hand"—and was by

trade—a blacksmith! In 1770 we have the following illustration of dress (Fig. 415) taken from the *Lady's Magazine,*
where the figure on the right is dressed in a bagwig, lace
ruffles, and a black solitaire, *i.e.* a broad black ribbon
worn round the neck, and extremely fashionable. In the
same year appeared the Nivernois; it was exceedingly
small, with the flaps fastened up to the shallow crown by
hooks and eyes. The corner worn in front was of the old

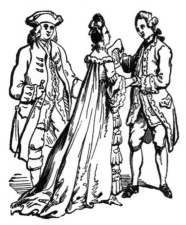 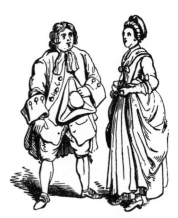

FIG. 415.—Costumes, 1770.   FIG. 416.—Country folk, 1772.

spout shape and stiffened out by wire. The gentleman
seen upon the left is in a bobwig, cocked hat, top-boots,
and the loose dress of a country squire. The plain
country folk of 1772 are shown in Fig. 416, where the man's
dress is remarkable as fitting only where it touches. There
are heavy folds in every part of the dress, no wig, and the
neckcloth has a loose twist—the habit altogether speaks of
capacious easiness.

The founding of the Macaroni Club in London marks
an epoch in the evolution of English dress. A number of

young men of the fashionable world, who had been travelling in Italy, formed this association in 1772, in opposition to the well-known Beef-Steak Club, and the devotees of this association were known as Macaronies. The peculiarities of the male and also the female *genus* of the Macaroni species may be seen in Fig. 417. The hair is drawn up-wards in a large toupee with rolled curls at the sides;

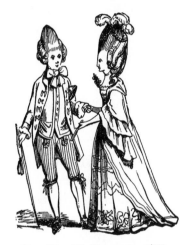
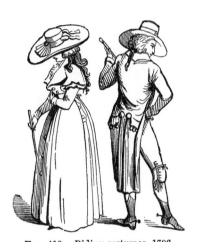

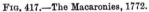

FIG. 417.—The Macaronies, 1772.   FIG. 418.—Riding costumes, 1786.

behind, it was made into an enormous knob which rested upon the back of the neck, and upon the whole of it the extremely small hat was worn. Round the neck a large white scarf was tied in a bow, from beneath which the protruding frills of the shirt appeared. The waistcoat was much shortened, as was also the coat, which was edged with lace or braid, and was decorated with frog buttons, tassels, and embroidery. The breeches shown are of striped silk, with bunches of strings at the knee. Silk stockings and small shoes were worn, while two watches were carried, one in each waistcoat pocket, from which depended large bunches of seals. In 1786 we find another fashion introduced, as seen in Fig. 418, where an exceedingly long sparrow-tailed coat, tight breeches, and a round broad-

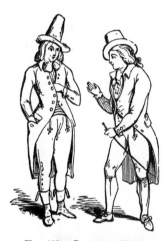

brimmed hat are the chief points. The next great change in gentlemen's dress after the Macaroni style, is that which was introduced at the time of the French Revolution, and is delineated in Fig. 419. The personage upon the left is habited in immaculate Parisian style, even to the sugar-loaf hat; his flowing hair is powdered, and he wears a loose cravat, frilled shirt, a white waistcoat with horizontal stripes, and a coat with wide and long skirts; the breeches,

FIG. 419.—Costumes, 1793.

which are tight, reach to the ankles, being buttoned up at the sides to mid-thigh. Low top-boots are worn. The second figure has the cone of the hat truncated, and the loose hair is tied in a club behind; the ruffles are very small, and his knee-breeches are of buckskin. The shoes are tied with laces, buckles having gone out of fashion.

THE WOMEN

At the beginning of the reign of George III. the ladies dressed very simply, even their hoops being of unpretending dimensions. Fig. 420 represents the costume of 1760. She wears a long-waisted gown laced over the stomacher, with

short sleeves to the elbow, where very full ruffles are displayed. Upon her head is a small "gipsy hat." Referring
to Fig. 415, which dates from 1770 (ten years later), the
lady is shown in the leading fashion; she wears a very
simple form of head-dress, a plain toupee turned up in a
club behind, and secured to the crown of the head by a
large bow of ribbon; round her neck is a tie of puffed
ribbon, a very fashionable orna-
ment. The gown, or polonese,
as it was termed, is open in

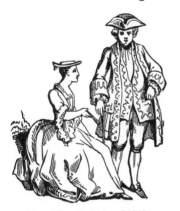 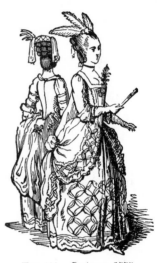

Fig. 420.—Costume of 1760.   Fig. 421.—Costume, 1775.

front, and, setting out fully behind, shows the petticoat,
which is covered with rows of furbelows beneath it. The
sleeve is short, having deep lace depending from it. Another
good example of the polonese may be seen in Fig. 421, where
it is looped up at the sides, thus showing the elaborate petticoat more clearly. It is easily seen that the polonese is
simply a modification of the sacque worn during the previous
reign. The sacque is distinctly seen in the larger figure.
The bodice is worn high behind, and low in the front, and

decorated with twists of gold and silver.   It is tightly
confined in corsets, strengthened with steel "busks."   It
was the fashion to educate girls in stiffness of manner at
all public schools, and particularly to cultivate a fall in
the shoulders, and an upright set of the bust.   The place
of the bunch of flowers in the above example was occupied
at schools by a long stocking-needle, to prevent girls from
spoiling their shapes by stooping too much over their work,
for the point of the needle ran into the chin if the head
was bent.   The sleeves worn by the second lady will be
seen to be decorated with rows of plaited ribbon of a
different colour from the gown; bows of silk ribbon tie
up the dress behind ; and it will be perceived that smaller
hoops are worn by both ladies.

In the *Lady's Magazine*, 1774, we are told, "The hair
is dressed very backward and low, with large flat puffs
on the top ; toupee not so low.   A bag, but rather more
round.   Three long curls, or about six small puffs, down
the sides.   Powder almost universal.   Pearl pins and Italian
lappets filigreed with flowers, which give them a very
becoming look.   This is quite a new fancy of Lady
Almeria C—— (Almeria Carpenter, a famous leader of
fashion).   Round the neck, German collars or pearls.   Sacques,
a beautiful new palish blue, or a kind of dark lilac satin.
Trimmings, large puffs down the sides with chenille, silver
or gold or blonde.   Stomacher crossed with silver or gold
cord.   Fine lace ruffles ; satin embroidered shoes, with
diamond roses ; small drop earrings ; Turkey handkerchiefs.
Trimming of the gown, white tissue or brown satin."

Head-dresses.—These were so many and varied, that
it would be a physical impossibility to enumerate them all.

The true Macaroni style, which appeared in 1772, will be distinctly seen upon referring back to Fig. 417, where the arrangement of the coiffure is almost identical with that of the gentleman. The hair was drawn over a very high cushion of wire, the top of the toupee being decorated with a plume or large feather, from the base of which depended festoons of *French curls* that resembled eggs strung on a wire. Behind, the hair was generally curled all over. The quantities of powder and pomatum required at this period to build up a lady's head, rendered it impossible to dress the hair every day. Frequently the coiffure remained untouched and perfect for a week, a fortnight, or more. One writer observes: "I consent, also, to the present fashion of curling the hair, so that it may stand a month without combing; though I must confess that I think three weeks, or a fortnight, might be a sufficient time. But I bar every application to those foreign artists who advertise that they have the secret of making up a lady's head for a quarter of a year." In a poem dated 1773, a lady's head-dress is described as

> " White as the covered Alps or wintry face
> Of snowy Lapland, her toupee uprear'd,
> Exhibits to the view a cumbrous mass
> Of curls high nodding o'er her polished brow."

The head-dresses worn by the ladies in Fig. 421 are curious. The first lady wears hers in a half-moon toupee, "brushed back tightly off the forehead, with large curls at the sides, and a very broad one under each ear ; a plume of stiff feathers surmounts the structure: "the fashion now is to erect the toupee into a high detached tuft like a cockatoo's crest, and this toupee they call the *physionomie*."

The other lady has her hair dressed in a great club, surmounted by rows of overhanging curls of large dimensions, above which an ornamental bandeau is placed, from
which hang two lace lappets.

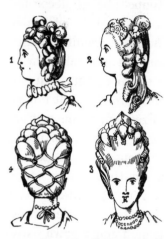

FIG. 422.—Coiffures.

1, 2, *circa* 1768.   3, 4, *circa* 1772.

In the *London Magazine*,
1775, we read that "the ladies'
hair was, with few exceptions,
a kind of half-moon toupee,
with two long curls, the second
depending opposite each other
below the ear; the hind part was
dressed as usual, for few ladies
had the addition of broad braided
bands crossing each other, as if
to confine as well as ornament
the back of the head which now
appears at inferior places of
public resort." This method of
decorating the back of the head
will be seen in Fig. 422, and, judging by the above, had
become vulgar.

But probably the most extraordinary invention for the
adornment of the head was that of the *capriole*. An old
poet thus speaks of this fantastical coiffure:

> " Here, on a fair one's head-dress, sparkling sticks,
>   Swinging on silver springs a coach and six;
>   There on a sprig or slop'd pourpon, you see
>   A chariot, pulky, chaise, or vis-à-vis."

And again in the same poem we read:

> " Nelly ! where is the creature fled ?
>   Put my post-chaise upon my head."

In a work written about 1760 we read: "Be it remembered that in this year many ladies of fortune and fashion, willing to set an example of prudence and economy to their inferior, did invent and make public, without a patent, a machine for the head, in form of a post-chaise and horses, and another imitating a chair and chairman, which were frequently worn by persons of distinction." Another description of this fashion is equally interesting: "Those heads which are not able to bear a coach and six so far act consistently as to make use of a post-chariot, or a single-horse chaise with a beau perching in the middle. . . . The vehicle itself was constructed of gold threads, and was drawn by six dapple greys of brown glass, with a coachman, postilion, and gentleman within, of the same brittle manufacture."

In the *Lady's Magazine* of 1776, the fashion writer notifies that "ladies' hair in front is high and thrown back; not so broad as has been worn; the hind hair in a puff bag with slab curls above it, and intermixed with white tiffany and beads. Turbans more the taste than caps, with large coloured roses. Lace and pearl feathers. Large wing caps; chip hats ornamented with lace, stars, roses, flowers, and fruit. . . . At Ranelagh many heads were lowered; and I with pleasure saw the Duchess of D.'s fine face ornamented more naturally, and with but three feathers instead of seven. Lady S.'s head was the most beyond the bounds of propriety, she having so many plates of fruit placed on the top pillar, and her hair being without powder it was not so delicate a mixture." Until 1785, the head-dress seems to have presented the most grotesque feature of a lady's dress, and to have constantly excited the ridicule of the press. Probably the maximum height of head-dress was attained in 1782, and one example is depicted in Fig. 423.

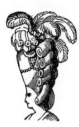

FIG. 423.—Head-dress, 1782.

In Fig. 424 is given a *calash* taken from a print dated 1780. It was made to work like the hood of a carriage, being pulled over the head by a string which was connected to the whalebone hoops. It was first introduced in 1765. No. 2 is a winter hat of black silk or other material, worn by women of the middle classes, and No. 1 gives us an idea of the ordinary flat hat of a country girl. It was trimmed with ribbon, and was worn by most women of the lower ranks. The last persons to discard this style were the fruit sellers and fisher women, to whom it was exceedingly convenient, as it allowed their baskets to repose safely upon the head. The whole process of hairdressing is given in the *London Magazine*, 1768. "False locks to supply deficiency of native hair, pomatum in profusion, greasy wool to bolster up the adopted locks, and grey powder to conceal dust." A lady was asked by her hairdresser, "How long it was since her head had been opened and repaired?" she answered, "not above nine week," to which he replied that, "that was as long as a head could well go in

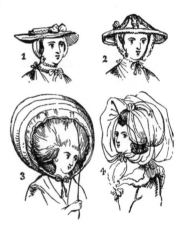

FIG. 424.

1. Country girl, 1773. 2. Winter hat of middle classes, 1773. 3. Lady's head-covering, 1780. 4. Lady's head-covering, 1786.

summer; and that therefore it was proper to deliver it now, as it began to be a little *hasardé*." The description of the opening of the hair, and the disturbance thereby occasioned to its numerous inhabitants, is too revolting for modern readers; but the various advertisements of poisonous compounds for their destruction, and the constant notice of these facts, prove that it is no exaggeration. Persons who are sceptical on many subjects of costume, and who doubt the accuracy of the old illuminators and sculptors in their representations of the female head-dress of their own times, would do well to consider whether any fashion more ugly or disgusting can be found than this, in vogue so very recently, or that looks more like caricature.

About the year 1786 the heads of the ladies began to lower, and the hair was allowed to fall down the back; a fashion attributed to the taste of the reigning portrait painters of the day, with Sir Joshua at their head. Hats were worn with tremendous brims both back and front, with flat crowns and plumes of feathers, having broad silk ribbons tied under the chin. Fig. 418 exhibits a lady in riding dress wearing such a hat, which is trimmed with large bows of silk ribbons round the crown; her hair is powdered and "frizzed" at the sides, but long curls repose on the shoulders and back. In 1788 the powdered wig, or natural hair, was arranged as wide as it was before high, in a series of large curls all round the head, the hair beneath at the back flowing down to the waist in loose curls.

In 1789 the ladies began to get tired of wearing such a mass of hair, and a fashion was introduced of frizzing it all over with pendent curls on the back and shoulders, and the high mob cap of the French peasants became a favourite. It was exceedingly ugly, as the lace with which it was trimmed fell over the features like a candle shade. An illustration of this mode is given in Fig. 425.

The fashionable riding dress of 1786 is shown in Fig. 418, which sufficiently explains itself. About 1790 the *buffont* was introduced, which consisted of white lawn or gauze, and projected to a great distance beneath the chin, like the breast of a pigeon (Fig. 425), while the little frilled

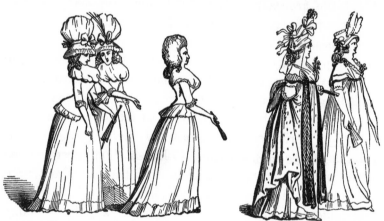

FIG. 425.—The buffont, 1790.   FIG. 426.—Costumes, 1796.

jacket and the tight sleeves showed what a lamentable lack of taste prevailed. No great novelty occurred in ladies' dress between the time when the Macaroni was introduced and the occurrence of the French Revolution; but shortly after the latter had commenced, we find that a distinctive style was evolved, of which the preceding illustration gives examples (Fig. 426). It will be seen that the waist appears under the arms, and a periodical at the time gives in its " Fashionable Information for Ladies in the Country," that the present fashion is " the most easy and graceful imaginable—it is simply this, the petticoat is tied round the neck and the arms put through the pocket holes."

Although at that time (1796) the hoop had been discarded in everyday life, it appeared regularly at court, and one noble lady of that time is represented in Fig. 427.

The costumes and head-gear which characterised the latter half of the eighteenth century were so multitudinous in varieties, and so Protean in shape, that we have only been able to indicate briefly their salient features. To go fully into details, and to accurately describe the changes, as we hope we have done in the Mediæval Period, is impossible in the limited space at our disposal; while to deal with the dress of the nineteenth century, and attempt to do justice to it, would necessitate a separate volume. Luckily for those

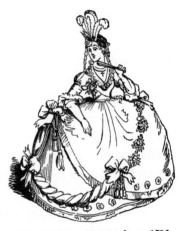

Fig. 427.—Lady's court dress, 1796.

who are interested in late costumes, abundant sources of supply are to hand, in many fashion plates and illustrated periodicals, which are to be found preserved in numberless local museums and libraries, not to speak of those embodied in family household treasures. Thus, having brought the student to the threshold of the nineteenth century, so far as civil costume is concerned, we say "Farewell," feeling sure that the examples of development in dress as traced in the past will prove of material assistance in comprehending those of later dates.

SECOND PART

ECCLESIASTICAL DRESS

CHAPTER XXV

THE SAXON PERIOD

The rule introduced by St. Augustine into England was the Benedictine, he being a Prior of a continental monastery under that order. But many missionaries came from the great foundation at Iona and subsequently from Lindisfarne, and consequently we find that, until the ninth century, the numerous monasteries which sprang up in England were under various rules. At that time, however, St. Dunstan reduced them all to the rule of St. Benedict, which became practically universal in the southern part of England. The vestments of the clergy were, during the early part of the Saxon Period, characterised by their simplicity and the absence of colour, white prevailing in the majority of them. As a number of vestments occur in ecclesiastical dress, we append the following notice of each.

The Cap.—During the Saxon Period, a low round cap of white linen, encircled by a band of embroidery, was the covering for the head, but no particular name for it has been preserved. At times the infulæ are shown, which were two pendent bands of embroidered material hanging down on either side at the back and attached to the cap. The evolution of the mitre from this primitive cap will be dealt with in subsequent pages.

The Alb.—The most ancient of the vestments was the Alb, of white linen, which enveloped the entire person of the wearer; it did not open in front like a surplice, but was girded round the loins; the sleeves were comparatively tight. It derived its name from *tunica alba*, and when first used was a dignified white robe, though later it was made in various colours, fitting loosely to the person; during the ninth century, however, its flowing proportions became much curtailed, and it began to fit closer, until finally it assumed the dimensions which distinguished it in the Middle Ages. In the later form it was confined round the waist by a narrow girdle.

The Dalmatic.—This vestment surmounts the Alb, from which it differs only in the greater width of its sleeves and in reaching half-way between the knees and the ground, but as years went on it became a little shorter. It was originally white, but in the ninth century it was made in various colours, and subsequently followed that of the chasuble.

The Stole.—In the early Saxon Period this was termed the *orarium*, and was a narrow scarf adjusted about the neck so as to hang down in front nearly to the feet. It was originally of a white woollen material, but later was made in various colours, and much enriched with ornaments. It was worn directly over the alb, so that only the ends were exposed if the dalmatic were worn. If the latter vestment were omitted, the stole is seen in early examples to cross upon the chest, and to be tucked through the girdle on either side. The primitive use of the stole, as the word *orarium* signifies, was a handkerchief to wipe the face.

The Maniple.—This was a short species of stole depending from the left hand, being clasped between the thumb and first finger during the early periods; it was originally substituted to fulfil the purpose to which the stole itself had been applied. The " Golden Legend " says of St. Peter, that "he bare always a sudary (or maniple) with which he wiped the tears that ran from his eyes." The maniple, however, like the stole, soon became a mere decorative enrichment of the costume; it was accounted a badge of honour as early as the sixth century; in the ninth it was common to priests and deacons, and conceded to the sub-deacon in the eleventh.

The Chasuble.—This vestment was nearly circular in shape, being slightly pointed before and behind; it had an aperture in the middle for the head, and its ample folds rested on either side upon the arms: it was worn over the other vestments, and was always constructed of rich materials. In the earlier Saxon Period it was termed the *Planeta*, and is recorded as having been an ecclesiastical vestment as early as the sixth century. It is important to remember that the chasuble was essentially the Eucharistic vestment, and was only worn at mass.

The Amice.—This was an oblong piece of fine linen, having on one of its lateral edges an embroidered collar, which was turned over and brought round the neck, the ends of the amice itself being visible only where they crossed each other in front of the throat.

The Pallium or Pall.—This was a narrow scarf composed of fine lambswool, which was worn over the chasuble by archbishops only. It was embroidered with purple crosses patée fitchée: these crosses probably are derived from the series of small fibulæ or brooches with which the pall was originally attached to the chasuble. It was precisely the same both back and front, and may be described as a circle which fitted upon the shoulders with two depending bands.

The Ring was of very large proportions, and when gloves had been adopted was worn over them, being always shown upon the right hand. It probably dates from the seventh century or earlier.

The Sandals.—During the Saxon Period sandals were generally in use among the ecclesiastics, boots or shoes being the adoptions of a subsequent period.

The Crozier at this early date consisted of a small cross upon a staff; the pastoral staff of a bishop or abbot was surmounted by a simple crook.

The Monks.—In the illuminations of the Anglo-Saxon MSS. before the ninth century the monks are represented in gowns of different colours—dark brown, black, grey, &c.; when, however, in the ninth century St. Dunstan reduced them all to the rule of St. Benedict, the habit of that order naturally prevailed. It consisted of a white cassock, over which was worn a black gown reaching to the feet, with an ample hood attached to the collar. Subsequently a black scapular was added.

One of the most interesting manuscripts in the British Museum is that marked Harl. 2908, an illumination in which represents Abbot Elfnoth (died A.D. 980) presenting his book of prayer to St. Augustine, one of the patron saints of the monastery (Fig. 428, Pl.). The Saint is represented as an archbishop wearing the pallium over a purple chasuble, the high collar seen being probably the amice. Under the chasuble is a white dalmatic, which shows the wide sleeves very clearly. The two ends of the stole appear beneath the dalmatic, and particular attention should be paid to their shape. This excessive widening of the ends is characteristic of the Saxon Period.

The last vestment to be noticed is the *Alb*, which is of a blue colour.

Abbot Elfnoth wears a blue chasuble and a white amice and dalmatic, with a blue alb. The stockings worn were very high, and reached to the thighs. The deacon bearing the Abbot's pastoral staff is habited in a garment befitting his rank, namely, the dalmatic over the alb, the former being white, and the latter blue. The attendant deacons shown behind the Archbishop have green and crimson dalmatics respectively.

EARLY NORMAN PERIOD: WILLIAM I.

The dress of the clergy of this period is chiefly distinguished by the increase of ornamentation upon the robes of the superior ecclesiastics, and sumptuary laws were enacted to restrain this extravagance. It does not appear, however, that they were very effectual.

The Mitre.—During the Saxon Period the covering for the head consisted merely of a cap, as we have seen, but which, in this period, assumed much larger dimensions, and for the first time prominence is given to the infulæ. In later times these were frequently made of metal, and fixed by hinges. There can be no doubt that these infulæ originated in a band affixed to the lower part of the cap; by being brought round to the back and tied there, they kept the cap in position. A curious example is given by

Willemin, which will be sufficiently explained by the illustration (Fig. 429). The pendent ribbons attached to the glengarry, and also to the sailor's cap, in every probability had a similar origin. The mitre in its incipient form may be seen in Fig. 430, Pl., from Cott. MS. Nero C iv., where a depression in the centre has caused a small knob to become apparent on either side, which subsequently became the horns.

The Alb.—In this period the alb for the first time appears with orphreys, consisting of narrow bands round the hem of the garment, and also round the sleeves, which were often of very elaborate needlework.

FIG. 429.—Primitive infulæ.

The Dalmatic.—A variation in this garment from that of the Saxon occurred in the Norman Period, namely, the openings more or less wide, which were made at the sides. They formed a very distinctive feature. Encircling these openings, and also passing round the hem, a rich orphrey was introduced, and this was also used round the openings of the bell-shaped sleeves. The garment thus lost its original primitive simplicity, and was further enriched by embroidery of a decorative character, covering the whole of the vestment (Fig. 428, Pl.).

The Stole and the *Chasuble* differ but little from those of the Saxon Period, except in bearing more ornamentation. They were essentially garments pertaining to the deacon.

The Tunicle was the garment appropriated to the subdeacon; it was similar to the dalmatic, but rather shorter and less ornamented.

The Amice.—A novelty occurs occasionally in the

apparel of the amice, which forms an ornamental collar round the neck. The original use of the amice as a capuchon or hood may be mentioned; it was customary in France to wear it on the head from the Feast of All Saints until Easter, letting it fall back upon the shoulders during the Gospel; ecclesiastics also were in the habit of holding it for a second or two over their heads, at the time of putting it on, thus symbolising the helmet of the Christian knight.

THE MONASTIC ORDERS

The Clugniacs, founded in 910, at Cluny, in France, were first introduced into England at Lewes, in Sussex, where a priory was founded in 1077. This was one of the alien monasteries, once so prevalent in England, and generally governed by foreigners. Being a reformed order of Benedictines, the Clugniacs retained the black dress.

The Carthusians, founded in 1084, were habited entirely in a white cassock and hood, over which was worn a white scapular, with two very prominent bands, joining the front and back portions. The cloak, if worn, was of black material. The order was introduced into England during the Norman Period, but never became of great importance.

The Cistercians, founded in 1098, built their first monastery in England in the early part of the twelfth century, and though one of the reformed Benedictine orders, they wore a white cassock with cape and a small hood; when at public prayer, a white gown was thrown over these, and when abroad, a black one.

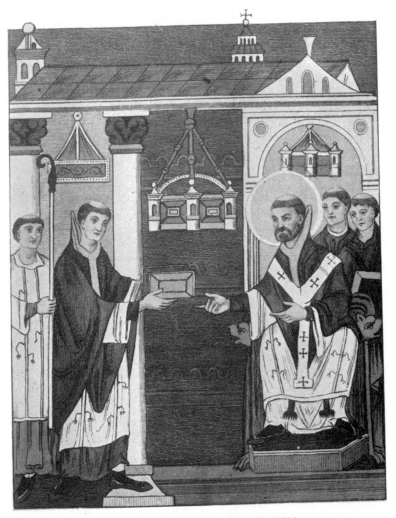

Fig. 428.—Abbot Elfnoth. (Harl. MS. 2908.)

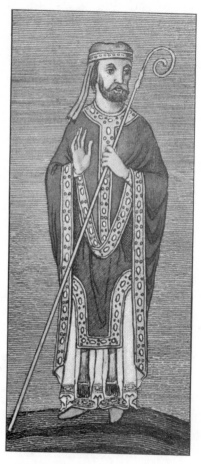

Fig. 430.—Development of the mitre.
(Cott. MS. Nero C iv.)

The Canons Regular of St. Augustine, or, briefly, the Augustinian Canons, founded about 1060, wore a white full-sleeved tunic, under which was a black cassock. The cloak and hood were also black; a leather girdle passed round the waist, and a square cap was upon the head. They did not wear a beard like the secular canons. They appear to have come into England during the time of Henry I., when they settled at Colchester, but subsequently over two hundred houses were under their sway.

The Præmonstratensian Canons, founded about 1130, sometimes termed the White Canons, were habited in cassock and tunic and round cap, with a long cloak and hood—all of them white. The abbots did not use any episcopal insignia; the nuns did not sing in church, and they were ordered to pray in silence. Less than forty houses of this order were founded in England, the chief being at Welbeck.

The Gilbertines, founded in 1139. The monks were dressed in black cassock and hood and white cloak; the nuns in black tunic, cloak, and hood. The cloak, in the first case, and the hood in the second, were lined with lambskin. The monks followed the Augustinian rule, the nuns the Cistercian. Less than thirty houses were of this order.

WILLIAM II., 1087–1100. HENRY I., 1100–1135
STEPHEN, 1135–1154

The seal of St. Anselm presents but few particulars of the habit of an Archbishop during the time of Rufus. There are some points, however, which are valuable. The crozier is no longer a Tau cross, but a crook; the pallium passes round the upper arms, and the band depending down the front almost reaches the ground. With the humility which characterised the man he is represented only in chasuble and alb; the maniple is extremely interesting, as it shows the original form from which it was derived,

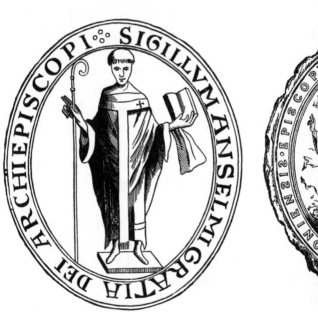

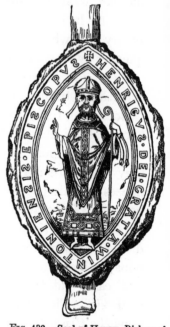

FIG. 431.—Seal of St. Anselm, Archbishop, 1093.

FIG. 432.—Seal of Henry, Bishop of Winchester, *temp.* King Stephen.

and is depicted as a towel hanging over the left wrist (Fig. 431).

The seal of Henry, Bishop of Winchester in the time of King Stephen, affords us a much better example of ecclesiastical dress. The mitre is of a peculiar form, as shown in Fig. 432. The prelate is habited in amice, chasuble, dalmatic, and alb, all richly ornamented; the orphrey of the alb consists of a very wide band. The head of the episcopal staff is not ornamented, and the maniple appears as a narrow band.

Perhaps the best example afforded us of the dress of the priest is a representation of the dream of Henry I., before passing over to Normandy in 1130, from the hands

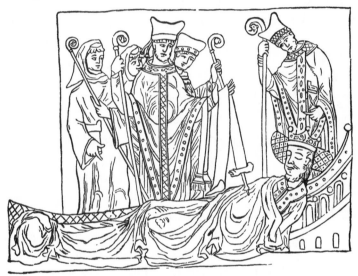

Fig. 433.—Clerical dress, *temp*. Henry I.

of Florence of Worcester, which is preserved in Corpus Christi College.   There are three illuminations of the dream, showing the sleeping monarch being upbraided by the clergy, the knights, and the husbandmen, the three greatest potentialities in the realm.   Probably the excessive taxation and rapacity to which all classes were subjected occasioned the dream, from which the King awoke with loud cries of fear.

The priests (Fig. 433) wear an incipient mitre with low

horns on either side; around the forehead in two cases appear ornamental bands, from which depend the infulæ fringed at the ends. They are habited in chasubles; the maniple is shown in a much developed form, with spreading ends and deep fringe. The pastoral staves of the Bishops now show traces of the ornamentation which subsequently distinguish them, and one dating from the early part of the twelfth century is shown in Fig. 434. Cott.

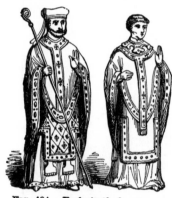

FIG. 434.—Ecclesiastical costume.
(Cott. MS. Nero C iv.)

MS. Nero C iv., of early twelfth century, is an Anglo-Norman version of the Psalter, and an illustration of the Last Judgment; it gives us an excellent idea of ecclesiastical and other costume. Fig. 435, Pl., represents five churchmen, three of whom are taken from the group on the right hand of the Deity, and the expression upon their ascetic faces sufficiently represents their self-conscious virtue. The clergy upon the left side are clean shaven, sleek, and fat; they wear their rich garments as objects of pride and ostentation; the absence of the mitre, pastoral staff, and stole indicate their degradation, while the physiognomical character of their expression does not represent any joyful expectancy. The colours used are green, red, blue, and purple.

An extremely interesting representation of three grades of the clergy of the twelfth century is shown in Fig. 436, Pl., taken from carved stone effigies in the cathedral at Chartres. The archbishop wears a remarkable mitre; the amice is

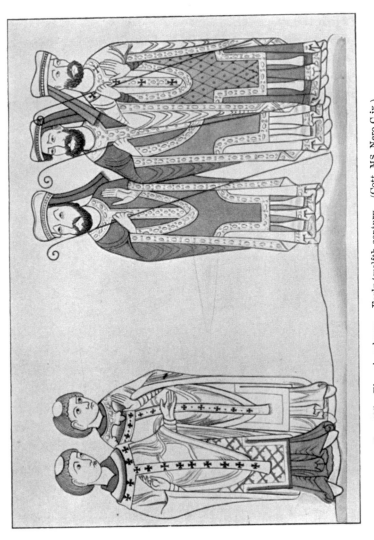

Fig. 435.—Five churchmen. Early twelfth century. (Cott. MS. Nero C iv.)

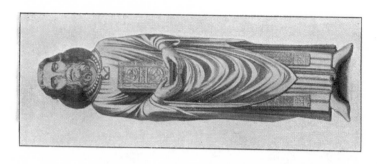

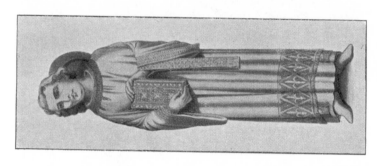

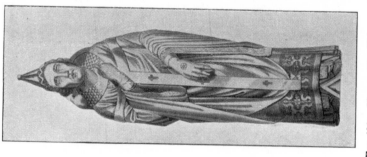

FIG. 436.—Clergy of twelfth century, taken from carved stone effigies in cathedral at Chartres. The priest is carrying a book of the Gospels.

quilted in chequers; the wide sleeves of the dalmatic appear below the chasuble; while the pallium, worn very low on the arms, exhibits crosses of a very plain character. The richly ornamented shoes, and also a portion of the apparel of the dalmatic, are also apparent. The second effigy represents a deacon in his appropriate dress of dalmatic and alb; the orphrey work decorating the dalmatic is of an extremely rich character. He wears the maniple and stole, and carries a beautifully bound Evangelisterium. The third figure is very simply dressed in chasuble, alb, and stole; he represents the ordinary priest, and bears a book of the Gospels.

CHAPTER XXVI

ANGEVIN PERIOD

HENRY II., 1154–1189.   RICHARD I., 1189–1199.   JOHN,
1199–1216.   HENRY III., 1216–1272

THE ecclesiastical vestments of this period did not differ
essentially from that of the preceding.   The chief point of
interest is the development
of the *Mitre*, which in this
period began to assume the
shape, but not the dimen-
sions, which subsequently distinguished it.   The seal of St.
Thomas à Becket shows us a
mitre with the blunt horns of
the previous period now rising
on either side to points (Fig.
437).   In a manuscript preserved in Trinity College,
Cambridge, the prelate is
shown in a cap which is
almost flat (Fig. 438, Pl.),
but the mitre preserved at
Sens, and traditionally said
to have belonged to him, is
shown in Fig. 439, Pl., and

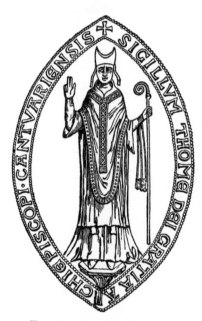

FIG. 437.—Seal of St. Thomas of
Canterbury, *temp.* Henry II.

presents a totally different aspect.   The horns would appear
front and back like the modern mitre, with the infulæ

344

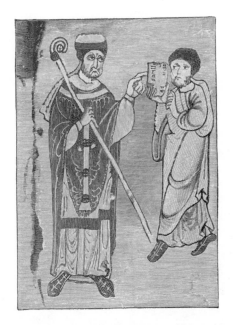

FIG. 438.—St. Thomas of Canterbury and his secretary.
(MS. Trinity College, Cambridge, B v. 4.)

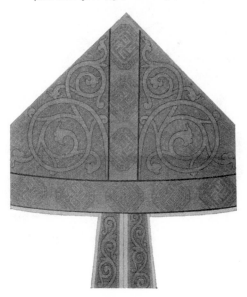

FIG. 439.—Mitre of St. Thomas of Canterbury.

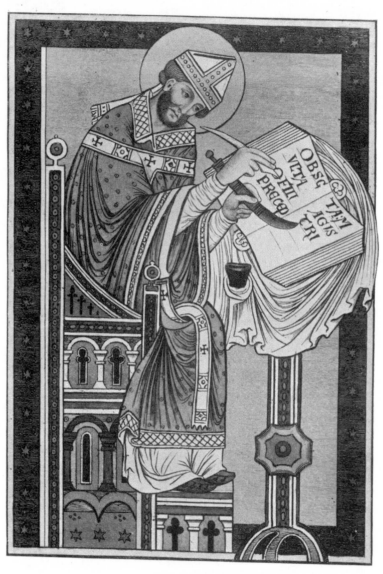

F<small>IG</small>. 440.—St. Dunstan. (Roy. MS. 10 A xiii.)

depending down the back. It is of most elaborate needle-work, a grey ground with a design of scarlet and gold.

In Roy. MS. 10 A xiii., dating from the end of the twelfth century, Dunstan, Archbishop of Canterbury, is depicted (Fig. 440, Pl.), and the artist being ignorant of Saxon archiepiscopal dress had perforce to array him in the archbishop's dress of the period. The mitre is almost pre-cisely the same shape as that preserved of St. Thomas (Fig. 439, Pl.). A feature of the dress is the plain apparel of the amice, the same pattern appearing upon the orphrey of the dalmatic. No apparels are shown upon the alb, but the pall has an extra decoration alternating with the crosses. The colours for the chasuble and dalmatic are blue and red respectively. In Harl. MS. Roll Y vi., dated from *c.* 1200, being the life of St. Guthlac, we have a number of illustra-tions of contemporary ecclesiastics. The mitre is shown more ornamented if possible than that of St. Thomas, a narrow orphrey encircles the wrists of the alb, and the dalmatic is represented richly embroidered. The pastoral staff is ornamented, but not elaborately. The priest bearing the cup wears the chasuble and alb, while the figure behind him is habited in a cope fastened with a large morse, the orphrey being blue in colour on the white garment. During the reign of Henry III. the red hat of the cardinal is said to have been first introduced; it was not flat as at the present time, but had a wide brim gradually rising to a shallow crown. The reign is notable for the intro-duction of the two great Orders of Friars, the Dominicans and the Franciscans.

The Dominicans, or *Black Friars*, or *Preaching Friars*, founded in 1215. They were habited in a white tunic fastened with a white girdle, over which appeared a white scapulary; the super garment was a black mantle and hood, while the shoes also were black. The lay brothers wore a black scapulary.

The Franciscans, founded in 1208, and first introduced into England in 1223, at Canterbury. They were usually termed Grey Friars, or Friars-Minor, from the colour of their dress, but sometimes Cordeliers from the knotted cord which formed their girdles. The dress consisted of a grey tunic, long and loose, girded with the cord, and a hood, or cowl, and cloak of the same colour. In the fifteenth century the colour of the habit was altered to a dark brown. The feet were always bare or only protected by sandals. The Franciscan Nuns, or Poor Clares, as they were at times called from St. Clare the foundress of the Order, wore the same habit as the monks, but with a black veil instead of a hood.

The Carmelites, or *White Friars*, founded in 1209, were introduced into England during the reign of Henry III., and ultimately owned about fifty houses. Their first habit was white throughout, but during the later half of the thirteenth century their cloaks were parti-coloured, white and red; these, however, changed again to white.

The Austin Friars, or "*Eremites*," or *Black Canons*, were founded in the middle of the thirteenth century, and owned about forty-five houses in England. Their exterior habit was a black gown with broad sleeves, held with a leather belt, and a black cloth hood; the under dress was a white cassock.

The Crutched Friars, or *Crossed Friars*, founded at the same time, were so called because they wore a red cross on the back and breast of their blue habit. They finally had ten houses here.

The Trinitarian Friars, or *Maturines,* were dressed in white, with an eight-pointed cross of blue and red.

The Friars de Pœnitentia, or *the Friars of the Sack,* had nine houses in England.

It should be remembered that the whole of these minor orders of friars, together with five or six others not mentioned, were abolished by the Council of Lyons in 1370, when only the four great orders, the Franciscans, Dominicans, Augustinians, and the Carmelites, were formally recognised.

The vestments which developed during this period had mostly seen their inception earlier, but in a very modest form. They were:—

The Cope, which had originally been a voluminous cloak with a hood attached, covered the head and the entire person of the wearer. It now, however, became much curtailed in its proportions, and finally resolved itself into the most gorgeous of mediæval ecclesiastical garments. Its use became essentially associated with processions and all ceremonies of an elaborate and dignified character, apart from the ministrations at the altar, when the chasuble was used. Made in every conceivable colour, and heavily adorned with the richest gold-work encrusted with jewels, they formed the highest type of gorgeous Church vestments then in vogue. The shape when spread out flat was a perfect semicircle. It was fastened across the breast by a morse, or clasp, but sometimes by a band of the same material as the cope.

The border apparels of the cope seen upon many brasses

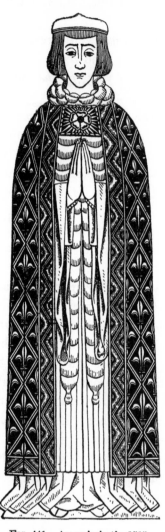

FIG. 441.—An ecclesiastic, 1515.
Queen's College, Oxford.

and effigies frequently represent canopied figures of saints, while heraldic devices, mystical crosses, &c., are often introduced. A famous cope, the Syon, may be viewed at the South Kensington Museum, while another may be seen at Ely. It may be mentioned that the hood was in some cases removable, to allow of special hoods of different shape, material, and colour being worn at various seasons.

The Almuce, or *Aumuce*, was introduced in the thirteenth century. It was a furred hood with long ends hanging down in front, which afforded warmth to the clergy when officiating in church during cold weather, or participating in outdoor processions. It is commonly found on the brasses of canons during the fifteenth century, having a cape and pendants of fur attached (Fig 441).

The Surplice.—This white outer garment was derived from the alb, and the name *super pelliceum* implies that a

furred garment was worn beneath it. Originally the surplice
was confined to the elder clergy who sat in the choir or to
those who had to move about in
the church. It was made full,
and reached nearly to the feet,
with large sleeves which widened
towards the hands. No opening
appeared in front, a round hole at
the top admitting the head.
Occasionally it was worn at ceremonials and in processions. At
Cowfold, in Sussex, the brass of
Thomas Nelond, Prior of Lewes,
furnishes the finest example of an
ecclesiastic wearing a surplice
(Fig. 442). It dates from 1433.

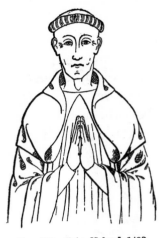

FIG. 442.—Prior Nelond, 1433.
Cowfold, Sussex.

The Mitre (Fig. 443).—At the
beginning of the twelfth century the mitre began to be
made of rich material, and to be adorned with costly

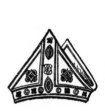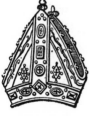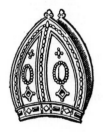

FIG. 443.

Archbishop Grenfeld,   Archbishop Goodrich,   Archbishop Harsnett,
1315.   York.   1554.   Ely.   1611.   Chigwell.

ornamentation. In the thirteenth century one acutely
pointed form was adopted, and the circlet at the base

was extremely narrow, as seen in Fig. 444. At the beginning of this century the points of the mitre were reversed, and instead of being seen on either side of the head they appeared at the front and back, as seen in the illustration (Fig. 445). With very little alteration this form continued during the fourteenth century, as observed upon the effigy of Godfrey Giffard, Bishop of Worcester, *d.* 1301 (Fig. 446). For the form of the mitre about the middle of the century we may refer to the brass of Abbot de la Mare (Fig. 447). Pugin gives three forms

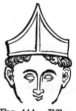 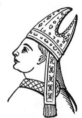 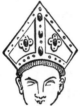

Fig. 444.—Effigy, Temple Church, 13th century.

Fig. 445.—Infulæ shown on the brass of John Boothe, Bishop of Exeter, 1470.

Fig. 446.—Bishop Giffard, 1301.

of mitres as used by the clergy—one of plain white linen; another, the *aurifrigiata*, which was ornamented with gold orphreys; and a third, the *pretiosa*, which, as its name suggests, was richly decorated and used upon special occasions. The De la Mare example is of the third description. The colour of the bishop's mitre was usually white; in an abbot's, varied.

The Crozier and the Pastoral Staff (Fig. 448, Pl.).—In the thirteenth century, the head of the pastoral staff became decorated with ornamental foliation (Fig. 450). The crozier was the special dignity of an archbishop, and was always surmounted by a cross. A prior's pastoral staff was

a silver wand with a ball at
the top.

As a general rule the
crozier was held by the archbishop in the left hand;
bishops held the pastoral staff
also in the left hand, with
the crook outwards. Abbots
held the staff in the right
hand, with the crook turned
inwards. Some abbots en-
joying episcopal jurisdiction
are at times distinguished
by holding the staff after
the manner of bishops (Fig.
451).

The Vexillum was a scarf
affixed to the crozier or the
pastoral staff immediately
below the cross head or the
crook, and was in use as early
as the tenth century. It is
well shown upon the brass
of John Yong, Bishop and
Warden, New College Chapel,
Oxford (Fig. 449).

The Humeral was an
oblong scarf worn round the
shoulders at certain portions
of the mass, and used in the
elevation of the host to prevent contamination by the
fingers of the officiating priest.

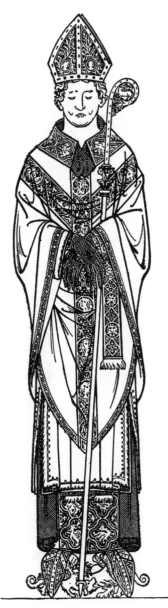

Fig. 447.—Abbot de la Mare, St. Albans
Abbey, *d.* 1396; brass *c.* 1375.

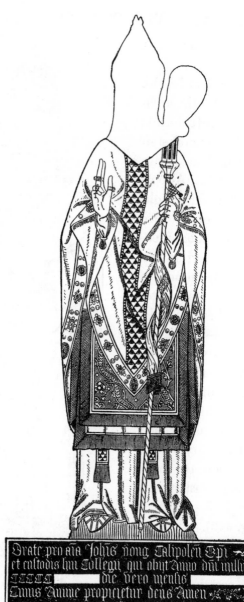

FIG. 449.—John Yong, Bishop and Warden, 1526.
New College Chapel, Oxford.

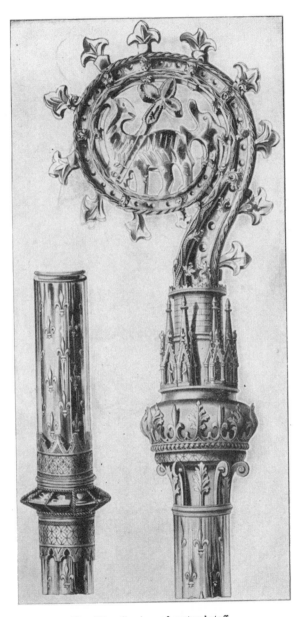

Fig. 448.—Crozier and pastoral staff.

The Pall, or *Pallium* (Fig. 454), worn only by archbishops, has been previously described (*vide* p. 334). During the mediæval period many chasubles were decorated with an apparel which closely resembled the pallium (Fig. 455) in form and appearance, but was a part of the garment, thus differing from the pallium.

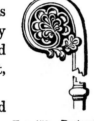

FIG. 450.—Pastoral staff, 1263.

The Chimere.—The garment distinguished by this name was a cope slightly modified.

The Rochet was a vestment apparently in use only by bishops; it somewhat resembled the alb, but was shorter, and open at the sides towards the bottom.

The Alb (*vide* p. 337).—In the mediæval period the alb was always decorated with apparels, which were placed on the skirt before and behind, upon the wrist of each sleeve, and sometimes, but not always, upon the back and breast. They consisted of pieces of cloth of gold, or other rich material, or of goldsmith's work (Figs. 452, 453).

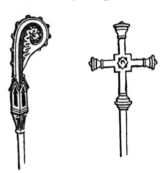

FIG. 451.

Pastoral staff, Abbot Esteney, 1498. Westminster Abbey.

Crozier, Archbishop Waldeby, 1397. Westminster Abbey.

The earliest brass of an ecclesiastic is that of De Bacon, 1310 (Fig. 456), in Oulton Church, Suffolk; and from that period down to the Reformation and later, brasses of archbishops, bishops, abbots, and priests are of frequent occurrence. A number of these are here reproduced, and a careful study will enable the student to readily recognise the different ecclesiastical vest-

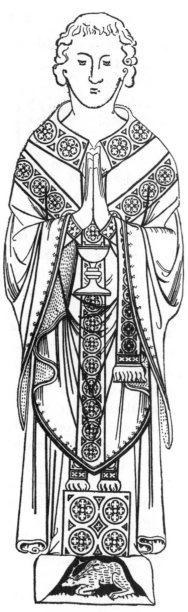

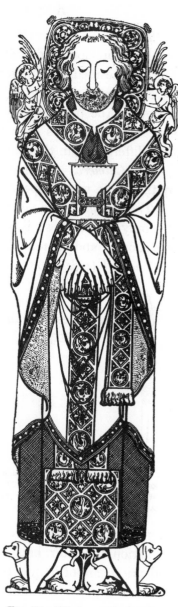

FIG. 452.—Priest, *c.* 1360. North Mimms
Church, Hertfordshire.

FIG. 453.—Priest, *c.* 1360. Wensley
Church, Yorkshire.

ments which we have described, while the various modifications which they underwent are faithfully shown in these representations.

We are so accustomed in this twentieth century to readily recognise an ecclesiastic, when not engaged in the ministration of his office, by some distinctive dress, according to the denomination to which he belongs, that we unconsciously suppose the same to have obtained during the Middle Ages. This, however, was far from being the case, for, omitting the friars, no particular habit was adopted to differentiate between the clergy and the laity. The chief dignitaries of the Church insisted upon the tonsure being worn and a sober habit

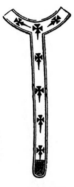

FIG. 454.—The pallium.

of dress, but these regulations were invariably neglected. They were ordered to wear garments not too gay in colour,

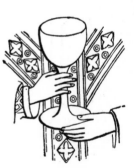

FIG. 455.—Ornamentation of chasuble.

and not to imitate any extravagances of fashion; also to abstain from excess in jewellery, and to refrain from the carrying of lethal weapons. We find that these rules were more observed in the breach than in the observance. The Archbishop of Canterbury, in 1342, speaks of ecclesiastics being dressed more like military persons than clericals, and having at times knives attached to their girdles, after the fashion of swords, green shoes with crackowes, and slashed belts studded with precious stones, gowns lined or turned up with fur or silk, rings upon the fingers, hoods with

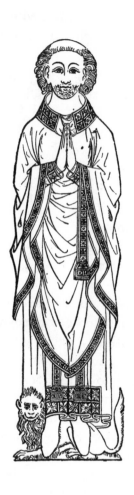

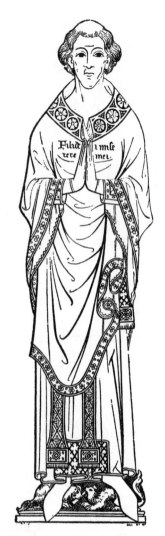

Fig. 456.—De Bacon, c. 1310.
Oulton Church, Suffolk.

Amice, Alb, Stole, Maniple, Chasuble.

Fig. 457.—Lawrence Seymour, 1337. Higham
Ferrers Church, Northamptonshire.

Amice, Alb, Stole, Maniple, Chasuble.

liripipes of wondrous development, and hair of effeminate

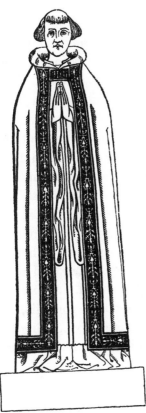

FIG. 458.—Ecclesiastic habited in Cope, c. 1400. Hitchin Church, Herts.

Cope, Surplice with hanging sleeves, Alb.

(The first ecclesiastic vested in a cope, and shown upon a brass, is William de Foulbourn, Foulbourn, Cambridge, 1370.)

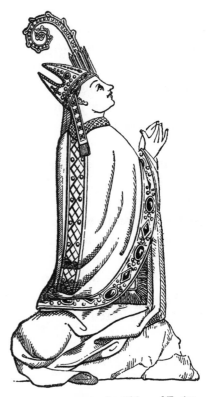

FIG. 459.—John Boothe, Bishop of Exeter, 1478, East Horsley, Surrey.

Alb, Dalmatic, Chasuble, Mitre.

length—in fact, all the extravagances affected by the exquisites of the day. In the middle of the fourteenth century some priests in the diocese of York were proceeded against for wearing ornamental tunics elaborately trimmed, and carrying baselards at their girdles. In the illuminated MSS. we constantly find them represented in ordinary civil costume. Even when engaged in the ministration of their office, the red and blue robes of everyday wear at times appear under the vestments, while an illustration from Harl. MS. 4425 represents a priest confessing a lady in church, and wearing his complete civilian dress without any attempt to cover it by a vestment. We also find from mediæval MSS. that where a particular vestment was ordained by the canons to be of a certain colour, these laws were disregarded, and the vestments made of any substance and colour that suited the fancy. Thus blue gowns and hoods, claret-coloured gowns, blue-grey gowns, with blue under-robe, and red shoes—in fact, every colour and combination that can be imagined—are discovered. By far the best examples, and most brilliantly executed portraits, are those preserved in the priceless MS. Nero D vii., being the Book of Benefactors of St. Albans Abbey, to which we have previously referred.

GLOSSARY

Alamode.—A plain silk, thick and loosely woven, mentioned in the Act for the better encouragement of the silk trade in England passed in the year 1692.

Armazine.—A strong corded silk used during the sixteenth century for ladies' gowns and gentlemen's waistcoats.

Baudekyn.—An extremely rich fabric composed of silk interwoven with threads of gold, much resembling the modern brocade. It is said to have derived its name from Baldeck or Babylon, where it was said to have been first manufactured. Henry III. appears to have been the first English monarch to wear cloth of baudekyn, but it was probably known upon the Continent some time before it was brought to England.

Bergamot.—A tapestry made of goat's or cow's hair mixed with hemp; worn by the lower classes.

Broella.—A coarse cloth used for ordinary dresses of countrymen in the Middle Ages.

Buckram.—A very stiff cloth, worn as early as the thirteenth century.

Calico.—The art of calico printing was invented and practised in England in 1676. It is a cotton material originally manufactured at Calicut, in India.

Cambric.—This material obtains its name from Cambrai, in France, where it was first manufactured. It is a thin kind of fine linen, introduced during the reign of Queen Elizabeth, and much used for the making of ruffs, collars, shirts, and handkerchiefs.

Camlet.—A material made of wool and silk, expensive, but of lasting wear. It was originally manufactured of the hair of the camel, and from thence its name is derived. Much worn during the time of Elizabeth and James I.

Cammaka.—A species of cloth; during the reign of Edward III. the church vestments were made of this material.

Canvas.—A very coarse kind of material, mentioned in 1611.

Cashmere.—A soft, fine material, half cotton and half wool; named after the country from whence it was first imported into Europe.

Cotton.—A material originally manufactured in the East. It was used in this country at an early date.

Crape.—A thin gauze-like material used only for mourning purposes.

Cyprus.—Resembles the modern crêpe de chine, and was used extensively for veiling, and winding round hats during the Tudor Period.

Diaper.—Linen cloth woven in slightly defined figures. Peacham says, "Diapering is a term in drawing; it chiefly serveth to counterfeit cloth of gold, silver, damask branch't velvet, camblet, etc."—*Compl. Gent.,* p. 345. Anderson, in his "History of Commerce," conjectures that diaper, a species of printed linen, took its name from the city of Ypres in Flanders, where it was first made, being originally called "d'ipre."

Dimity.—A stout linen cloth, named from its first manufacture at Damietta—the Dimyat of the Arabs.

Dowlas.—Coarse linen cloth, used by the lower classes, chiefly made in Brittany.

Drugget.—A stuff of the nature of baize, usually all wool, sometimes half wool and silk. It was formerly used for coarse clothing.

Ducape.—A corded silk of moderate fineness.

Duffel.—A coarse woollen cloth mentioned by De Foe as made at Witney and exported to America for winter wear.

Dunster.—A broad cloth made in Somersetshire, mentioned in an Act of the third year of Edward III.

Durance, or Duretty.—A strong kind of material, used in the sixteenth and seventeenth centuries. Nares says it obtained the name of *durance* from the everlasting strength of its texture.

Frieze.—A thick woollen cloth, much worn by the lower classes, and frequently mentioned by writers of the sixteenth century. Fuller, in his "Worthies," speaks of it as a coarse kind of cloth, made in Wales, "than which none warmer to be worn in winter, and the finest sort thereof very fashionable and genteele. Prince Henry [son of James I.] has a frieze suit."

Fustian.—A cotton material much used by the Normans, more especially by the clergy for the making of their chasubles. The Cistercians were forbidden to wear them made of anything but linen or fustian. It was first manufactured in this country at Norwich, during the reign of Edward VI. *Woollen* fustians were made at Norwich as early at 1336.

Gauze.—A thin, transparent stuff, of silk or cotton.

Gazzatum.—A fine kind of silk or linen stuff, after the manner of gauze, supposed to have taken its name from the city of Gaza, in Palestine, where it was manufactured.

Holland cloth.—A material made of linen, as much in use during the Middle Ages as at the present time.

Hurden.—A kind of canvas made of very coarse hemp.

Kendal or Kendal-green.—A cloth manufactured at Kendal, in Westmorland, where it was first made. It is mentioned in a statute of the reign of Richard II., 1389.

Kersey.—Generally a coarse narrow woollen cloth, but at times of fine fabric, and used for better purposes.

Marry-Muffe.—A coarse common cloth.

Muslin.—A thin fabric of Eastern manufacture, which, according to Marco Polo, takes its name from Mosul or Moosul, a large town in Turkish Asia, where it was first made.

Mustardevelin, or *Mustardevillers.*—A mixed grey woollen cloth, often mentioned by writers of the fifteenth and sixteenth centuries. Mustardevillers and mustardevillin are noticed in writings of the Middle Ages; and Meyrick says that Elmham mentions a town near Harfleur, which he calls by a similar name, and which is probably Montiguliers, where it was first manufactured. Moustier de Villiers, near Harfleur, is the town mentioned in the accounts of the wars of Henry V. In Stow's "Survey" mustard villars is spoken of as a colour now out of use.

Nankeen.—A cloth imported from China, and named from Nankin, where it was largely manufactured. It was of a yellow colour, natural to the wool of which it was made. It was introduced into America in 1823 from Sicily.

Oldham.—A coarse kind of cloth, so called from its original place of manufacture, a town in Norfolk. Norwich became the principal place of its fabrication. It was used during the time of Richard II.

Osnaburg.—A coarse linen manufactured at and named from that province in Hanover.

Paduasoy.—A material made of silk very strong, much used for ladies' gowns during the eighteenth century. It obtained its name from Padua, the place where it was first manufactured.

Pall.—A fine cloth used for the robes of nobles. In Warton's "History of English Poetry" (1840), volume i. p. 169, we are told that "anciently pallium, as did purpura, signifies in general any rich cloth." Thus there were saddles de pallis et ebore, a bed de pallis, a cope de pallis, &c.

Perpetuana.—A woollen material which derived its name from its supposed durable nature. It is mentioned in "Cynthia's Revels," 1601; and from a passage in Dekker's "Satiromastic," 1602, it was a glossy kind of stuff like parchment.

Persian.—A thin silk used only for linings.

Plush.—A coarse kind of silk velvet with a thick nap.

Poldavis.—A coarse linen. In "Eastward Hoe," 1605, the tailor is called by this name.

Rash.—A species of inferior silk, or silk and wool manufacture.

Ratteen.—A rough woollen cloth, chiefly used for travelling coats, &c. Howell's Dictionary makes *rash* the same as the French *burail*, which again, according to a French dictionary, was a kind of ratine. From this it is highly probable that *burel, ratteen,* and *rash* were all names for a coarse woollen stuff. "*Ratteen* frocks" were fashionable for gentlemen in 1774.—*Westminster Magazine.*

Ray.—A striped cloth which was brought over from Flanders. It is mentioned in the reign of King John in the Domesday of Gippeswich:

> " And each of them a good mantell
> Of scarlet and of *raye*."
>
> ROBIN HOOD.

Raynes (Cloth of).—Very fine linen which took its name from the city of Rennes, in Bretagne, where it was originally manufactured. It was chiefly used for bed-sheets or for shirts. It is mentioned by Chaucer, and in the older romances. Joane, Lady Abergavenny, in 1434, bequeaths to Sir James, son of the Earl of Ormond, "two pair *sheets of raynes*."

Rug.—A coarse woollen material, worn by the poorer classes. "Dame Niggardise in a sage rugge kirtle," 1592. "Like a subsister [a beggar] in a gowne of rug," 1592. "Judas yonder that walks in rug" is mentioned by Dekker.

Russell.—A black woollen cloth, something like baize with knots over the surface, first made at Norwich; mentioned time of Henry VIII.

Sagathy.—A light woollen material, after the fashion of serge.

Samite.—A very rich silk, interwoven with gold, or worked in embroidery.

Sarcenet.—A thin silk much used for linings, first used in the thirteenth century.

Sarciatus or Sarcilis.—A woollen cloth worn only by the lowest classes; mentioned during the thirteenth century.

Satin.—A thick closely-woven silk, mentioned in the thirteenth century.

Say.—A woollen cloth. During the reign of Rufus a pair of stockings made of this material were valued at 3s. It was used for external garments during the time of Elizabeth: " Both hood and gown of green and yellow saye," 1578.

Sendall.—A thin silk.

Sergedusoy.—A coarse silken stuff. Used for coats during the eighteenth century, considered rather better than cloth.

Shag.—A shaggy cloth, with a velvet nap on one side, sometimes of silk, though generally of worsted.

Shalloon.—A woollen stuff imported from Chalons, in France.

Shanks.—A common kind of fur used by ordinary people for trimming their gowns in the sixteenth century. Sheepskin.

Silk.—In A.D. 551 we find the silkworm was brought by two monks to Constantinople from Bokhara, but the manufacture of silk was confined to the Greek Empire till the year 1130. In the thirteenth century Bruges was the principal market for this commodity.

INDEX

FIRST PART : CIVIL

SECOND PART : ECCLESIASTICAL

THE END

A CATALOG OF SELECTED
DOVER BOOKS
IN ALL FIELDS OF INTEREST

A CATALOG OF SELECTED DOVER
BOOKS IN ALL FIELDS OF INTEREST

CONCERNING THE SPIRITUAL IN ART, Wassily Kandinsky. Pioneering work by father of abstract art. Thoughts on color theory, nature of art. Analysis of earlier masters. 12 illustrations. 80pp. of text. 5⅜ x 8½.   23411-8 Pa. $4.95

ANIMALS: 1,419 Copyright-Free Illustrations of Mammals, Birds, Fish, Insects, etc., Jim Harter (ed.). Clear wood engravings present, in extremely lifelike poses, over 1,000 species of animals. One of the most extensive pictorial sourcebooks of its kind. Captions. Index. 284pp. 9 x 12.   23766-4 Pa. $14.95

CELTIC ART: The Methods of Construction, George Bain. Simple geometric techniques for making Celtic interlacements, spirals, Kells-type initials, animals, humans, etc. Over 500 illustrations. 160pp. 9 x 12. (Available in U.S. only.)   22923-8 Pa. $9.95

AN ATLAS OF ANATOMY FOR ARTISTS, Fritz Schider. Most thorough reference work on art anatomy in the world. Hundreds of illustrations, including selections from works by Vesalius, Leonardo, Goya, Ingres, Michelangelo, others. 593 illustrations. 192pp. 7⅛ x 10¼.   20241-0 Pa. $9.95

CELTIC HAND STROKE-BY-STROKE (Irish Half-Uncial from "The Book of Kells"): An Arthur Baker Calligraphy Manual, Arthur Baker. Complete guide to creating each letter of the alphabet in distinctive Celtic manner. Covers hand position, strokes, pens, inks, paper, more. Illustrated. 48pp. 8¼ x 11.   24336-2 Pa. $3.95

EASY ORIGAMI, John Montroll. Charming collection of 32 projects (hat, cup, pelican, piano, swan, many more) specially designed for the novice origami hobbyist. Clearly illustrated easy-to-follow instructions insure that even beginning papercrafters will achieve successful results. 48pp. 8¼ x 11.   27298-2 Pa. $3.50

THE COMPLETE BOOK OF BIRDHOUSE CONSTRUCTION FOR WOOD-WORKERS, Scott D. Campbell. Detailed instructions, illustrations, tables. Also data on bird habitat and instinct patterns. Bibliography. 3 tables. 63 illustrations in 15 figures. 48pp. 5¼ x 8½.   24407-5 Pa. $2.50

BLOOMINGDALE'S ILLUSTRATED 1886 CATALOG: Fashions, Dry Goods and Housewares, Bloomingdale Brothers. Famed merchants' extremely rare catalog depicting about 1,700 products: clothing, housewares, firearms, dry goods, jewelry, more. Invaluable for dating, identifying vintage items. Also, copyright-free graphics for artists, designers. Co-published with Henry Ford Museum & Greenfield Village. 160pp. 8¼ x 11.   25780-0 Pa. $12.95

HISTORIC COSTUME IN PICTURES, Braun & Schneider. Over 1,450 costumed figures in clearly detailed engravings–from dawn of civilization to end of 19th century. Captions. Many folk costumes. 256pp. 8⅜ x 11¾.   23150-X Pa. $12.95

STICKLEY CRAFTSMAN FURNITURE CATALOGS, Gustav Stickley and L. & J. G. Stickley. Beautiful, functional furniture in two authentic catalogs from 1910. 594 illustrations, including 277 photos, show settles, rockers, armchairs, reclining chairs, bookcases, desks, tables. 183pp. 6½ x 9¼. 23838-5 Pa. $11.95

AMERICAN LOCOMOTIVES IN HISTORIC PHOTOGRAPHS: 1858 to 1949, Ron Ziel (ed.). A rare collection of 126 meticulously detailed official photographs, called "builder portraits," of American locomotives that majestically chronicle the rise of steam locomotive power in America. Introduction. Detailed captions. xi+129pp. 9 x 12. 27393-8 Pa. $13.95

AMERICA'S LIGHTHOUSES: An Illustrated History, Francis Ross Holland, Jr. Delightfully written, profusely illustrated fact-filled survey of over 200 American lighthouses since 1716. History, anecdotes, technological advances, more. 240pp. 8 x 10¾. 25576-X Pa. $12.95

TOWARDS A NEW ARCHITECTURE, Le Corbusier. Pioneering manifesto by founder of "International School." Technical and aesthetic theories, views of industry, economics, relation of form to function, "mass-production split" and much more. Profusely illustrated. 320pp. 6⅛ x 9¼. (Available in U.S. only.) 25023-7 Pa. $10.95

HOW THE OTHER HALF LIVES, Jacob Riis. Famous journalistic record, exposing poverty and degradation of New York slums around 1900, by major social reformer. 100 striking and influential photographs. 233pp. 10 x 7⅞. 22012-5 Pa. $11.95

FRUIT KEY AND TWIG KEY TO TREES AND SHRUBS, William M. Harlow. One of the handiest and most widely used identification aids. Fruit key covers 120 deciduous and evergreen species; twig key 160 deciduous species. Easily used. Over 300 photographs. 126pp. 5⅜ x 8½. 20511-8 Pa. $3.95

COMMON BIRD SONGS, Dr. Donald J. Borror. Songs of 60 most common U.S. birds: robins, sparrows, cardinals, bluejays, finches, more—arranged in order of increasing complexity. Up to 9 variations of songs of each species. Cassette and manual 99911-4 $8.95

ORCHIDS AS HOUSE PLANTS, Rebecca Tyson Northen. Grow cattleyas and many other kinds of orchids—in a window, in a case, or under artificial light. 63 illustrations. 148pp. 5⅜ x 8½. 23261-1 Pa. $7.95

MONSTER MAZES, Dave Phillips. Masterful mazes at four levels of difficulty. Avoid deadly perils and evil creatures to find magical treasures. Solutions for all 32 exciting illustrated puzzles. 48pp. 8¼ x 11. 26005-4 Pa. $2.95

MOZART'S DON GIOVANNI (DOVER OPERA LIBRETTO SERIES), Wolfgang Amadeus Mozart. Introduced and translated by Ellen H. Bleiler. Standard Italian libretto, with complete English translation. Convenient and thoroughly portable—an ideal companion for reading along with a recording or the performance itself. Introduction. List of characters. Plot summary. 121pp. 5¼ x 8½. 24944-1 Pa. $3.95

TECHNICAL MANUAL AND DICTIONARY OF CLASSICAL BALLET, Gail Grant. Defines, explains, comments on steps, movements, poses and concepts. 15-page pictorial section. Basic book for student, viewer. 127pp. 5⅜ x 8½. 21843-0 Pa. $4.95

THE CLARINET AND CLARINET PLAYING, David Pino. Lively, comprehensive work features suggestions about technique, musicianship, and musical interpretation, as well as guidelines for teaching, making your own reeds, and preparing for public performance. Includes an intriguing look at clarinet history. "A godsend," *The Clarinet,* Journal of the International Clarinet Society. Appendixes. 7 illus. 320pp. 5⅜ x 8½. 40270-3 Pa. $9.95

HOLLYWOOD GLAMOR PORTRAITS, John Kobal (ed.). 145 photos from 1926-49. Harlow, Gable, Bogart, Bacall; 94 stars in all. Full background on photographers, technical aspects. 160pp. 8⅜ x 11¼. 23352-9 Pa. $12.95

THE ANNOTATED CASEY AT THE BAT: A Collection of Ballads about the Mighty Casey/Third, Revised Edition, Martin Gardner (ed.). Amusing sequels and parodies of one of America's best-loved poems: Casey's Revenge, Why Casey Whiffed, Casey's Sister at the Bat, others. 256pp. 5⅜ x 8½. 28598-7 Pa. $8.95

THE RAVEN AND OTHER FAVORITE POEMS, Edgar Allan Poe. Over 40 of the author's most memorable poems: "The Bells," "Ulalume," "Israfel," "To Helen," "The Conqueror Worm," "Eldorado," "Annabel Lee," many more. Alphabetic lists of titles and first lines. 64pp. 5 3/16 x 8¼. 26685-0 Pa. $1.00

PERSONAL MEMOIRS OF U. S. GRANT, Ulysses Simpson Grant. Intelligent, deeply moving firsthand account of Civil War campaigns, considered by many the finest military memoirs ever written. Includes letters, historic photographs, maps and more. 528pp. 6⅛ x 9¼. 28587-1 Pa. $12.95

ANCIENT EGYPTIAN MATERIALS AND INDUSTRIES, A. Lucas and J. Harris. Fascinating, comprehensive, thoroughly documented text describes this ancient civilization's vast resources and the processes that incorporated them in daily life, including the use of animal products, building materials, cosmetics, perfumes and incense, fibers, glazed ware, glass and its manufacture, materials used in the mummification process, and much more. 544pp. 6⅛ x 9¼. (Available in U.S. only.) 40446-3 Pa. $16.95

RUSSIAN STORIES/PYCCKNE PACCKA3bl: A Dual-Language Book, edited by Gleb Struve. Twelve tales by such masters as Chekhov, Tolstoy, Dostoevsky, Pushkin, others. Excellent word-for-word English translations on facing pages, plus teaching and study aids, Russian/English vocabulary, biographical/critical introductions, more. 416pp. 5⅜ x 8½. 26244-8 Pa. $9.95

PHILADELPHIA THEN AND NOW: 60 Sites Photographed in the Past and Present, Kenneth Finkel and Susan Oyama. Rare photographs of City Hall, Logan Square, Independence Hall, Betsy Ross House, other landmarks juxtaposed with contemporary views. Captures changing face of historic city. Introduction. Captions. 128pp. 8¼ x 11. 25790-8 Pa. $9.95

AIA ARCHITECTURAL GUIDE TO NASSAU AND SUFFOLK COUNTIES, LONG ISLAND, The American Institute of Architects, Long Island Chapter, and the Society for the Preservation of Long Island Antiquities. Comprehensive, well-researched and generously illustrated volume brings to life over three centuries of Long Island's great architectural heritage. More than 240 photographs with authoritative, extensively detailed captions. 176pp. 8¼ x 11. 26946-9 Pa. $14.95

NORTH AMERICAN INDIAN LIFE: Customs and Traditions of 23 Tribes, Elsie Clews Parsons (ed.). 27 fictionalized essays by noted anthropologists examine religion, customs, government, additional facets of life among the Winnebago, Crow, Zuni, Eskimo, other tribes. 480pp. 6⅛ x 9¼. 27377-6 Pa. $10.95

FRANK LLOYD WRIGHT'S DANA HOUSE, Donald Hoffmann. Pictorial essay of residential masterpiece with over 160 interior and exterior photos, plans, elevations, sketches and studies. 128pp. 9¼ x 10¾.   29120-0 Pa. $14.95

THE MALE AND FEMALE FIGURE IN MOTION: 60 Classic Photographic Sequences, Eadweard Muybridge. 60 true-action photographs of men and women walking, running, climbing, bending, turning, etc., reproduced from rare 19th-century masterpiece. vi + 121pp. 9 x 12.   24745-7 Pa. $12.95

1001 QUESTIONS ANSWERED ABOUT THE SEASHORE, N. J. Berrill and Jacquelyn Berrill. Queries answered about dolphins, sea snails, sponges, starfish, fishes, shore birds, many others. Covers appearance, breeding, growth, feeding, much more. 305pp. 5¼ x 8¼.   23366-9 Pa. $9.95

ATTRACTING BIRDS TO YOUR YARD, William J. Weber. Easy-to-follow guide offers advice on how to attract the greatest diversity of birds: birdhouses, feeders, water and waterers, much more. 96pp. 5³⁄₁₆ x 8¼.   28927-3 Pa. $2.50

MEDICINAL AND OTHER USES OF NORTH AMERICAN PLANTS: A Historical Survey with Special Reference to the Eastern Indian Tribes, Charlotte Erichsen-Brown. Chronological historical citations document 500 years of usage of plants, trees, shrubs native to eastern Canada, northeastern U.S. Also complete identifying information. 343 illustrations. 544pp. 6½ x 9¼.   25951-X Pa. $12.95

STORYBOOK MAZES, Dave Phillips. 23 stories and mazes on two-page spreads: Wizard of Oz, Treasure Island, Robin Hood, etc. Solutions. 64pp. 8¼ x 11.
                    23628-5 Pa. $2.95

AMERICAN NEGRO SONGS: 230 Folk Songs and Spirituals, Religious and Secular, John W. Work. This authoritative study traces the African influences of songs sung and played by black Americans at work, in church, and as entertainment. The author discusses the lyric significance of such songs as "Swing Low, Sweet Chariot," "John Henry," and others and offers the words and music for 230 songs. Bibliography. Index of Song Titles. 272pp. 6½ x 9¼.   40271-1 Pa. $10.95

MOVIE-STAR PORTRAITS OF THE FORTIES, John Kobal (ed.). 163 glamor, studio photos of 106 stars of the 1940s: Rita Hayworth, Ava Gardner, Marlon Brando, Clark Gable, many more. 176pp. 8⅜ x 11¼.   23546-7 Pa. $14.95

BENCHLEY LOST AND FOUND, Robert Benchley. Finest humor from early 30s, about pet peeves, child psychologists, post office and others. Mostly unavailable elsewhere. 73 illustrations by Peter Arno and others. 183pp. 5⅜ x 8½. 22410-4 Pa. $6.95

YEKL and THE IMPORTED BRIDEGROOM AND OTHER STORIES OF YIDDISH NEW YORK, Abraham Cahan. Film Hester Street based on *Yekl* (1896). Novel, other stories among first about Jewish immigrants on N.Y.'s East Side. 240pp. 5⅜ x 8½.   22427-9 Pa. $7.95

SELECTED POEMS, Walt Whitman. Generous sampling from *Leaves of Grass*. Twenty-four poems include "I Hear America Singing," "Song of the Open Road," "I Sing the Body Electric," "When Lilacs Last in the Dooryard Bloom'd," "O Captain! My Captain!"–all reprinted from an authoritative edition. Lists of titles and first lines. 128pp. 5³⁄₁₆ x 8¼.   26878-0 Pa. $1.00

CATALOG OF DOVER BOOKS

THE BEST TALES OF HOFFMANN, E. T. A. Hoffmann. 10 of Hoffmann's most important stories: "Nutcracker and the King of Mice," "The Golden Flowerpot," etc. 458pp. 5⅜ x 8½. 21793-0 Pa. $9.95

FROM FETISH TO GOD IN ANCIENT EGYPT, E. A. Wallis Budge. Rich detailed survey of Egyptian conception of "God" and gods, magic, cult of animals, Osiris, more. Also, superb English translations of hymns and legends. 240 illustrations. 545pp. 5⅜ x 8½. 25803-3 Pa. $13.95

FRENCH STORIES/CONTES FRANÇAIS: A Dual-Language Book, Wallace Fowlie. Ten stories by French masters, Voltaire to Camus: "Micromegas" by Voltaire; "The Atheist's Mass" by Balzac; "Minuet" by de Maupassant; "The Guest" by Camus, six more. Excellent English translations on facing pages. Also French-English vocabulary list, exercises, more. 352pp. 5⅜ x 8½. 26443-2 Pa. $9.95

CHICAGO AT THE TURN OF THE CENTURY IN PHOTOGRAPHS: 122 Historic Views from the Collections of the Chicago Historical Society, Larry A. Viskochil. Rare large-format prints offer detailed views of City Hall, State Street, the Loop, Hull House, Union Station, many other landmarks, circa 1904-1913. Introduction. Captions. Maps. 144pp. 9⅜ x 12¼. 24656-6 Pa. $12.95

OLD BROOKLYN IN EARLY PHOTOGRAPHS, 1865-1929, William Lee Younger. Luna Park, Gravesend race track, construction of Grand Army Plaza, moving of Hotel Brighton, etc. 157 previously unpublished photographs. 165pp. 8⅞ x 11¾. 23587-4 Pa. $13.95

THE MYTHS OF THE NORTH AMERICAN INDIANS, Lewis Spence. Rich anthology of the myths and legends of the Algonquins, Iroquois, Pawnees and Sioux, prefaced by an extensive historical and ethnological commentary. 36 illustrations. 480pp. 5⅜ x 8½. 25967-6 Pa. $10.95

AN ENCYCLOPEDIA OF BATTLES: Accounts of Over 1,560 Battles from 1479 B.C. to the Present, David Eggenberger. Essential details of every major battle in recorded history from the first battle of Megiddo in 1479 B.C. to Grenada in 1984. List of Battle Maps. New Appendix covering the years 1967-1984. Index. 99 illustrations. 544pp. 6½ x 9¼. 24913-1 Pa. $16.95

SAILING ALONE AROUND THE WORLD, Captain Joshua Slocum. First man to sail around the world, alone, in small boat. One of great feats of seamanship told in delightful manner. 67 illustrations. 294pp. 5⅜ x 8½. 20326-3 Pa. $6.95

ANARCHISM AND OTHER ESSAYS, Emma Goldman. Powerful, penetrating, prophetic essays on direct action, role of minorities, prison reform, puritan hypocrisy, violence, etc. 271pp. 5⅜ x 8½. 22484-8 Pa. $8.95

MYTHS OF THE HINDUS AND BUDDHISTS, Ananda K. Coomaraswamy and Sister Nivedita. Great stories of the epics; deeds of Krishna, Shiva, taken from puranas, Vedas, folk tales; etc. 32 illustrations. 400pp. 5⅜ x 8½. 21759-0 Pa. $12.95

THE TRAUMA OF BIRTH, Otto Rank. Rank's controversial thesis that anxiety neurosis is caused by profound psychological trauma which occurs at birth. 256pp. 5⅜ x 8½. 27974-X Pa. $7.95

A THEOLOGICO-POLITICAL TREATISE, Benedict Spinoza. Also contains unfinished Political Treatise. Great classic on religious liberty, theory of government on common consent. R. Elwes translation. Total of 421pp. 5⅜ x 8½. 20249-6 Pa. $10.95

MY BONDAGE AND MY FREEDOM, Frederick Douglass. Born a slave, Douglass became outspoken force in antislavery movement. The best of Douglass' autobiographies. Graphic description of slave life. 464pp. 5⅜ x 8½. 22457-0 Pa. $8.95

FOLLOWING THE EQUATOR: A Journey Around the World, Mark Twain. Fascinating humorous account of 1897 voyage to Hawaii, Australia, India, New Zealand, etc. Ironic, bemused reports on peoples, customs, climate, flora and fauna, politics, much more. 197 illustrations. 720pp. 5⅜ x 8½. 26113-1 Pa. $15.95

THE PEOPLE CALLED SHAKERS, Edward D. Andrews. Definitive study of Shakers: origins, beliefs, practices, dances, social organization, furniture and crafts, etc. 33 illustrations. 351pp. 5⅜ x 8½. 21081-2 Pa. $12.95

THE MYTHS OF GREECE AND ROME, H. A. Guerber. A classic of mythology, generously illustrated, long prized for its simple, graphic, accurate retelling of the principal myths of Greece and Rome, and for its commentary on their origins and significance. With 64 illustrations by Michelangelo, Raphael, Titian, Rubens, Canova, Bernini and others. 480pp. 5⅜ x 8½. 27584-1 Pa. $10.95

PSYCHOLOGY OF MUSIC, Carl E. Seashore. Classic work discusses music as a medium from psychological viewpoint. Clear treatment of physical acoustics, auditory apparatus, sound perception, development of musical skills, nature of musical feeling, host of other topics. 88 figures. 408pp. 5⅜ x 8½. 21851-1 Pa. $11.95

THE PHILOSOPHY OF HISTORY, Georg W. Hegel. Great classic of Western thought develops concept that history is not chance but rational process, the evolution of freedom. 457pp. 5⅜ x 8½. 20112-0 Pa. $9.95

THE BOOK OF TEA, Kakuzo Okakura. Minor classic of the Orient: entertaining, charming explanation, interpretation of traditional Japanese culture in terms of tea ceremony. 94pp. 5⅜ x 8½. 20070-1 Pa. $3.95

LIFE IN ANCIENT EGYPT, Adolf Erman. Fullest, most thorough, detailed older account with much not in more recent books, domestic life, religion, magic, medicine, commerce, much more. Many illustrations reproduce tomb paintings, carvings, hieroglyphs, etc. 597pp. 5⅜ x 8½. 22632-8 Pa. $12.95

SUNDIALS, Their Theory and Construction, Albert Waugh. Far and away the best, most thorough coverage of ideas, mathematics concerned, types, construction, adjusting anywhere. Simple, nontechnical treatment allows even children to build several of these dials. Over 100 illustrations. 230pp. 5⅜ x 8½. 22947-5 Pa. $8.95

THEORETICAL HYDRODYNAMICS, L. M. Milne-Thomson. Classic exposition of the mathematical theory of fluid motion, applicable to both hydrodynamics and aerodynamics. Over 600 exercises. 768pp. 6⅛ x 9¼. 68970-0 Pa. $20.95

SONGS OF EXPERIENCE: Facsimile Reproduction with 26 Plates in Full Color, William Blake. 26 full-color plates from a rare 1826 edition. Includes "TheTyger," "London," "Holy Thursday," and other poems. Printed text of poems. 48pp. 5¼ x 7. 24636-1 Pa. $4.95

OLD-TIME VIGNETTES IN FULL COLOR, Carol Belanger Grafton (ed.). Over 390 charming, often sentimental illustrations, selected from archives of Victorian graphics–pretty women posing, children playing, food, flowers, kittens and puppies, smiling cherubs, birds and butterflies, much more. All copyright-free. 48pp. 9¼ x 12¼. 27269-9 Pa. $9.95

PERSPECTIVE FOR ARTISTS, Rex Vicat Cole. Depth, perspective of sky and sea, shadows, much more, not usually covered. 391 diagrams, 81 reproductions of drawings and paintings. 279pp. 5⅜ x 8½. 22487-2 Pa. $9.95

DRAWING THE LIVING FIGURE, Joseph Sheppard. Innovative approach to artistic anatomy focuses on specifics of surface anatomy, rather than muscles and bones. Over 170 drawings of live models in front, back and side views, and in widely varying poses. Accompanying diagrams. 177 illustrations. Introduction. Index. 144pp. 8⅜ x11¼. 26723-7 Pa. $9.95

GOTHIC AND OLD ENGLISH ALPHABETS: 100 Complete Fonts, Dan X. Solo. Add power, elegance to posters, signs, other graphics with 100 stunning copyright-free alphabets: Blackstone, Dolbey, Germania, 97 more–including many lower-case, numerals, punctuation marks. 104pp. 8⅛ x 11. 24695-7 Pa. $9.95

HOW TO DO BEADWORK, Mary White. Fundamental book on craft from simple projects to five-bead chains and woven works. 106 illustrations. 142pp. 5⅜ x 8. 20697-1 Pa. $5.95

THE BOOK OF WOOD CARVING, Charles Marshall Sayers. Finest book for beginners discusses fundamentals and offers 34 designs. "Absolutely first rate . . . well thought out and well executed."–E. J. Tangerman. 118pp. 7¾ x 10⅝. 23654-4 Pa. $7.95

ILLUSTRATED CATALOG OF CIVIL WAR MILITARY GOODS: Union Army Weapons, Insignia, Uniform Accessories, and Other Equipment, Schuyler, Hartley, and Graham. Rare, profusely illustrated 1846 catalog includes Union Army uniform and dress regulations, arms and ammunition, coats, insignia, flags, swords, rifles, etc. 226 illustrations. 160pp. 9 x 12. 24939-5 Pa. $12.95

WOMEN'S FASHIONS OF THE EARLY 1900s: An Unabridged Republication of "New York Fashions, 1909," National Cloak & Suit Co. Rare catalog of mail-order fashions documents women's and children's clothing styles shortly after the turn of the century. Captions offer full descriptions, prices. Invaluable resource for fashion, costume historians. Approximately 725 illustrations. 128pp. 8⅜ x 11¼. 27276-1 Pa. $12.95

THE 1912 AND 1915 GUSTAV STICKLEY FURNITURE CATALOGS, Gustav Stickley. With over 200 detailed illustrations and descriptions, these two catalogs are essential reading and reference materials and identification guides for Stickley furniture. Captions cite materials, dimensions and prices. 112pp. 6½ x 9¼. 26676-1 Pa. $9.95

EARLY AMERICAN LOCOMOTIVES, John H. White, Jr. Finest locomotive engravings from early 19th century: historical (1804–74), main-line (after 1870), special, foreign, etc. 147 plates. 142pp. 11⅜ x 8¼. 22772-3 Pa. $12.95

THE TALL SHIPS OF TODAY IN PHOTOGRAPHS, Frank O. Braynard. Lavishly illustrated tribute to nearly 100 majestic contemporary sailing vessels: Amerigo Vespucci, Clearwater, Constitution, Eagle, Mayflower, Sea Cloud, Victory, many more. Authoritative captions provide statistics, background on each ship. 190 black-and-white photographs and illustrations. Introduction. 128pp. 8⅞ x 11¾. 27163-3 Pa. $14.95

LITTLE BOOK OF EARLY AMERICAN CRAFTS AND TRADES, Peter Stockham (ed.). 1807 children's book explains crafts and trades: baker, hatter, cooper, potter, and many others. 23 copperplate illustrations. 140pp. 4⁵/₈ x 6.
23336-7 Pa. $4.95

VICTORIAN FASHIONS AND COSTUMES FROM HARPER'S BAZAR, 1867–1898, Stella Blum (ed.). Day costumes, evening wear, sports clothes, shoes, hats, other accessories in over 1,000 detailed engravings. 320pp. 9⅜ x 12¼.
22990-4 Pa. $16.95

GUSTAV STICKLEY, THE CRAFTSMAN, Mary Ann Smith. Superb study surveys broad scope of Stickley's achievement, especially in architecture. Design philosophy, rise and fall of the Craftsman empire, descriptions and floor plans for many Craftsman houses, more. 86 black-and-white halftones. 31 line illustrations. Introduction 208pp. 6½ x 9¼.
27210-9 Pa. $9.95

THE LONG ISLAND RAIL ROAD IN EARLY PHOTOGRAPHS, Ron Ziel. Over 220 rare photos, informative text document origin (1844) and development of rail service on Long Island. Vintage views of early trains, locomotives, stations, passengers, crews, much more. Captions. 8⅞ x 11¾.
26301-0 Pa. $14.95

VOYAGE OF THE LIBERDADE, Joshua Slocum. Great 19th-century mariner's thrilling, first-hand account of the wreck of his ship off South America, the 35-foot boat he built from the wreckage, and its remarkable voyage home. 128pp. 5⅜ x 8½.
40022-0 Pa. $5.95

TEN BOOKS ON ARCHITECTURE, Vitruvius. The most important book ever written on architecture. Early Roman aesthetics, technology, classical orders, site selection, all other aspects. Morgan translation. 331pp. 5⅜ x 8½.   20645-9 Pa. $9.95

THE HUMAN FIGURE IN MOTION, Eadweard Muybridge. More than 4,500 stopped-action photos, in action series, showing undraped men, women, children jumping, lying down, throwing, sitting, wrestling, carrying, etc. 390pp. 7⅞ x 10⅝.
20204-6 Clothbd. $29.95

TREES OF THE EASTERN AND CENTRAL UNITED STATES AND CANADA, William M. Harlow. Best one-volume guide to 140 trees. Full descriptions, woodlore, range, etc. Over 600 illustrations. Handy size. 288pp. 4½ x 6⅜.
20395-6 Pa. $6.95

SONGS OF WESTERN BIRDS, Dr. Donald J. Borror. Complete song and call repertoire of 60 western species, including flycatchers, juncoes, cactus wrens, many more–includes fully illustrated booklet.   Cassette and manual 99913-0 $8.95

GROWING AND USING HERBS AND SPICES, Milo Miloradovich. Versatile handbook provides all the information needed for cultivation and use of all the herbs and spices available in North America. 4 illustrations. Index. Glossary. 236pp. 5⅜ x 8½.
25058-X Pa. $7.95

BIG BOOK OF MAZES AND LABYRINTHS, Walter Shepherd. 50 mazes and labyrinths in all–classical, solid, ripple, and more–in one great volume. Perfect inexpensive puzzler for clever youngsters. Full solutions. 112pp. 8⅛ x 11.
22951-3 Pa. $5.95

PIANO TUNING, J. Cree Fischer. Clearest, best book for beginner, amateur. Simple repairs, raising dropped notes, tuning by easy method of flattened fifths. No previous skills needed. 4 illustrations. 201pp. 5$\frac{3}{8}$ x 8$\frac{1}{2}$. 23267-0 Pa. $6.95

HINTS TO SINGERS, Lillian Nordica. Selecting the right teacher, developing confidence, overcoming stage fright, and many other important skills receive thoughtful discussion in this indispensible guide, written by a world-famous diva of four decades' experience. 96pp. 5$\frac{3}{8}$ x 8$\frac{1}{2}$. 40094-8 Pa. $4.95

THE COMPLETE NONSENSE OF EDWARD LEAR, Edward Lear. All nonsense limericks, zany alphabets, Owl and Pussycat, songs, nonsense botany, etc., illustrated by Lear. Total of 320pp. 5$\frac{3}{8}$ x 8$\frac{1}{2}$. (Available in U.S. only.) 20167-8 Pa. $7.95

VICTORIAN PARLOUR POETRY: An Annotated Anthology, Michael R. Turner. 117 gems by Longfellow, Tennyson, Browning, many lesser-known poets. "The Village Blacksmith," "Curfew Must Not Ring Tonight," "Only a Baby Small," dozens more, often difficult to find elsewhere. Index of poets, titles, first lines. xxiii + 325pp. 5$\frac{5}{8}$ x 8$\frac{1}{4}$. 27044-0 Pa. $12.95

DUBLINERS, James Joyce. Fifteen stories offer vivid, tightly focused observations of the lives of Dublin's poorer classes. At least one, "The Dead," is considered a masterpiece. Reprinted complete and unabridged from standard edition. 160pp. 5$\frac{3}{16}$ x 8$\frac{1}{4}$. 26870-5 Pa. $1.50

GREAT WEIRD TALES: 14 Stories by Lovecraft, Blackwood, Machen and Others, S. T. Joshi (ed.). 14 spellbinding tales, including "The Sin Eater," by Fiona McLeod, "The Eye Above the Mantel," by Frank Belknap Long, as well as renowned works by R. H. Barlow, Lord Dunsany, Arthur Machen, W. C. Morrow and eight other masters of the genre. 256pp. 5$\frac{3}{8}$ x 8$\frac{1}{2}$. (Available in U.S. only.) 40436-6 Pa. $8.95

THE BOOK OF THE SACRED MAGIC OF ABRAMELIN THE MAGE, translated by S. MacGregor Mathers. Medieval manuscript of ceremonial magic. Basic document in Aleister Crowley, Golden Dawn groups. 268pp. 5$\frac{3}{8}$ x 8$\frac{1}{2}$. 23211-5 Pa. $9.95

NEW RUSSIAN-ENGLISH AND ENGLISH-RUSSIAN DICTIONARY, M. A. O'Brien. This is a remarkably handy Russian dictionary, containing a surprising amount of information, including over 70,000 entries. 366pp. 4$\frac{1}{2}$ x 6$\frac{1}{8}$. 20208-9 Pa. $10.95

HISTORIC HOMES OF THE AMERICAN PRESIDENTS, Second, Revised Edition, Irvin Haas. A traveler's guide to American Presidential homes, most open to the public, depicting and describing homes occupied by every American President from George Washington to George Bush. With visiting hours, admission charges, travel routes. 175 photographs. Index. 160pp. 8$\frac{1}{4}$ x 11. 26751-2 Pa. $13.95

NEW YORK IN THE FORTIES, Andreas Feininger. 162 brilliant photographs by the well-known photographer, formerly with *Life* magazine. Commuters, shoppers, Times Square at night, much else from city at its peak. Captions by John von Hartz. 181pp. 9$\frac{1}{4}$ x 10$\frac{3}{4}$. 23585-8 Pa. $13.95

INDIAN SIGN LANGUAGE, William Tomkins. Over 525 signs developed by Sioux and other tribes. Written instructions and diagrams. Also 290 pictographs. 111pp. 6$\frac{1}{8}$ x 9$\frac{1}{4}$. 22029-X Pa. $3.95

ANATOMY: A Complete Guide for Artists, Joseph Sheppard. A master of figure drawing shows artists how to render human anatomy convincingly. Over 460 illustrations. 224pp. 8⅜ x 11¼. 27279-6 Pa. $11.95

MEDIEVAL CALLIGRAPHY: Its History and Technique, Marc Drogin. Spirited history, comprehensive instruction manual covers 13 styles (ca. 4th century through 15th). Excellent photographs; directions for duplicating medieval techniques with modern tools. 224pp. 8⅜ x 11¼. 26142-5 Pa. $12.95

DRIED FLOWERS: How to Prepare Them, Sarah Whitlock and Martha Rankin. Complete instructions on how to use silica gel, meal and borax, perlite aggregate, sand and borax, glycerine and water to create attractive permanent flower arrangements. 12 illustrations. 32pp. 5⅜ x 8½. 21802-3 Pa. $1.00

EASY-TO-MAKE BIRD FEEDERS FOR WOODWORKERS, Scott D. Campbell. Detailed, simple-to-use guide for designing, constructing, caring for and using feeders. Text, illustrations for 12 classic and contemporary designs. 96pp. 5⅜ x 8½. 25847-5 Pa. $3.95

SCOTTISH WONDER TALES FROM MYTH AND LEGEND, Donald A. Mackenzie. 16 lively tales tell of giants rumbling down mountainsides, of a magic wand that turns stone pillars into warriors, of gods and goddesses, evil hags, powerful forces and more. 240pp. 5⅜ x 8½. 29677-6 Pa. $6.95

THE HISTORY OF UNDERCLOTHES, C. Willett Cunnington and Phyllis Cunnington. Fascinating, well-documented survey covering six centuries of English undergarments, enhanced with over 100 illustrations: 12th-century laced-up bodice, footed long drawers (1795), 19th-century bustles, 19th-century corsets for men, Victorian "bust improvers," much more. 272pp. 5⅝ x 8¼. 27124-2 Pa. $9.95

ARTS AND CRAFTS FURNITURE: The Complete Brooks Catalog of 1912, Brooks Manufacturing Co. Photos and detailed descriptions of more than 150 now very collectible furniture designs from the Arts and Crafts movement depict davenports, settees, buffets, desks, tables, chairs, bedsteads, dressers and more, all built of solid, quarter-sawed oak. Invaluable for students and enthusiasts of antiques, Americana and the decorative arts. 80pp. 6½ x 9¼. 27471-3 Pa. $8.95

WILBUR AND ORVILLE: A Biography of the Wright Brothers, Fred Howard. Definitive, crisply written study tells the full story of the brothers' lives and work. A vividly written biography, unparalleled in scope and color, that also captures the spirit of an extraordinary era. 560pp. 6⅛ x 9¼. 40297-5 Pa. $17.95

THE ARTS OF THE SAILOR: Knotting, Splicing and Ropework, Hervey Garrett Smith. Indispensable shipboard reference covers tools, basic knots and useful hitches; handsewing and canvas work, more. Over 100 illustrations. Delightful reading for sea lovers. 256pp. 5⅜ x 8½. 26440-8 Pa. $8.95

FRANK LLOYD WRIGHT'S FALLINGWATER: The House and Its History, Second, Revised Edition, Donald Hoffmann. A total revision–both in text and illustrations–of the standard document on Fallingwater, the boldest, most personal architectural statement of Wright's mature years, updated with valuable new material from the recently opened Frank Lloyd Wright Archives. "Fascinating"–*The New York Times*. 116 illustrations. 128pp. 9¼ x 10¾. 27430-6 Pa. $12.95

PHOTOGRAPHIC SKETCHBOOK OF THE CIVIL WAR, Alexander Gardner. 100 photos taken on field during the Civil War. Famous shots of Manassas Harper's Ferry, Lincoln, Richmond, slave pens, etc. 244pp. 10⅝ x 8¼.   22731-6 Pa. $10.95

FIVE ACRES AND INDEPENDENCE, Maurice G. Kains. Great back-to-the-land classic explains basics of self-sufficient farming. The one book to get. 95 illustrations. 397pp. 5⅜ x 8½.   20974-1 Pa. $7.95

SONGS OF EASTERN BIRDS, Dr. Donald J. Borror. Songs and calls of 60 species most common to eastern U.S.: warblers, woodpeckers, flycatchers, thrushes, larks, many more in high-quality recording.   Cassette and manual 99912-2 $9.95

A MODERN HERBAL, Margaret Grieve. Much the fullest, most exact, most useful compilation of herbal material. Gigantic alphabetical encyclopedia, from aconite to zedoary, gives botanical information, medical properties, folklore, economic uses, much else. Indispensable to serious reader. 161 illustrations. 888pp. 6½ x 9¼. 2-vol. set. (Available in U.S. only.)   Vol. I: 22798-7 Pa. $10.95
Vol. II: 22799-5 Pa. $10.95

HIDDEN TREASURE MAZE BOOK, Dave Phillips. Solve 34 challenging mazes accompanied by heroic tales of adventure. Evil dragons, people-eating plants, blood-thirsty giants, many more dangerous adversaries lurk at every twist and turn. 34 mazes, stories, solutions. 48pp. 8¼ x 11.   24566-7 Pa. $2.95

LETTERS OF W. A. MOZART, Wolfgang A. Mozart. Remarkable letters show bawdy wit, humor, imagination, musical insights, contemporary musical world; includes some letters from Leopold Mozart. 276pp. 5⅜ x 8½.   22859-2 Pa. $9.95

BASIC PRINCIPLES OF CLASSICAL BALLET, Agrippina Vaganova. Great Russian theoretician, teacher explains methods for teaching classical ballet. 118 illustrations. 175pp. 5⅜ x 8½.   22036-2 Pa. $6.95

THE JUMPING FROG, Mark Twain. Revenge edition. The original story of The Celebrated Jumping Frog of Calaveras County, a hapless French translation, and Twain's hilarious "retranslation" from the French. 12 illustrations. 66pp. 5⅜ x 8½.   22686-7 Pa. $4.95

BEST REMEMBERED POEMS, Martin Gardner (ed.). The 126 poems in this superb collection of 19th- and 20th-century British and American verse range from Shelley's "To a Skylark" to the impassioned "Renascence" of Edna St. Vincent Millay and to Edward Lear's whimsical "The Owl and the Pussycat." 224pp. 5⅜ x 8½.   27165-X Pa. $5.95

COMPLETE SONNETS, William Shakespeare. Over 150 exquisite poems deal with love, friendship, the tyranny of time, beauty's evanescence, death and other themes in language of remarkable power, precision and beauty. Glossary of archaic terms. 80pp. 5³⁄₁₆ x 8¼.   26686-9 Pa. $1.00

THE BATTLES THAT CHANGED HISTORY, Fletcher Pratt. Eminent historian profiles 16 crucial conflicts, ancient to modern, that changed the course of civilization. 352pp. 5⅜ x 8½.   41129-X Pa. $9.95

THE WIT AND HUMOR OF OSCAR WILDE, Alvin Redman (ed.). More than 1,000 ripostes, paradoxes, wisecracks: Work is the curse of the drinking classes; I can resist everything except temptation; etc. 258pp. $5\frac{3}{8} \times 8\frac{1}{2}$. 20602-5 Pa. $6.95

SHAKESPEARE LEXICON AND QUOTATION DICTIONARY, Alexander Schmidt. Full definitions, locations, shades of meaning in every word in plays and poems. More than 50,000 exact quotations. 1,485pp. $6\frac{1}{2} \times 9\frac{1}{4}$. 2-vol. set.
Vol. 1: 22726-X Pa. $17.95
Vol. 2: 22727-8 Pa. $17.95

SELECTED POEMS, Emily Dickinson. Over 100 best-known, best-loved poems by one of America's foremost poets, reprinted from authoritative early editions. No comparable edition at this price. Index of first lines. 64pp. $5\frac{3}{16} \times 8\frac{1}{4}$.
26466-1 Pa. $1.00

THE INSIDIOUS DR. FU-MANCHU, Sax Rohmer. The first of the popular mystery series introduces a pair of English detectives to their archnemesis, the diabolical Dr. Fu-Manchu. Flavorful atmosphere, fast-paced action, and colorful characters enliven this classic of the genre. 208pp. $5\frac{3}{16} \times 8\frac{1}{4}$. 29898-1 Pa. $2.00

THE MALLEUS MALEFICARUM OF KRAMER AND SPRENGER, translated by Montague Summers. Full text of most important witchhunter's "bible," used by both Catholics and Protestants. 278pp. $6\frac{5}{8} \times 10$. 22802-9 Pa. $12.95

SPANISH STORIES/CUENTOS ESPAÑOLES: A Dual-Language Book, Angel Flores (ed.). Unique format offers 13 great stories in Spanish by Cervantes, Borges, others. Faithful English translations on facing pages. 352pp. $5\frac{3}{8} \times 8\frac{1}{2}$.
25399-6 Pa. $9.95

GARDEN CITY, LONG ISLAND, IN EARLY PHOTOGRAPHS, 1869–1919, Mildred H. Smith. Handsome treasury of 118 vintage pictures, accompanied by carefully researched captions, document the Garden City Hotel fire (1899), the Vanderbilt Cup Race (1908), the first airmail flight departing from the Nassau Boulevard Aerodrome (1911), and much more. 96pp. $8\frac{7}{8} \times 11\frac{3}{4}$. 40669-5 Pa. $12.95

OLD QUEENS, N.Y., IN EARLY PHOTOGRAPHS, Vincent F. Seyfried and William Asadorian. Over 160 rare photographs of Maspeth, Jamaica, Jackson Heights, and other areas. Vintage views of DeWitt Clinton mansion, 1939 World's Fair and more. Captions. 192pp. $8\frac{7}{8} \times 11$. 26358-4 Pa. $14.95

CAPTURED BY THE INDIANS: 15 Firsthand Accounts, 1750-1870, Frederick Drimmer. Astounding true historical accounts of grisly torture, bloody conflicts, relentless pursuits, miraculous escapes and more, by people who lived to tell the tale. 384pp. $5\frac{3}{8} \times 8\frac{1}{2}$. 24901-8 Pa. $9.95

THE WORLD'S GREAT SPEECHES (Fourth Enlarged Edition), Lewis Copeland, Lawrence W. Lamm, and Stephen J. McKenna. Nearly 300 speeches provide public speakers with a wealth of updated quotes and inspiration–from Pericles' funeral oration and William Jennings Bryan's "Cross of Gold Speech" to Malcolm X's powerful words on the Black Revolution and Earl of Spenser's tribute to his sister, Diana, Princess of Wales. 944pp. $5\frac{3}{8} \times 8\frac{3}{8}$. 40903-1 Pa. $15.95

THE BOOK OF THE SWORD, Sir Richard F. Burton. Great Victorian scholar/adventurer's eloquent, erudite history of the "queen of weapons"–from prehistory to early Roman Empire. Evolution and development of early swords, variations (sabre, broadsword, cutlass, scimitar, etc.), much more. 336pp. $6\frac{1}{8} \times 9\frac{1}{4}$.
25434-8 Pa. $9.95

AUTOBIOGRAPHY: The Story of My Experiments with Truth, Mohandas K. Gandhi. Boyhood, legal studies, purification, the growth of the Satyagraha (nonviolent protest) movement. Critical, inspiring work of the man responsible for the freedom of India. 480pp. 5⅜ x 8½. (Available in U.S. only.)   24593-4 Pa. $9.95

CELTIC MYTHS AND LEGENDS, T. W. Rolleston. Masterful retelling of Irish and Welsh stories and tales. Cuchulain, King Arthur, Deirdre, the Grail, many more. First paperback edition. 58 full-page illustrations. 512pp. 5⅜ x 8½.   26507-2 Pa. $9.95

THE PRINCIPLES OF PSYCHOLOGY, William James. Famous long course complete, unabridged. Stream of thought, time perception, memory, experimental methods; great work decades ahead of its time. 94 figures. 1,391pp. 5⅜ x 8½. 2-vol. set.
Vol. I: 20381-6 Pa. $14.95
Vol. II: 20382-4 Pa. $16.95

THE WORLD AS WILL AND REPRESENTATION, Arthur Schopenhauer. Definitive English translation of Schopenhauer's life work, correcting more than 1,000 errors, omissions in earlier translations. Translated by E. F. J. Payne. Total of 1,269pp. 5⅜ x 8½. 2-vol. set.
Vol. 1: 21761-2 Pa. $12.95
Vol. 2: 21762-0 Pa. $12.95

MAGIC AND MYSTERY IN TIBET, Madame Alexandra David-Neel. Experiences among lamas, magicians, sages, sorcerers, Bonpa wizards. A true psychic discovery. 32 illustrations. 321pp. 5⅜ x 8½. (Available in U.S. only.)   22682-4 Pa. $9.95

THE EGYPTIAN BOOK OF THE DEAD, E. A. Wallis Budge. Complete reproduction of Ani's papyrus, finest ever found. Full hieroglyphic text, interlinear transliteration, word-for-word translation, smooth translation. 533pp. 6½ x 9¼.
21866-X Pa. $12.95

MATHEMATICS FOR THE NONMATHEMATICIAN, Morris Kline. Detailed, college-level treatment of mathematics in cultural and historical context, with numerous exercises. Recommended Reading Lists. Tables. Numerous figures. 641pp. 5⅜ x 8½.
24823-2 Pa. $11.95

PROBABILISTIC METHODS IN THE THEORY OF STRUCTURES, Isaac Elishakoff. Well-written introduction covers the elements of the theory of probability from two or more random variables, the reliability of such multivariable structures, the theory of random function, Monte Carlo methods of treating problems incapable of exact solution, and more. Examples. 502pp. $5^{3}/_{8}$ x $8^{1}/_{2}$.   40691-1 Pa. $16.95

THE RIME OF THE ANCIENT MARINER, Gustave Doré, S. T. Coleridge. Doré's finest work; 34 plates capture moods, subtleties of poem. Flawless full-size reproductions printed on facing pages with authoritative text of poem. "Beautiful. Simply beautiful."–*Publisher's Weekly.* 77pp. 9¼ x 12.   22305-1 Pa. $7.95

NORTH AMERICAN INDIAN DESIGNS FOR ARTISTS AND CRAFTSPEOPLE, Eva Wilson. Over 360 authentic copyright-free designs adapted from Navajo blankets, Hopi pottery, Sioux buffalo hides, more. Geometrics, symbolic figures, plant and animal motifs, etc. 128pp. 8⅜ x 11. (Not for sale in the United Kingdom.)   25341-4 Pa. $9.95

SCULPTURE: Principles and Practice, Louis Slobodkin. Step-by-step approach to clay, plaster, metals, stone; classical and modern. 253 drawings, photos. 255pp. 8⅛ x 11.
22960-2 Pa. $11.95

THE INFLUENCE OF SEA POWER UPON HISTORY, 1660–1783, A. T. Mahan. Influential classic of naval history and tactics still used as text in war colleges. First paperback edition. 4 maps. 24 battle plans. 640pp. 5⅜ x 8½.   25509-3 Pa. $14.95

THE STORY OF THE TITANIC AS TOLD BY ITS SURVIVORS, Jack Winocour (ed.). What it was really like. Panic, despair, shocking inefficiency, and a little heroism. More thrilling than any fictional account. 26 illustrations. 320pp. 5⅜ x 8½.
20610-6 Pa. $8.95

FAIRY AND FOLK TALES OF THE IRISH PEASANTRY, William Butler Yeats (ed.). Treasury of 64 tales from the twilight world of Celtic myth and legend: "The Soul Cages," "The Kildare Pooka," "King O'Toole and his Goose," many more. Introduction and Notes by W. B. Yeats. 352pp. 5⅜ x 8½.   26941-8 Pa. $8.95

BUDDHIST MAHAYANA TEXTS, E. B. Cowell and others (eds.). Superb, accurate translations of basic documents in Mahayana Buddhism, highly important in history of religions. The Buddha-karita of Asvaghosha, Larger Sukhavativyuha, more. 448pp. 5⅜ x 8½.   25552-2 Pa. $12.95

ONE TWO THREE . . . INFINITY: Facts and Speculations of Science, George Gamow. Great physicist's fascinating, readable overview of contemporary science: number theory, relativity, fourth dimension, entropy, genes, atomic structure, much more. 128 illustrations. Index. 352pp. 5⅜ x 8½.   25664-2 Pa. $9.95

EXPERIMENTATION AND MEASUREMENT, W. J. Youden. Introductory manual explains laws of measurement in simple terms and offers tips for achieving accuracy and minimizing errors. Mathematics of measurement, use of instruments, experimenting with machines. 1994 edition. Foreword. Preface. Introduction. Epilogue. Selected Readings. Glossary. Index. Tables and figures. 128pp. $5^{3}/_{8}$ x $8^{1}/_{2}$.
40451-X Pa. $6.95

DALÍ ON MODERN ART: The Cuckolds of Antiquated Modern Art, Salvador Dalí. Influential painter skewers modern art and its practitioners. Outrageous evaluations of Picasso, Cézanne, Turner, more. 15 renderings of paintings discussed. 44 calligraphic decorations by Dalí. 96pp. 5⅜ x 8½. (Available in U.S. only.)   29220-7 Pa. $5.95

ANTIQUE PLAYING CARDS: A Pictorial History, Henry René D'Allemagne. Over 900 elaborate, decorative images from rare playing cards (14th–20th centuries): Bacchus, death, dancing dogs, hunting scenes, royal coats of arms, players cheating, much more. 96pp. 9¼ x 12¼.   29265-7 Pa. $12.95

MAKING FURNITURE MASTERPIECES: 30 Projects with Measured Drawings, Franklin H. Gottshall. Step-by-step instructions, illustrations for constructing handsome, useful pieces, among them a Sheraton desk, Chippendale chair, Spanish desk, Queen Anne table and a William and Mary dressing mirror. 224pp. 8⅛ x 11¼.
29338-6 Pa. $16.95

THE FOSSIL BOOK: A Record of Prehistoric Life, Patricia V. Rich et al. Profusely illustrated definitive guide covers everything from single-celled organisms and dinosaurs to birds and mammals and the interplay between climate and man. Over 1,500 illustrations. 760pp. 7½ x 10⅛.   29371-8 Pa. $29.95

Prices subject to change without notice.

Available at your book dealer or write for free catalog to Dept. GI, Dover Publications, Inc., 31 East 2nd St., Mineola, N.Y. 11501. Dover publishes more than 500 books each year on science, elementary and advanced mathematics, biology, music, art, literary history, social sciences and other areas.